Revascularization and Replantation in the Hand

Editors

KYLE R. EBERLIN
NEAL C. CHEN

HAND CLINICS

www.hand.theclinics.com

Consulting Editor
KEVIN C. CHUNG

May 2019 • Volume 35 • Number 2

ELSEVIER

1600 John F. Kennedy Boulevard • Suite 1800 • Philadelphia, Pennsylvania, 19103-2899

http://www.theclinics.com

HAND CLINICS Volume 35, Number 2
May 2019 ISSN 0749-0712, ISBN-13: 978-0-323-67843-8

Editor: Lauren Boyle
Developmental Editor: Kristen Helm

Hand Clinics (ISSN 0749-0712) is published quarterly by Elsevier Inc., 360 Park Avenue South, New York, NY 10010-1710. Months of publication are February, May, August, and November. Business and Editorial Offices: 1600 John F. Kennedy Blvd., Ste. 1800, Philadelphia, PA 19103-2899. Customer Service Office: 3251 Riverport Lane, Maryland Heights, MO 63043. Periodicals postage paid at New York, NY and at additional mailing offices. Subscription price is $435.00 per year (domestic individuals), $813.00 per year (domestic institutions), $100.00 per year (domestic students/residents), $501.00 per year (Canadian individuals), $947.00 per year (Canadian institutions), $546.00 per year (international individuals), $947.00 per year (international institutions), and $256.00 per year (international and Canadian students/residents). Foreign air speed delivery is included in all *Clinics* subscription prices. All prices are subject to change without notice. **POSTMASTER:** Send address changes to *Hand Clinics*, Elsevier Health Sciences Division, Subscription Customer Service, 3251 Riverport Lane, Maryland Heights, MO 63043. Customer Service (orders, claims, online, change of address): Elsevier Health Sciences Division, Subscription **Customer Service, 3251 Riverport Lane, Maryland Heights, MO 63043. Tel: 1-800-654-2452 (U.S. and Canada); 314-447-8871 (outside U.S. and Canada). Fax: 314-447-8029. E-mail: journalscustomerservice-usa@elsevier.com (for print support); journalsonlinesupport-usa@elsevier.com (for online support).**

Reprints. For copies of 100 or more of articles in this publication, please contact the Commercial Reprints Department, Elsevier Inc., 360 Park Avenue South, New York, New York 10010-1710. Tel.: 212-633-3874; Fax: 212-633-3820; E-mail: reprints@elsevier.com.

Hand Clinics is covered in *MEDLINE/PubMed (Index Medicus), Current Contents/Clinical Medicine, EMBASE/Excerpta Medica,* and *ISI/BIOMED.*

Contributors

CONSULTING EDITOR

KEVIN C. CHUNG, MD, MS
Chief of Hand Surgery, University of Michigan Health System, Charles B.G. de Nancrede Professor of Plastic Surgery and Orthopaedic Surgery, Department of Surgery, Assistant Dean for Faculty Affairs, Associate Director of Global REACH, University of Michigan Medical School, Director of University of Michigan Comprehensive Hand Center, Ann Arbor, Michigan, USA

EDITORS

KYLE R. EBERLIN, MD
Plastic Surgery, Hand Surgery, and Peripheral Nerve Surgery, Assistant Professor of Surgery, Associate Director, MGH Hand Surgery Fellowship, Associate Program Director, Harvard Plastic Surgery Residency Program, Division of Plastic and Reconstructive Surgery, Harvard Medical School, Massachusetts General Hospital, Boston, Massachusetts, USA

NEAL C. CHEN, MD
Interim Chief, Hand and Arm Center, Program Director, Hand Surgery Fellowship Program, Assistant Professor of Orthopaedic Surgery, Harvard Medical School, Massachusetts General Hospital, Boston, Massachusetts, USA

AUTHORS

BRIAN H. CHO, MD
Plastic Surgery Resident, Curtis National Hand Center, Baltimore, Maryland, USA

HOYUNE E. CHO, MD
T32 Postdoctoral Research Fellow, Section of Plastic Surgery, Department of Surgery, University of Michigan Medical School, Ann Arbor, Michigan, USA

KEVIN C. CHUNG, MD, MS
Chief of Hand Surgery, University of Michigan Health System, Charles B.G. de Nancrede Professor of Plastic Surgery and Orthopaedic Surgery, Department of Surgery, Assistant Dean for Faculty Affairs, Associate Director of Global REACH, University of Michigan Medical School, Director of University of Michigan Comprehensive Hand Center, Ann Arbor, Michigan, USA

BRIAN C. DROLET, MD
Associate Residency Program Director and Assistant Professor, Departments of Plastic Surgery and Biomedical Informatics, Center for Biomedical Ethics and Society, Vanderbilt University Medical Center, Nashville, Tennessee, USA

KYLE R. EBERLIN, MD
Plastic Surgery, Hand Surgery, and Peripheral Nerve Surgery, Assistant Professor of Surgery, Associate Director, MGH Hand Surgery Fellowship, Associate Program Director, Harvard Plastic Surgery Residency Program, Division of Plastic and Reconstructive Surgery, Harvard Medical School, Massachusetts General Hospital, Boston, Massachusetts, USA

JEFFREY B. FRIEDRICH, MD, MC, FACS
Professor of Surgery, Orthopaedics, Division of Plastic Surgery, University of Washington, Harborview Medical Center, Seattle Children's Hospital, Seattle, Washington, USA

DANIEL J. GITTINGS, MD
Orthopedic Surgery Resident, University of Pennsylvania, Philadelphia, Pennsylvania, USA

MARK A. GREYSON, MD
Resident, Division of Plastic and Reconstructive Surgery, Harvard Medical School, Massachusetts General Hospital, Massachusetts, USA

MITSUNOBU HARIMA, MD
Lecturer, Department of Plastic and Reconstructive Surgery, Graduate School of Medicine, The University of Tokyo, Tokyo, Japan

JAMES P. HIGGINS, MD
Chief of Hand Surgery, The Curtis National Hand Center at MedStar Union Memorial Hospital, Baltimore, Maryland, USA

HIROFUMI IMAI, MD
Lecturer, International Center for Lymphedema, Hiroshima University Hospital, Hiroshima City, Japan

MATTHEW L. IORIO, MD
Associate Professor, Co-Director of Hand Surgery and of Extremity Microsurgery, Department of Surgery, Division of Plastic and Reconstructive Surgery, Department of Orthopedics, University of Colorado, Anschutz Medical Center, Aurora, Colorado, USA

SHEPARD P. JOHNSON, MBBS
Resident, Plastic and Reconstructive Surgery, Vanderbilt University Medical Center, Nashville, Tennessee, USA

JIN SOO KIM, MD, PhD
Attending Physician, Department of Plastic and Reconstructive Surgery, Gwangmyeong Sungae General Hospital, Gwangmyeong, Gyeonggi-do, South Korea

YONG WOO KIM, MD
Senior Resident, Department of Plastic and Reconstructive Surgery, Gwangmyeong Sungae General Hospital, Gwangmyeong, Gyeonggi-do, South Korea

JASON H. KO, MD
Associate Professor of Surgery (Plastic Surgery) and Orthopaedic Surgery, Northwestern University School of Medicine, Chicago, Illinois, USA

ISAO KOSHIMA, MD
Professor and Chief, International Center for Lymphedema, Hiroshima University Hospital, Hiroshima City, Japan

SANDRA V. KOTSIS, MPH
Research Coordinator, Section of Plastic Surgery, Department of Surgery, University of Michigan Medical School, Ann Arbor, Michigan, USA

DONG CHUL LEE, MD
Attending Physician, Department of Plastic and Reconstructive Surgery, Gwangmyeong Sungae General Hospital, Gwangmyeong, Gyeonggi-do, South Korea

KYUNG JIN LEE, MD
Attending Physician, Department of Plastic and Reconstructive Surgery, Gwangmyeong Sungae General Hospital, Gwangmyeong, Gyeonggi-do, South Korea

L. SCOTT LEVIN, MD, FACS
Chairman of the Department of Orthopedic Surgery, University of Pennsylvania, Philadelphia, Pennsylvania, USA

SHAUN D. MENDENHALL, MD
Hand Surgeon, Division of Plastic and Reconstructive Surgery, Department of Surgery, University of Utah School of Medicine, Salt Lake City, Utah, USA

HARUKI MIZUTA, MD
Lecturer, Department of Plastic and Reconstructive Surgery, Graduate School of Medicine, The University of Tokyo, Tokyo, Japan

SHOGO NAGAMATSU, MD
Lecturer, Plastic and Reconstructive Surgery, Hiroshima University Hospital, Hiroshima City, Japan

MITCHELL A. PET, MD
Assistant Professor of Surgery (Plastic Surgery), Washington University School of Medicine, St Louis, Missouri, USA

BRENT B. PICKRELL, MD
Resident, Division of Plastic and Reconstructive Surgery, Harvard Medical School, Massachusetts General Hospital, Boston, Massachusetts, USA

ADNAN PRSIC, MD
Assistant Professor, Plastic and Reconstructive Surgery, Yale School of Medicine, New Haven, Connecticut, USA

SI YOUNG ROH, MD, PhD
Attending Physician, Department of Plastic and Reconstructive Surgery, Gwangmyeong Sungae General Hospital, Gwangmyeong, Gyeonggi-do, South Korea

BAUBACK SAFA, MD, MBA
The Buncke Clinic, San Francisco, California, USA

AYANO SASAKI, MD
Lecturer, Plastic and Reconstructive Surgery, Hiroshima University Hospital, Hiroshima City, Japan

AMIR H. TAGHINIA, MD, MPH, MBA
Staff Surgeon, Department of Plastic and Oral Surgery, Boston Children's Hospital, Assistant Professor, Harvard Medical School, Boston, Massachusetts, USA

JYUNSUKE TASHIRO, MD
Lecturer, Department of Plastic and Reconstructive Surgery, Graduate School of Medicine, The University of Tokyo, Tokyo, Japan

SHUJI YAMASHITA, MD
Assistant Professor, Department of Plastic and Reconstructive Surgery, Graduate School of Medicine, The University of Tokyo, Tokyo, Japan

KAZUNORI YOKOTA, MD
Professor and Chief, Plastic and Reconstructive Surgery, Hiroshima University Hospital, Hiroshima City, Japan

SHUHEI YOSHIDA, MD
Lecturer, International Center for Lymphedema, Hiroshima University Hospital, Hiroshima City, Japan

Contents

defect is performed. In this article, the authors present and discuss the venous free flap, thenar free flap, toe plantar free flap, free style perforator flap, hypothenar free flap, and anconeus muscle free flap.

Revascularization and Replantation in the Hand: Ectopic Banking and Replantation **199**

Brian H. Cho and James P. Higgins

Traumatic amputation of the upper extremity remains a challenging problem for reconstructive hand surgeons. Temporary ectopic banking of amputated parts for subsequent replantation is an innovative and valuable surgical technique for patients who would otherwise be poor candidates for replantation. The applications of ectopic banking have evolved and expanded to include various clinical scenarios. Although there is considerable variability within the literature, this article summarizes the optimal banking locations and duration, while also highlighting several treatment considerations when performing this technique.

Outcomes Following Replantation/Revascularization in the Hand **207**

Hoyune E. Cho, Sandra V. Kotsis, and Kevin C. Chung

The variability in reported outcomes and outcome measures used in digit replantation makes it difficult to compare results among studies. This article reviews the principles of measuring functional and patient-reported outcomes after replantation, and describes the recommended instruments to use and ways to report results.

Postoperative Management and Rehabilitation of the Replanted or Revascularized Digit **221**

Adnan Prsic and Jeffrey B. Friedrich

Postoperative care of amputated digits begins before replantation. Detailed informed consent should be obtained and completion amputation discussed if revascularization is not ultimately successful. Complications and failure of the replanted digit should also be addressed. Postoperative pharmacologic treatment should consist of aspirin, at minimum. Complications, such as venous congestion or occlusion, and arterial thrombosis, should be dealt with expediently. Digital motion rehabilitation should start after 5 to 7 days of digital viability and splinting of the affected digit. Early protective motion protocol is implemented to maintain digital motion with emphasis on tendon glide and joint motion.

Secondary Surgery Following Replantation and Revascularization **231**

Brent B. Pickrell and Kyle R. Eberlin

Secondary surgery following digital replantation and revascularization is common and is often performed to improve range of motion, tendon gliding, sensibility, and/or contour. In this article, the authors present the most common secondary procedures performed after digital replantation or revascularization and discuss current techniques. The importance of patient selection and postoperative compliance with ongoing hand therapy is paramount to achieving good outcomes.

HAND CLINICS

FORTHCOMING ISSUES

August 2019
Current Concepts and Controversies in Scaphoid Fracture Management
Steven L. Moran, *Editor*

November 2019
Global Hand Surgery: Learning and Contributing in the Developing World
Kevin C. Chung, *Editor*

February 2020
Soft Tissue Reconstruction for Digital Defects
Sandeep J. Sebastin and David M.K. Tan, *Editors*

RECENT ISSUES

February 2019
Global Advances in Wide Awake Hand Surgery
Don Lalonde and Jin Bo Tang, *Editors*

November 2018
Management of Spastic Conditions of the Upper Extremity
Joshua M. Adkinson, *Editor*

August 2018
Dupuytren Disease
Steven C. Haase and Kevin C. Chung, *Editors*

Preface
Revascularization and Replantation in the Hand

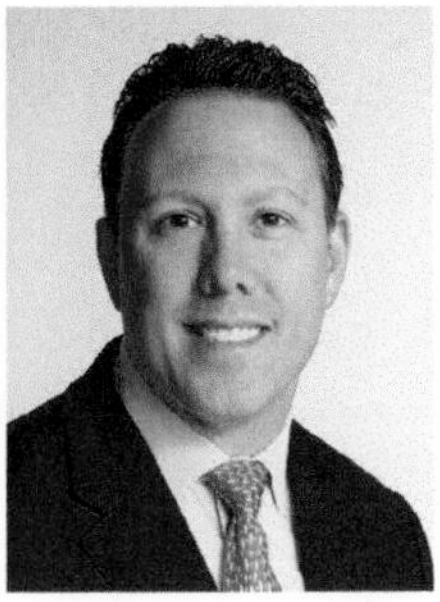
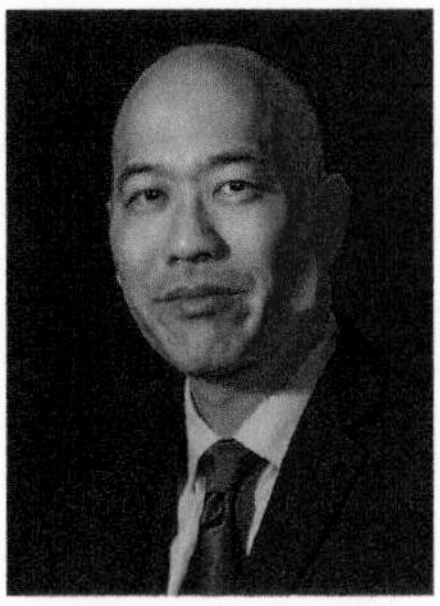

Kyle R. Eberlin, MD   Neal C. Chen, MD
Editors

The development of upper extremity replantation in the 1960s and 1970s provided a momentous advance in the care of traumatic injuries to the hand and digits. The expansion of novel microsurgical techniques and instruments ushered in a new era of hand surgery, in which operative procedures were performed for many amputation injuries with a modicum of success. This was initially followed by a growing enthusiasm for replantation surgery throughout the world. However, some of this excitement has waned over subsequent decades given the understandable focus on functional outcomes over the pure viability of the replanted part.

Modern microsurgical techniques, hand therapy protocols, and the interest in centralizing regional care for traumatic hand injuries have led to a renewed vigor and enthusiasm for hand and digital replantation. There are many new reconstructive tools in the hand surgery armamentarium, including distal replantation, artery-only protocols, and venous flaps for soft tissue coverage. These procedures have resulted in a "renaissance" of sorts for replantation, with a burgeoning interest among trainees to learn these techniques and incorporate them into their future clinical practice.

As contemporary hand surgeons in the twenty-first century, it is our charge to balance the desire for technical advances with the need to perform operations that have demonstrable functional benefit for our patients. It is our obligation to offer sophisticated surgical procedures with a healthy dose of practicality, knowing that these procedures most often involve a lengthy recovery with frequent and dedicated hand therapy. The swinging pendulum of enthusiasm for replantation provides an apt analogy; we must carefully consider the most prudent intervention, if at all, based on the myriad factors that are involved in this complex shared decision-making process.

This issue presents modern indications, techniques, and outcomes for replantation and revascularization in the hand, with updated protocols and options for the most challenging cases. We believe that this issue will allow hand surgeons to better understand current strategies for the care of these devastating injuries.

We appreciate your continued interest in *Hand Clinics*. Please share topics that you would like discussed in future issues.

Kyle R. Eberlin, MD
Plastic Surgery, Hand Surgery, and Peripheral Nerve Surgery
MGH Hand Surgery Fellowship
Massachusetts General Hospital
Harvard Medical School
55 Fruit Street, Wang Building 435
Boston, MA 02114, USA

Neal C. Chen, MD
Hand & Arm Center
Massachusetts General Hospital
Harvard Medical School
55 Fruit Street, Yawkey Building 2100
Boston, MA 02114, USA

E-mail addresses:
keberlin@mgh.harvard.edu (K.R. Eberlin)
nchen1@partners.org (N.C. Chen)

Hand Clin 35 (2019) xi
https://doi.org/10.1016/j.hcl.2019.01.005
0749-0712/19/© 2019 Published by Elsevier Inc.

hand.theclinics.com

A Decade of Progress Toward Establishing Regional Hand Trauma Centers in the United States

Daniel J. Gittings, MD[a], Shaun D. Mendenhall, MD[b],
L. Scott Levin, MD[a,*]

KEYWORDS

• Replantation • Revascularization • Microsurgery • Regional hand trauma centers

KEY POINTS

- There is a need for designated centers that provide high-quality emergent microvascular surgical treatment in the United States.
- Barriers to emergent microvascular surgical treatment include a highly fragmented, overburdened, and underspecialized health system.
- Changes in health policy and pilot programs that show value in establishing regional hand trauma centers will provide accessible high-quality emergent microsurgical care.

HISTORY OF MICROVASCULAR AND REPLANTATION SURGERY

Replantation surgery has a rich history that closely parallels the history of vascular and microvascular surgery.[1] Starting more than a century ago with Alexis Carrel's description of an end-to-end vascular anastomosis in 1902, the disciplines of vascular, microvascular, and transplantation surgery were born.[2] Two other key advancements that led to the development of microvascular surgery include the discovery of heparin in 1916 by McLean, Howell, and Holt, and the description of using an operative microscope to perform a microvascular anastomosis by Jacobson and Suarez in 1960.[3–5] Once these fundamentals of vascular surgery were in place, advancements in microsurgical instrumentation, sutures, and needles led to the beginnings of the modern microsurgical era.[1]

The era of clinical replantation officially commenced with the report of a successful arm replant in a child by Malt and McKhann in 1963.[6] This was followed by the first successful thumb replantation by Komatsu and Tamai in 1965.[7] These early reports were met with enthusiasm and paralleled the establishment of microsurgical research centers around the world, leading to the first free tissue transfers and toe-to-hand transfers in addition to replantation of amputated parts.[1] Since that time, replantation and the treatment of microsurgical emergencies has gone through multiple distinct phases (**Table 1**).

Disclosures: The authors have not received any financial support for the work. Dr D.J. Gittings and Dr S.D. Mendenhall certify that they have no commercial associations (eg, consultancies, stock ownership, equity interest, patent/licensing arrangements, etc) that might pose a conflict of interest in connection with the submitted article.

[a] University of Pennsylvania, 3737 Market Street, 6th Floor, Philadelphia, PA 19104, USA; [b] Division of Plastic and Reconstructive Surgery, Department of Surgery, University of Utah School of Medicine, 50 North Medical Drive, Salt Lake City, UT 84132, USA
* Corresponding author.
E-mail address: lawrence.levin2@uphs.upenn.edu

Hand Clin 35 (2019) 103–108
https://doi.org/10.1016/j.hcl.2018.12.001

Table 1
Key eras for replantation and microsurgical hand trauma in the United States

1960s	Era of beginnings
1970s	Era of discovery
1980s	Era of enthusiasm and refinement
1990s	Era of outcomes
2000s	Era of decline
2010s	Era of refusal
2020s	Era of revitalization and regionalization

The 1970s may be thought of as the era of "discovery" in microsurgery and replantation. During this time pioneers such as Taylor, Buncke, O'Brien, Tamai, and Kleinert introduced techniques and basic principles of replantation followed by free tissue transfer and built successful programs throughout the world. This was also a time of advancement for microneural surgery characterized by pioneering work in fascicular nerve repair and nerve grafting by Millesi, Terzis, Brunelli, and others.[1] The 1980s were an era of "enthusiasm" and "refinement" as microsurgical centers expanded and promoted technical modifications to improve outcomes. The era included descriptions of microsurgical procedures such as ring avulsion replantation, toe wrap around flaps, scapular flaps, early perforator flaps such as the deep inferior epigastric perforator flap, and functional muscle transfers. This experience in microsurgery paralleled the evolution of microsurgical procedures in hand trauma. The 1990s ushered in an era of "outcomes" during which functional outcomes of extremity replantation and free tissue transfer were scrutinized and indications were revised. The era also marked the beginning of vascularized composite allotransplantation of hands from deceased donors to those who lost limbs previously.[8]

The 2000s marked an era of "decline" in replantation and urgent microsurgical reconstruction. During this decade there was a trend of fewer and fewer replantation attempts and a decreasing success rate of replantations in the United States.[9] Poor reimbursement, unpredictable timing of microsurgical emergencies, lack of institutional support, and decreased microsurgical training for hand surgeons made replantation less appealing and likely contributed to this trend.[10,11] This situation continued to worsen in the 2010s, which became the era of "refusal" by surgeons to perform replantation services, likely because of surgeon inexperience, poor reimbursement from patients being uninsured or underinsured, and risk of litigation. Misra and colleagues[12] found that self-pay and Medicaid insurance were independent predictors of transfer to bypass other Level I centers.

Hand surgeons should not abandon replantation surgery. As a specialty, we have an ethical obligation to help patients with these problems based on our knowledge, understanding of indications and contraindications, and unique surgical skills. We owe it to our patients, colleagues, and specialty to do better in the upcoming decade. It is our hope and goal that the 2020s will become the era of "revitalization" and "regionalization" by establishing regional hand trauma centers throughout the United States.

BARRIERS TO ACCESSIBLE HAND TRAUMA COVERAGE

In 2006, the Institute of Medicine emphasized a need for accountable and equitable emergency care system in the United States.[13] However, only 47% of Level I and 29% of Level II trauma centers had emergent microsurgery and replantation services available 24 hours a day, 7 days a week, 365 days a year in 2010.[14] As a response to the shortage of hand microsurgery coverage, the American College of Surgeons (ACS) has partnered with the American Society for Surgery of the Hand (ASSH) and American Association of Hand Surgery to identify the obstacles to improve access to emergent microsurgical care. It was found that several barriers to change existed, which included the policies guiding the accreditation of trauma centers and the hurdles encountered by individual hand surgeons and the hospitals where they deliver care.

The ACS Committee on Trauma has developed a system of policies entitled *Resources for the Optimal Care of the Injured Patient*.[15] These policies are used to delineate the services provided by Level I trauma centers. Specifically, before 2010 the guidelines originally stated that "hand surgery… capabilities must be present at Level I trauma centers."[16] However, this policy did not specify a requirement for microvascular replantation services necessary for hand trauma call. This ambiguous policy contributes to the current heterogeneity in emergent hand microsurgical services and, ultimately, hand replantation services are inconsistent among Level I trauma centers. In a survey of Level I trauma centers performed in 2010, Peterson and colleagues[14] found 47% of Level I trauma centers provide continuous microsurgical replantation services while the other centers offer part-time replantation services based on hand surgeon call schedule. Furthermore, this study discusses how Level II trauma centers have less consistent coverage, citing how these centers provide hand replantation services 50% to 80% of the time without a clearly defined call schedule.

Inconsistent hand replantation coverage among trauma centers results in delay of care resulting from patient transfers. Patients may spend precious hours with prolonged ischemia times waiting for initial providers to identify a trauma center with a specialized hand surgeon who is capable and willing to accept the patient for microvascular care.[17,18] Emergency medicine physicians without readily available emergent microsurgical coverage in their hospitals struggle to identify another institution with a specialized hand microvascular surgeon who is willing to provide care. Often patients are transferred long distances, bypassing multiple Level I trauma centers before arriving at the facility that provides definitive treatment. Misra and colleagues[12] found that median of 4 Level I trauma centers were bypassed during patient transfer to their institution for emergent microsurgical care. Access to centers with specialized emergent hand microsurgical care is challenging for patients and emergency providers because of a lack of a clear identification of hand trauma centers.

In addition to access to emergent hand microsurgical care, another barrier to care is appropriate transfer criteria. The Emergency Medical Treatment and Active Labor Act (EMTALA) requires a hospital that is unable to treat a trauma patient to stabilize and transfer the patient to a Level I or II trauma center.[17] However, patients who are managed without an experienced hand trauma specialist may undergo a completion amputation in a situation whereby replantation was feasible and possibly the optimal treatment. Disability may be reduced if the patient is transported to the appropriate specialized hand trauma center in a timely fashion.[18,19] Patients with amputations who are treated in large urban academic hospitals have a higher likelihood of undergoing replantation than revision amputation at smaller rural nonteaching hospitals.[20]

Inappropriate transfers that are within the scope of practice of the transferring facility also occur. Vulnerable populations such as patients who are uninsured or underinsured, minorities, and those living in rural areas may encounter numerous hurdles to accessing appropriate hand trauma care.[21,22] These economically vulnerable patients are more likely to have their care delayed because they are transferred to referral centers whether or not they require care provided by a specialized hand surgeon.[23] Inappropriate transfers increase the cost of trauma care and delay treatment.[19] The lack of guidelines for transferring patients with acute hand trauma creates inefficiencies within the American health care system. The overuse of the trauma system increases health care costs and may both negatively affect the patient who undergoes an unnecessary transfer and potentially limit access to other patients who need specialty care at the same time. In addition to the issues with the health system, a shortage of hand surgeons available to take emergency call further exacerbates inaccessibility to care.[10,24]

Several recent studies have identified multiple factors that have contributed to the decreasing number of hand surgeons who provide emergent microsurgical hand call coverage.[10,24] A 2007 survey of ASSH members with a 45% response rate (561 of 1238 members) reported that 29% of respondents do not take emergency hand call and 44% did not provide emergent hand trauma microsurgical services. Moreover, 74% of the surgeons perceived a decrease in replantation performed over the previous decade. Of the providers that performed replantation, 62% (196 of 316) carried out fewer than 5 replantations per year.[10] In a national database study by Chung and colleagues,[24] 15% (136 of 906) hospitals performed finger replantation. Of the hospitals that performed replants, only 2% performed 10 or more cases in 1 year during which 60% performed only 1 procedure. The shortage of specialized hand trauma surgeons is due to several factors that include busy elective schedules, declining reimbursement, and inadequate surgeon confidence in performing replantation. Furthermore, improved occupational safety mechanisms with fewer amputation injuries, more stringent indications for surgical replantation, and patient preference for revision amputation for quicker return to activity may also account for the diminished volume of replantation procedures. Ultimately, the majority of replantations performed by a select number of specialized individual surgeons supports the concept of centralization or regionalization of emergent hand trauma microsurgical care. This regionalization may improve patient outcomes and health system efficiency. The hand trauma center is a concept that has emerged to meet the needs for emergent hand trauma microsurgical services.

Hand trauma centers may provide resources for improved patient outcomes with efficiency. These centers have experienced surgeons in replantation surgery who may provide outcomes superior to those by inexperienced surgeons, for several reasons. Experienced surgeons have a better understanding of the indications and outcomes associated with replantation versus revision amputation. By contrast, an inexperienced surgeon may have less success in attempting replantation and or have an inherent bias for revision amputation given a lack of technical expertise for replantation. Inexperienced surgeons may also inappropriately waste resources when incorrectly identifying candidates for emergent transfer of care. Clear identification of hand trauma centers may improve efficiency in providing timely care. Multiple studies have described prolonged transfer times in patients requiring digital replantation.[25,26] Ozer and colleagues[25] reported a mean transport time of 5 hours (range 1–24 hours) for patients transferred for digital replantation. In another study, 40% of patient transfers took more than 3 hours.[26] A system in which hand trauma centers are designated can provide guidance to inexperienced providers and may improve outcomes and optimize utilization of resources.

ACTIONS TAKEN TO IMPROVE ACCESSIBLE HAND TRAUMA COVERAGE

Over the past decade there have been many steps taken to improve hand trauma coverage. A taskforce led by the ASSH with the support of ACS, the American Academy of Orthopedic Surgery, and the American Society of Plastic Surgeons has paved the way for revolutionizing the way emergent upper extremity trauma will be provided in the United States. These changes have included changes to health policy, a pilot program of a system of hand trauma centers, and prospective data collection to demonstrate the value of these centers.

In 2010, the ASSH drafted a white paper to the ACS to request a change to the *Resources for the Optimal Care of the Injured Patient* guidelines, also known as the "green book." In 2011, the green book policies specifically defined 24-hour a day/7 days a week/365 days a year coverage of hand, microvascular, and replantation emergencies for all Level I trauma centers and, if those services are unavailable, that transfer agreements are required.[16] These changes in policy have assisted in identifying centers best equipped to provide emergent upper extremity microsurgical care with contact information more accessible to emergency providers.

After identifying centers equipped to provide emergent upper extremity microsurgical care, a pilot program for hand trauma centers began. These centers are based on those established for other surgical subspecialties including burn centers, bariatric centers, and general trauma centers. Designated centers have previously been identified for other subspecialties based on the availability of their ability to provide accessible and efficient care with skilled personnel. The definition of hand trauma centers was created according to the following criteria:

1. All hand trauma centers are available 24/7/365 for hand trauma emergencies that include revascularization, replantation, and mutilating hand injuries.
2. A specific call list of physicians on call is available.
3. A center may include residents and fellows from plastic, orthopedic, and general Surgery.
4. The hand trauma center does NOT have to be a Level I ACS designated center as long as criterion #1 is fulfilled.
5. A director of the hand trauma center (or codirectors) is (are) needed to verify and report data with regard to treatment (number of patients seen, injury patterns).

After defining hand trauma centers, 33 institutions that met these criteria were identified to collect data to show proof of concept that this system demonstrates value to the American health system. Centers enrolled in the pilot program consisted centers that self-identified as 26 (79%) academic medical centers, 4 (13%) private practice centers, 1 (2%) hybrid academic/private practice center, and 2 (6%) others (**Fig. 1**). These centers have collected data during their enrollment in the program to include total number of hand trauma patients, replants, revascularizations, and mutilating hand injuries. After 5 months of data collection, 2252 hand trauma patients were evaluated, and 35 (1.6%) of that number underwent replantation surgery, 79 (3.5%) underwent revascularization surgery, and 357 (15.8%) presented with mutilating hand injuries.

Currently under way, the hand trauma centers in the pilot program are working to better refine transfer agreements. The basic tenet of a transfer

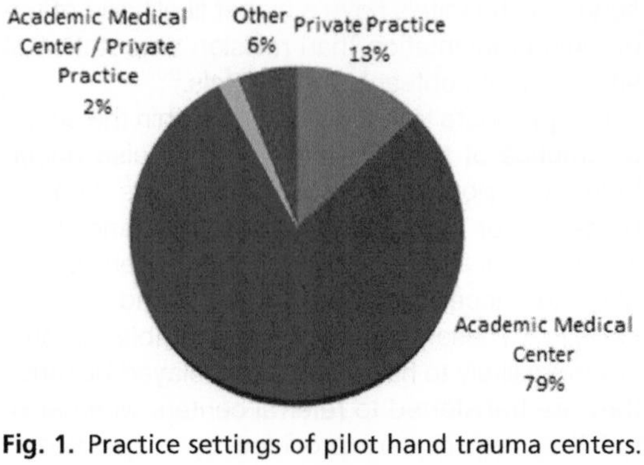

Fig. 1. Practice settings of pilot hand trauma centers.

agreement includes that a specific financial agreement exists between a referring hospital and the regional hand trauma center, that the centers have defined injuries appropriate for transfer, and more importantly have defined when transfer is inappropriate to avoid misuse of resources. Furthermore, programs to document and enforce the transfer agreement are under way. In future, these programs will evolve into a system to accredit and verify hand trauma centers and provide a mechanism to enforce an appropriate utilization of resources within health systems. Of the hand trauma centers within the pilot program, currently 86.5% of the centers have transfer agreements with other Level I trauma centers, and 13.5% of centers do not (**Fig. 2**).

Current and future work is focusing on how to reimburse hand trauma centers for their service of providing high-quality hand trauma microsurgical care. Ideally a specific reimbursement schema for centers and for on-call physicians working in the hand trauma centers would be established and endorsed by the ACS. At present, of the surgeons in the pilot hand trauma center program, 44% of surgeons are compensated to take call whereas 56% of surgeons are not (**Fig. 3**). Data collection from the hand trauma centers including clinically relevant outcomes and metrics demonstrating efficient high-quality care will be used to garner financial support and reimbursement to sustain these centers in the future. Ultimately, this pilot study will be used to designate a defined network of hand trauma centers that will readily accessible for facilities to refer microsurgical emergencies. The outcomes used in this study will be used to negotiate financially incentivized transfer agreements between referring facilities and the hand trauma centers. Furthermore, outcomes showing high-quality care may be used by ACS Fellows to lobby for additional governmental financial support to continue to provide this vital public service.

Are there transfer agreements with other Level I centers?

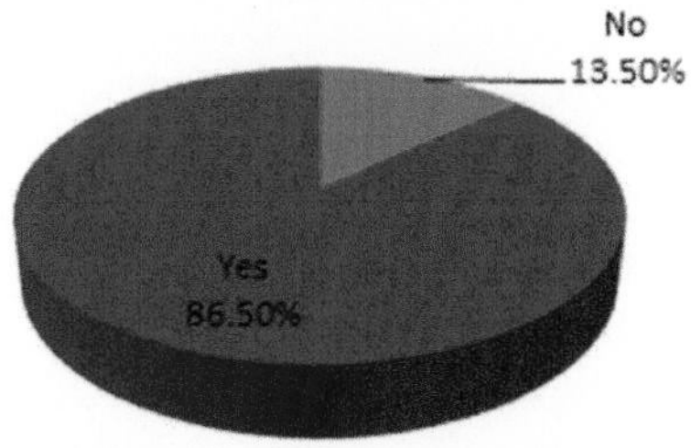

Fig. 2. Pilot hand trauma centers with transfer agreements.

Are surgeons compensated to take call?

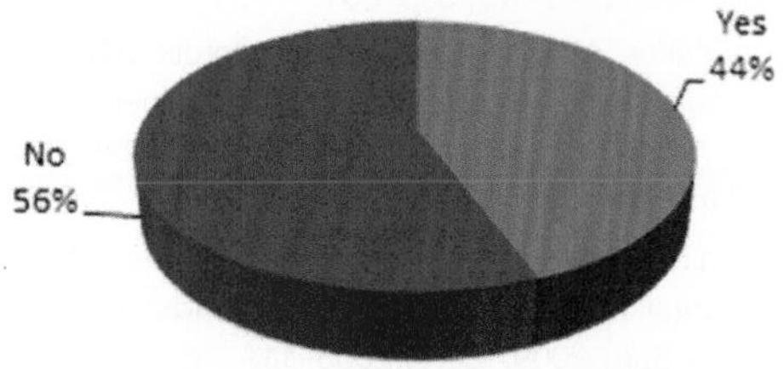

Fig. 3. Surgeons compensated at pilot hand trauma centers to take call.

In conclusion, over the past decade progress for access to hand trauma microsurgical expertise has included redefining policies for trauma center coverage with a more clear identification of specialized centers, a pilot program for regional hand trauma centers, and prospective data collection that demonstrates the value of these centers. Over the next several years, the focus will be on collecting data to demonstrate that the hand trauma centers and a regional network meet the public need. Furthermore, work is under way to financially incentivize both hospital systems and providers to provide this integral service.

REFERENCES

1. Tamai S. History of microsurgery. Plast Reconstr Surg 2009;124(6 Suppl):e282–94.
2. Carrel D. Operative technic of vascular anastomoses and visceral transplantation. Lyon Med 1964; 212:1561–8 [in French]. Available at: http://www.ncbi.nlm.nih.gov/pubmed/14253645. Accessed June 23, 2018.
3. McLean J. The thromboplastic action of cephalin. Am J Physiol 1916. https://doi.org/10.1152/ajplegacy.1916.41.2.250.
4. Howell WH, Holt E. Two new factors in blood coagulation—heparin and pro-antithrombin. Am J Physiol 1918;47:328–41.
5. Jacobson JH, Suarez EL. Microsurgery in anastomosis of small vessels. Surg Forum 1960;11:243–5.
6. Malt RA, McKhann C. Replantation of severed arms. JAMA 1964;189:716–22. Available at: http://www.ncbi.nlm.nih.gov/pubmed/14175645. Accessed June 23, 2018.
7. Komatsu S, Tamai S. Successful replantation of a completely cut off thumb. Plast Reconstr Surg 1968;42:374–7.
8. Dubernard J-M, Owen E, Herzberg G, et al. Human hand allograft: report on first 6 months. Lancet 1999; 353(9161):1315–20.
9. Hustedt JW, Bohl DD, Champagne L. The detrimental effect of decentralization in digital

replantation in the United States: 15 years of evidence from the national inpatient sample. J Hand Surg Am 2016;41(5):593–601.
10. Payatakes AH, Zagoreos NP, Fedorcik GG, et al. Current practice of microsurgery by members of the American Society for Surgery of the Hand. J Hand Surg Am 2007;32(4):541–7.
11. Chen MW, Narayan D. Economics of upper extremity replantation: national and local trends. Plast Reconstr Surg 2009;124(6):2003–11.
12. Misra S, Wilkens SC, Chen NC, et al. Patients transferred for upper extremity amputation: participation of regional trauma centers. J Hand Surg Am 2017;42(12):987–95.
13. Institute of Medicine. Emergency medical services at the crossroads 2007. Available at: https://www.nasemso.org/Projects/DomesticPreparedness/documents/EMS-at-Crossroads.pdf. Accessed May 20, 2018.
14. Peterson BC, Mangiapani D, Kellogg R, et al. Hand and microvascular replantation call availability study: a national real-time survey of level-I and level-II trauma centers. J Bone Joint Surg Am 2012;94(24):e185.
15. Commiittee on Trauma, American College of Surgeons. Chapter 1. Regional trauma systems: optimal elements, integration, and assessment. In: Rotondo MF, Cribari C, Smith SR, editors. Resources for optimal care of the injured patient. Chicago (IL): ACS; 2014. Available at: https://www.facs.org/~/media/files/quality programs/trauma/vrc resources/resources for optimal care.ashx. Accessed August 17, 2018.
16. Rotondo MF, Cribari C, Smith SR, editors. Resources for optimal care of the injured patient. Chicago (IL): ACS; 2014. Available at: https://www.facs.org/~/media/files/quality programs/trauma/vrc resources/resources for optimal care.ashx. Accessed May 19, 2018.
17. Hartzell TL, Kuo P, Eberlin KR, et al. The overutilization of resources in patients with acute upper extremity trauma and infection. J Hand Surg Am 2013;38(4):766–73.
18. Potini VC, Bratchenko W, Jacob G, et al. Repeat emergency room visits for hand and wrist injuries. J Hand Surg Am 2014;39(4):752–6.
19. Butala P, Fisher MD, Blueschke G, et al. Factors associated with transfer of hand injuries to a level 1 trauma center: a descriptive analysis of 1147 cases. Plast Reconstr Surg 2014;133(4):842–8.
20. Maroukis BL, Chung KC, MacEachern M, et al. Hand trauma care in the United States. Plast Reconstr Surg 2016;137(1):100e–11e.
21. Calfee RP, Shah CM, Canham CD, et al. The influence of insurance status on access to and utilization of a tertiary hand surgery referral center. J Bone Joint Surg Am 2012;94(23):2177–84.
22. Patterson JM, Boyer MI, Ricci WM, et al. Hand trauma: a prospective evaluation of patients transferred to a level I trauma center. Am J Orthop (Belle Mead NJ) 2010;39(4):196–200. Available at: http://www.ncbi.nlm.nih.gov/pubmed/20512173. Accessed May 27, 2018.
23. Eberlin KR, Hartzell TL, Kuo P, et al. Patients transferred for emergency upper extremity evaluation: does insurance status matter? Plast Reconstr Surg 2013;131(3):593–600.
24. Chung KC, Kowalski CP, Walters MR. Finger replantation in the United States: rates and resource use from the 1996 healthcare cost and utilization project. J Hand Surg Am 2000;25(6):1038–42.
25. Ozer K, Kramer W, Gillani S, et al. Replantation versus revision of amputated fingers in patients air-transported to a level 1 trauma center. J Hand Surg Am 2010;35(6):936–40.
26. Menchine MD, Baraff LJ. On-call specialists and higher level of care transfers in California emergency departments. Acad Emerg Med 2008;15(4):329–36.

Revascularization and Replantation in the Hand

Presurgical Preparation and Patient Transfer

Shepard P. Johnson, MBBS[a], Brian C. Drolet, MD[b,c,d,*]

KEYWORDS

• Digit amputation • Hand amputation • Transfer • Triage

KEY POINTS

- Current literature indicates that digit and hand replantation is more successful at centers with higher annual volumes.
- Given the movement for centralization of replantation at specialized centers, physicians and hospitals must be adept at triaging and transferring patients with amputations.
- Successful transfers of patients for replantation are predicated on (1) injury assessment, (2) communication, (3) preparing the patient (and amputated part) for surgery, and (4) providing a timely and safe disposition of the transfer.
- The critical, presurgical management of amputated digits includes preservation of all tissues, limiting warm ischemia time, imaging, and judicious use of tourniquets.
- The critical, presurgical management of patients with amputated digits includes maintenance of hemodynamic stability, update of vaccinations, and administration of antibiotics.

INTRODUCTION

Hand injuries are responsible for 10% to 30% of trauma-related emergency department visits,[1,2] and there are an estimated 45,000 digital amputations in the United States each year.[3,4] Although improvements in microvascular techniques have made digit salvage more successful, with reported replantation and revascularization rates as high as 80% to 90%, the decision to pursue salvage is complex and depends on several factors related to the injury, patient, surgeon, and health care system.[5–7] Furthermore, replantation requires a large investment of time, cost, and resources by numerous involved individuals, including the patient, family, surgeon, health care team (nursing, occupational therapy, and so forth), and treating institution (operating rooms [OR], intensive care facilities, and so forth). In contrast, completion amputation is simple, inexpensive, and has a shorter recovery with quicker return to work.[6,8,9] Therefore, the decision to pursue replantation must be carefully considered. For example, a healthy young patient with a clean, sharp thumb amputation in which there are functional and long-term economic benefits of replantation contrasts significantly with an index finger amputation in an older patient with multiple comorbidities.[9]

Despite advancement in microvascular surgery, there has been a decline in enthusiasm for digital replantation across the United States over the last 20 years.[10–13] This is likely related to several

[a] Plastic and Reconstructive Surgery, Vanderbilt University Medical Center, 1211 Medical Center Drive, Nashville, TN 37232, USA; [b] Department of Plastic Surgery, Vanderbilt University Medical Center, 1211 Medical Center Drive, Medical Center North, D-4219, Nashville, TN 37232, USA; [c] Department of Biomedical Informatics, Vanderbilt University Medical Center, 1211 Medical Center Drive, Medical Center North, D-4219, Nashville, TN 37232, USA; [d] Center for Biomedical Ethics and Society, Vanderbilt University Medical Center, 1211 Medical Center Drive, Medical Center North, D-4219, Nashville, TN 37232, USA
* Corresponding author. Department of Plastic Surgery, Vanderbilt University Medical Center, 1211 Medical Center Drive, Medical Center North, D-4219, Nashville, TN 37232.
E-mail address: brian.c.drolet@gmail.com

Hand Clin 35 (2019) 109–117
https://doi.org/10.1016/j.hcl.2018.12.002
0749-0712/19/

factors, including improved industrial standards and fewer injuries, lower reimbursement rates, the cost-benefit ratio of amputation versus replantation, and more selective indications for replantation.[13–17] In a recent national inpatient sample study, Hustedt and colleagues[10] found that referrals to specialized practice centers were diminishing, and concurrently, there were lower success rates of replants nationwide. Decreased volume may be related to decreased success, which further diminishes enthusiasm for replantation. In response to the decline in available microvascular expertise, there has been a movement to centralize the care of replantation at high-volume centers.[14,15] A growing body of literature indicates that outcomes of replantation at referral institutions are better with respect to digital survival, function, patient satisfaction, and aesthetic appearance.[14,15] This systematic change has now placed an emphasis on referring institutions to disposition patients safely and quickly to a tertiary institution.

Timely triage for digit and hand replantation depends on the interplay of several factors that are related to the amputated part and patient (**Fig. 1**, **Table 1**). However, before any consideration of replantation is made, the medical stability of the traumatically injured patient must be ensured. Under no circumstances should a patient be considered for transfer or replantation until the patient has undergone a complete trauma evaluation using Advanced Trauma Life Support (ATLS) protocols and any life-threatening medical issues have been managed. Then, assessment of the injured extremity should be performed with regard to the extent, mechanism, and timing of injury. A thorough evaluation of the injury is imperative to accurately communicate the expected functional outcomes of replantation versus amputation with the patient. If an attempt at replantation is reasonable, the patient should then be transferred to a specialized regional center. Although several public health policies and socioeconomic factors influence the triage and allocation of resources for traumatic amputations, this article focuses on the salient points of patient and part preparation that will assist health care providers in a successful replantation.

Assessment of Injury

Part-related factors

Accepted indications for replantation include thumb amputation, amputation at or proximal to the palm, any pediatric amputation, and involvement of multiple digits.[15,17–20] For some surgeons, single-digit amputation distal to the flexor digitorum superficialis tendon insertion is a relative indication, with more proximal amputations in the long finger being advocated by others.[2,17,21] Surgeons must consider that hand function may be impaired by a stiff, insensate, replanted finger or that other unaffected digits may become stiff and weak following immobilization of the hand postoperatively. Therefore, completion amputation may be indicated, particularly for the index finger proximal

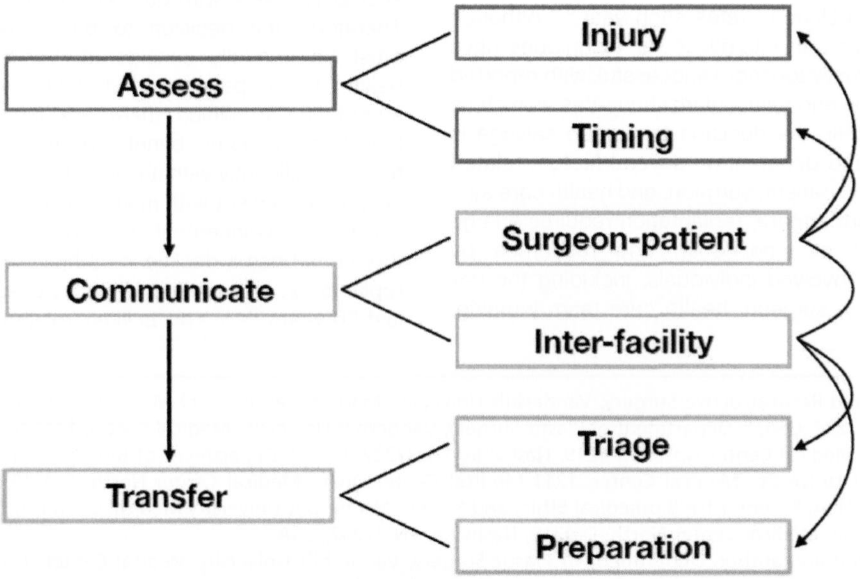

Fig. 1. Triaging patients with amputated digits. Referring physicians must (1) assess the injury and timing of events, (2) communicate with the patient and referral institution, and (3) prepare patients for replantation before transferring to a specialized, high-volume center.

Table 1
Part- and patient-related factors that must be considered when preparing patients for transfer to a tertiary center for digit or hand replantation

	Part-Related Factors	Patient-Related Factors
Assessment of the amputation		
Injury	Digit(s) and level Mechanism Condition of tissue	ATLS (airway, breathing, circulation) Life-threatening polytrauma Comorbidities
Timing	Warm/cold ischemia time Time to replantation	Tourniquet time
Communication regarding replantation (vs amputation)		
Surgeon-patient	Digit survival Functional & aesthetic outcomes Secondary surgeries	Socioeconomic implications Health care utilization Rehabilitation
Interfacility	Communicate assessment	Communicate assessment
Transferring the amputated part and patient		
Triage	Replants at tertiary centers	Health care utilization Mode of transport (ground)
Preparation	Transporting part Preserve all tissue Imaging	Resuscitation Antibiotics Tetanus prophylaxis

to flexor tendon zone I.[19] Distal digital replantation is technically more challenging owing to smaller vessels, but a systematic review by Sebastin and Chung[6] found no difference in survival between Tamai Classification zone I and zone II injuries. Although distal injuries have acceptable functional outcomes, in general, flexor tendon zone I and V replants have better range of motion than replantation involving zones II, III, and IV.[22] Replantation of injuries involving and proximal to the midpalm is encouraged given reasonable outcomes, but these injuries are also at high risk of incomplete nerve regeneration, and therefore, often lack protective sensation.[20]

Equally predictive of the success of replantation is the mechanism of injury, which has been shown to be strongly predictive of functional outcome.[20] Heavy contamination, crush injuries, and avulsion injuries are predictors of replant failure.[14] The success rate of replantation following avulsion and degloving injuries is estimated to be 66% and 50%, respectively.[23,24] In contrast, sharp amputations fare better given the smaller zone of injury on all structures involved, including bone, artery, tendons, and nerves. Few absolute contraindications to replantation have been described, but multilevel, mutilating, or blast injuries, which have resulted in severe articular and bony damage, should be strongly discouraged.

Patient-related factors

All patients with upper extremity amputations should be treated in accordance with American College of Surgery Advance Trauma Life Support guidelines.[25] Limb amputations are often associated with a high-energy mechanism, and therefore, maintenance of the patient's airway, breathing, and circulation takes precedence over extremity trauma. Physicians must be mindful of the condition of the patient, and pursuit of replantation of a digit or hand should only be made after the patient has been resuscitated and hemodynamically stabilized, and life-threatening injuries have been ruled out. In proximal hand amputations, hemorrhage can be significant, and transfusions may be necessary. Furthermore, microsurgeons must be cognizant that after large-volume resuscitation, patients are at risk of coagulopathy, termed acute traumatic coagulopathy, and revascularization can be compromised by abnormal clotting physiology.[26] Surgeons should also be mindful that patient comorbidities influence outcomes, and that smoking and diabetes are associated with a higher risk of failure.[21] Any patient who cannot undergo the significant physiologic stress of an extended surgery and recovery should not be considered for replantation. Finally, psychiatric and contextual factors must be considered as well. Patients often require extended recovery periods with frequent interventions (eg, leech therapy) in an intensive care unit and then months of laborious occupational therapy. If a patient is not adequately prepared for the postoperative psychological and socioeconomic stressors, then replantation may not be indicated.

Assessment of Timing

Part-related factors

Time to revascularization of an amputated digit is presumed to directly correlate with survival.[18] However, generally accepted guidelines are not strongly based on evidence, but rather anecdotal experience. Although reports have suggested successful replantation after 96 hours, warm and cold ischemia guideline times for digital replantation are typically 12 and 24 hours.[15,17,20,27] The ability of digits to survive longer ischemia time is attributed to the lack of muscle within the amputated segment. More proximal injuries carry a greater risk of myonecrosis and the sequelae of reperfusion (eg, acute tubular necrosis), and therefore, recommended maximum warm and cold ischemia times for hand amputations are 6 and 12 hours, respectively.[15,17,20] Perioperative intravenous hydration is critical in patients undergoing replantation of proximal upper extremity amputations to prevent the sequelae of reperfusion injury and reperfusion coagulopathy.[20]

Patient-related factors

Time from traumatic amputation to definitive replantation is less of an issue for the patient side (stump) of the injury, provided that it has maintained a healthy blood supply. Injuries involving wrist and forearm amputations may necessitate the use of a tourniquet for life-threatening hemorrhage. In this scenario, disciplined timekeeping and proper use are essential to preserving the tissues within the stump. Although a fail-safe tourniquet time does not exist, recommended continuous cuff inflation periods should not exceed 2 to 2.5 hours, without interval tourniquet-free periods of 10 to 20 minutes.[28,29] Evidence suggests that rest periods protect soft tissue structures by preventing the buildup of toxic metabolites (eg, oxygen free radicals) and overall depletion of adenosine triphosphate.[28–30] To prevent long tourniquet times, large vessels can be isolated and ligated, while being conscious of preserving length for eventual anastomosis. In addition, vasospasm and clotting of vessels may occur, so the injured extremity should be reevaluated whenever a tourniquet is released for adequate hemostasis in order to avoid unnecessary tourniquet time, which may be helpful later for efficient use of OR time during replantation.

Communication Between Surgeon and Patient

Part-related factors

In considering hand or digit completion amputation versus replantation, the most important determinants of patient satisfaction are education and informed consent. Before attempted replantation, the treating surgeon or other treating physician should provide clarity regarding the anticipated functional and aesthetic outcomes of a replant or amputated digit. Previous investigators have emphasized the importance of this discussion. Ozer and colleagues[21] advocate counseling (and consenting) each patient about digit survival (immediate and long-term), function of digit (and need for rehabilitation), the cost of replantation (10–15 times greater than amputation), and ensuring patients are aware that secondary surgeries are common. A fully informed patient is one that understands the benefits and consequences of both revascularization/replantation versus amputation. Although the formal consent discussion occurs with the surgeon performing amputation or replantation, a common message from transferring providers to patients is important in order to avoid discordance and dissatisfaction.

The assessment of the amputated injury can guide the surgeon in discussing potential outcomes after replantation. For example, the thumb provides approximately half the function of the hand, and therefore, thumb amputations are of greater consequence.[31,32] Furthermore, Sears and colleagues[9] found that thumb replantation resulted in greater quality-adjusted life-years than completion amputation. As previously mentioned, amputations through flexor tendon zone II are considered a relative contraindication to replantation, given that loss in range of motion is often in excess of 60%.[22,33] Assessment of the mechanism of injury is also informative of outcomes. Patients can be advised that 2-point discrimination in replanted digits is typically better following sharp injury (8 mm) than avulsion injury (15 mm).[34] To contrast the outcome of replantation, the expected functionality after completion amputations should also be explained.

The American Medical Association Guide predicts functional impairment after completion amputations based on anatomic level of injury within digits (**Fig. 2**).[3,35] In addition, multiple amputated digits combine to affect hand function more heavily. Importantly, the American Medical Association Guide rates complete transverse sensory loss as an equal impairment to amputation of the digit at that level, and therefore, an insensate digit may be no better than a failed replantation or completion amputation. Although this assessment represents functional outcomes, it does not capture all aspects of patient disability, which is more appropriately assessed through patient-reported outcomes measures, such as the Michigan Hand Questionnaire.[3] Although research is needed to truly understand the differences in functional

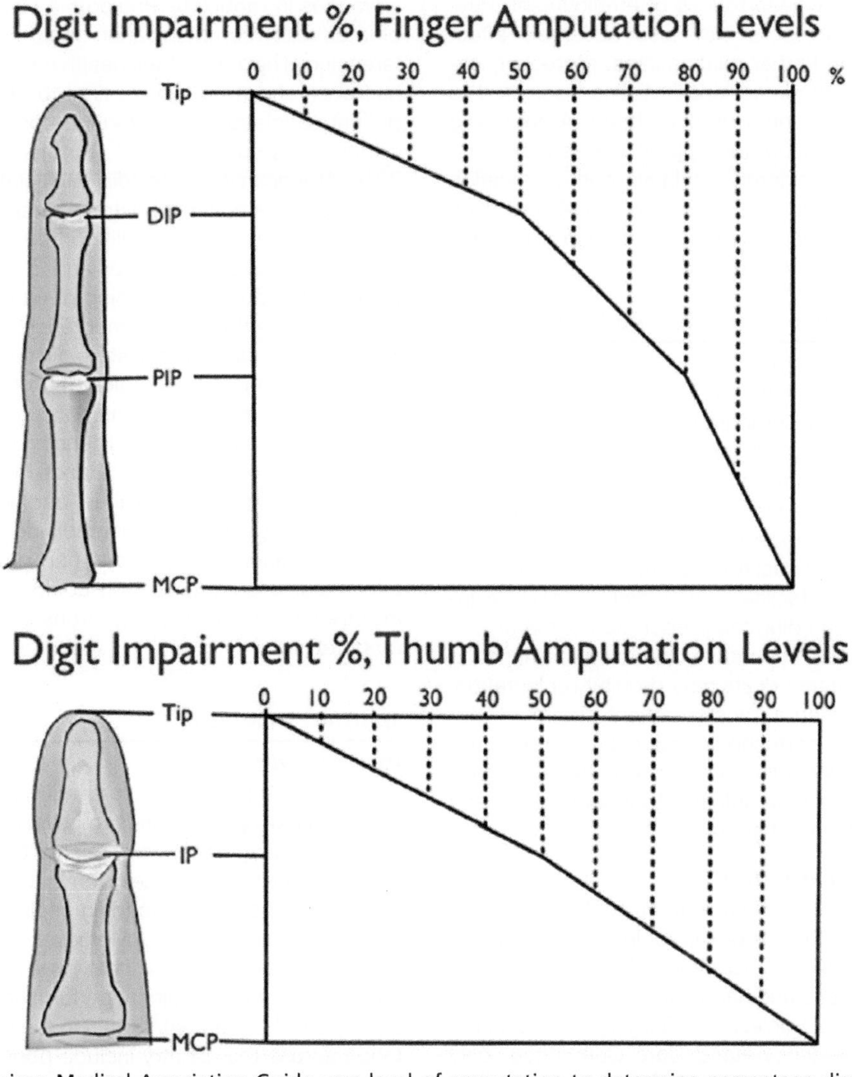

Fig. 2. American Medical Association Guide uses level of amputation to determine percentage disability from traumatic finger amputations. DIP, distal interphalangeal joint; MCP, metacarpophalangeal joint; PIP, proximal interphalangeal joint. (*From* Giladi AM, McGlinn EP, Shauver MJ, et al. Measuring outcomes and determining long-term disability after revision amputation for treatment of traumatic finger and thumb amputation injuries. Plast Reconstr Surg 2014;134(5):746e–55e; with permission.)

outcomes between completion amputation and replantation, surgeons can advise patients that completion amputation offers a more simple and expedient solution with considerably less recovery and rehabilitation. Furthermore, revision amputations can safely be performed in the emergency department without conferring an increased risk of secondary revision.[36]

Patient-related factors

In addition to understanding how the nature of injury dictates the functional outcome, patients must consider the global impact of digital replantation. Discussions should be conceptualized in a biopsychosocial context, such that patients comprehend how the injury will affect their physical health, mental health, and socioeconomic well-being. Patients who undergo replantation are commonly out of work for 4 to 12 months, whereas patients who elect for completion amputation often return to work within 1 to 2 months.[37] Fortunately, with distal digital replantation, 98% of patients return to work; 87% of patients with thumb amputation return to the same occupation.[6,33] If a patient is not prepared for the longer period of partial disability that follows replantation, then replantation may be considered relatively contraindicated. Multiple surgeries and absence from work may lead to loss of employment. Psychological stressors may also adversely affect marriages and other relationships. Moreover, understanding the importance of time dedicated to hand therapy cannot be overstated. A perceived lack of motivation for aggressive rehabilitation should be considered a relative contraindication to replant, given that if therapy is delayed even 14 days after injury, range of motion outcomes are significantly worse.[21]

Communication with Referring Facility

Part-related factors

Regional replantation centers are experienced with presurgical preparation of patients and the amputated part, but their successes are heavily influenced by the management of the patient before arrival at the receiving tertiary institution. A critical component of successful transfers is the content and quality of communication between the 2 treating facilities. In particular, precise instructions regarding the preparation of the amputated part are imperative, because mishandling of the amputated digits may prohibit replantation. When accepting a transfer patient, the microvascular replant team should request accurate timeline details, including time of amputation, warm/cold ischemia time, inflated tourniquet time, and anticipated time of arrival.

Patient-related factors

Problems with communication continue to exist between health care providers involved in interfacility transfers.[38–40] In a survey of emergency medicine physicians and hand surgeons conducted by the American Society for Surgery of the Hand (ASSH) Emergency Hand Care Committee, only half of hand surgeons reported that they frequently received direct communication from transferring providers.[39] Moreover, the reported diagnosis on arrival at the referral institution was frequently inaccurate. Thakur and colleagues[40] found that 97% of inappropriate orthopedic-related transfers were accepted by an emergency department physician, without the knowledge of the on-call orthopedist. The impact of unnecessary transfers, with regard to cost and resource utilization, is well documented in the literature and adds credence to the need for guidelines, protocols, and better communication during interfacility transfers. For digital amputations, direct communication between the referring physician and the hand surgeon at the receiving hospital maximizes efficiency and minimizes error.

Direct communication allows the surgeon to make an informed recommendation about disposition and provides guidance for transfer. Given advances in mobile technology, a valuable mode of interfacility communication could be videoconferencing. This form of telehealth (or telemedicine) has been shown to reduce time to care, improve patient satisfaction, and reduce cost in selected orthopedic populations.[41,42] Furthermore, at the 2016 American Orthopaedic Association Annual Meeting, a live poll demonstrated that 96% of participants believed in the utility of telehealth.[41] Unfortunately, the use of videos and images has not been adopted in the provision of care or transfer of hand patients in the emergency department. This is likely due to the systemic issues inhibiting the application of telemedicine in other medical settings, including governmental barriers (eg, Medicare restrictions, state licensing issues), concerns with HIPAA (Health Insurance Portability and Accountability Act) compliance, and narrow insurance coverage for the telemedicine services. If these bureaucratic limitations can be overcome, telemedicine communication could be beneficial in streamlining interfacility transfers of digital amputations.

Transfer: Triaging

Part-related factors

Traumatic amputations represent approximately 25% of hand injury transfers to Level I trauma centers,[42] and triage of these patients to specialized centers is likely to increase given that 1 out of every 20 hospitals stops performing replantation each year in the United States.[14] Moreover, a 2007 survey of ASSH members found that only 56% perform replantation, with a majority performing fewer than 5 per year.[13] Other contributors to the fall in replantation across the country include poor reimbursement rates and an unwillingness to provide emergency hand care. In fact, Butala and colleagues[43] recently showed that only half of Level I trauma centers had continuous access to microvascular expertise, even though this is a requirement for certification as a Level 1 trauma center by American College of Surgeons. Collectively, these factors have contributed to the 6% decline in replants performed per year in the United States.[14] Therefore, the American College of Surgeons and the ASSH have supported regionalizing hand and upper extremity trauma care given the improved outcomes at high-volume digit replant centers.[32]

At high-volume centers, digital replantation is more likely to be attempted and more likely to succeed.[6,14,15] Therefore, timely triage to a specialized center is imperative to optimize outcomes. To economically sustain this approach, there should be an emphasis on the referring institutions' ability to assess and triage digital amputations. Secondary overtriage (ie, unnecessary interfacility transfer of minimally injured patients) is an expected consequence of a system that has inadequate interfacility communication.[44] This has been seen in prior studies, which show that many patients transferred for specialty evaluation are rapidly discharged home (ie, revision amputation without admission).[38,45] To minimize secondary overtriage, referring and referral hospital must make a collaborative decision on the feasibility of replant. This strategy would avoid unnecessary transfers, because completion amputations could be performed by local surgeons on urgent but nonemergent basis.

Patient-related factors

Transfer time is a critical component for digital amputations that are candidates for replantation. Although emergency air transportation provides the fastest mode of transfer, it comes at a considerable cost, estimated $6000 more than ground transportation.[46] In 2006, the *Guidelines for Air Medical Dispatch*, published by the American College of Emergency Physicians, recommended that finger and thumb amputation not be qualifiers for air transportation. After publication of these guidelines, Nolte and colleagues[47] concluded from a 17-year retrospective database review that clinical outcomes and hospital volume were not affected by this policy.[46,48] Despite their findings, literature indicates that the guidelines are not strictly adhered to, and additionally, Ozer and colleagues[21] found that a considerable portion of patients (65%) transported by air for traumatic amputation does not undergo replantation. The most common reason for not replanting was injury characteristics, reinforcing that poor communication between the referring and referral hospitals is a major source of health care overutilization.

Transfer: Preparation

Part-related factors

Preparation of the amputated part for transfer and surgical replantation is simple, but critical. All amputated parts should be collected regardless of contamination or quality of tissue. Even if not suitable for replantation, spare parts (eg, skin) can be used for autologous grafting. Immediately after retrieval, the amputation should be cleaned, wrapped in saline-moistened gauze, and placed on ice in a labeled, sealed bag.[15] Placing the amputated part directly on ice results in freeze injuries and must be avoided. Radiographic images of the tissue proximal (stump) and distal (amputated part) are also important to assess bony injuries that require fixation or preclude replantation. Some surgeons advocate photographing the amputated digit and stump, because these documents can be important for medicolegal purposes in scenarios where replantation is not feasible.[49]

Patient-related factors

A standard ATLS trauma survey should not be overlooked. Adequate volume resuscitation can be monitored with a Foley catheter in patients with large-volume blood loss. Vasopressors are avoided if possible. Hospital infrastructure should be notified. If needed, a warm room or intensive care unit bed should be reserved. For proximal amputations, it is preferable if the OR has a room prepared before patient arrival. In patients with a proximal limb amputation, the blood bank at the receiving institution should be alerted that multiple transfusions may be needed; upon patient arrival, a blood bank sample should be acquired. While the patient is undergoing evaluation in the emergency department, the amputated digit or limb can be taken to the OR suite for exploration and preparation. If leeches are a possibility, the pharmacy should be notified as well.

After patients are hemodynamically stabilized, preoperative preparation of patients for replantation can take priority. With regard to the amputated stump, tourniquets should be removed, and preference should be placed on maintaining hemostasis with manual pressure, nonadherent pressure dressings, and targeted blood vessel clamping or ligation only when necessary. In digit and distal hand injuries, minor bleeding is typically self-limiting with a nonadherent dressing, gauze wrap, and soft compression using an elastic bandage. Amputations are Gustilo Grade IIIC open fractures (contaminated with vascular injury), and appropriate perioperative antibiotics should be given for prophylaxis (eg, cefazolin or ceftriaxone). If severe contamination is present, such as in farming injuries, then consideration can be given to covering gram-negative and anaerobic bacteria (eg, metronidazole or clindamycin).[50] Furthermore, tetanus prophylaxis should be initiated at arrival if the patient's immunization status is unknown or overdue.

SUMMARY

Success of digit replantation in the United States could be improved with triage systems that better identify patients appropriate for replantation and initiate presurgical preparation that ultimately improves functional outcomes. Educating health professionals on the best management of completion amputation and increasing interfacility communication are critical components to the future success of a health care system that emphasizes regionalization of amputation.

REFERENCES

1. Cohen S. The concentration of health care expenditures and related expenses for costly medical conditions, 2012. Rockville (MD): Agency for Healthcare Research and Quality; 2014. Statistical Brief #455.
2. Ootes D, Lambers KT, Ring DC. The epidemiology of upper extremity injuries presenting to the emergency department in the United States. Hand (N Y) 2012;7:18–22.
3. Giladi AM, McGlinn EP, Shauver MJ, et al. Measuring outcomes and determining long-term disability after revision amputation for treatment of traumatic finger and thumb amputation injuries. Plast Reconstr Surg 2014;134(5):746e–55e.
4. Maroukis BL, Chung KC, MacEachern M, et al. Hand trauma care in the United States: a literature review. Plast Reconstr Surg 2016;137(1):100e–11e.
5. Dec W. A meta-analysis of success rates for digit replantation. Tech Hand Up Extrem Surg 2006; 10(3):124e–9e.
6. Sebastin SJ, Chung KC. A systematic review of the outcomes of replantation of distal digital amputation. Plast Reconstr Surg 2011;128(3):723e–37e.
7. Agarwal JP, Trovato MJ, Agarwal S, et al. Selected outcomes of thumb replantation after isolated thumb amputation injury. J Hand Surg Am 2010;35(9): 1485e–90e.
8. Zhou H, Bao B, Zheng X. A Comparison of functional outcomes and therapeutic costs: Single-digit replantation versus revision amputation. Plast Reconstr Surg 2018;141(2):244e–93.
9. Sears ED, Shin R, Prosser LA, et al. Economic analysis of revision amputation and replantation treatment of finger amputation injuries. Plast Reconstr Surg 2014;133(4):827e–40e.
10. Hustedt JW, Bohl DD, Champagne L. The detrimental effect of decentralization in digital replantation in the United States: 15 years of evidence from the National Inpatient Sample. J Hand Surg Am 2016;41(5):593e–601e.
11. Richards WT, Barber MK, Richards WA, et al. Hand injuries in the state of Florida, are centers of excellence needed? J Trauma 2010;68(6):1480e–90e.
12. Fufa D, Calfee R, Wall L, et al. Digit replantation: experience of two U.S. academic level-I trauma centers. J Bone Joint Surg Am 2013;95(23): 2127e–34e.
13. Payatakes AH, Zagoreos NP, Fedorcik GG, et al. Current practice of microsurgery by members of the American Society for Surgery of the Hand. J Hand Surg Am 2007;32(4):541e–7e.
14. Reavey P, Stranix J, Muresan H, et al. Disappearing digits: analysis of national trends in amputation and replantation in the United States. Plast Reconstr Surg 2018;141(6):857e–67e.
15. Bueno RA, Battiston B, Ciclamini D, et al. Replantation: current concepts and outcomes. Clin Plast Surg 2014;14:385–95.
16. Brown M, Lu Y, Chung KC, et al. Annual hospital volume and success of digital replantation. Plast Reconstr Surg 2017;139(3):672–80.
17. Wolfe VM, Wange AA. Replantation of the upper extremity: current concepts. J Am Acad Orthop Surg 2015;23:373–81.
18. Breahna A, Siddiqui A, Fitzgerald O'Connor E, et al. Replantation of digits: a review of predictive factors for survival. J Hand Surg Eur Vol 2016;41(7):753–7.
19. Barbary S, Dap F, Dautel G. Finger replantation: surgical technique and indications. Chir Main 2013;32: 363–72.
20. Higgins JP. Chapter 42: replantation. In: Wolfe SW, Hotchkiss RN, Pederson WC, et al, editors. Green's operative hand surgery. 7th edition. Philadelphia: Elsevier; 2017. p. 1476–85.
21. Ozer K, Kramer W, Gillani S, et al. Replantation versus revision of amputated fingers in patients air-transported to a level 1 trauma center. J Hand Surg 2010;35A:936–40.
22. Ross DC, Manktelow RT, Wells MT, et al. Tendon function after replantation: Prognostic factors and strategies to enhance total active motion. Ann Plast Surg 2003;51(2):141–6.
23. Waikakul S, Sakkarnkosol S, Vanadurongwan V, et al. Results of 1018 digital replantations in 552 patients. Injury 2000;31(1):33–40.
24. Sears ED, Chung KC. Replantation of finger avulsion injuries: a systematic review of survival and functional outcomes. J Hand Surg Am 2011;36(4): 686–94.
25. Solarz MK, Thoder JJ, Rehman S. Management of major traumatic upper extremity amputations. Orthop Clin North Am 2016;47:127–36.
26. Maegele M, Schochl H, Cohen MJ. An update on the coagulopathy of trauma. Shock 2014;41:21–5.
27. Wei FC, Chang YL, Chen HC, et al. Three successful digital replantations in a patient after 84, 86, and 94 hours of cold ischemia time. Plast Reconstr Surg 1988;82(2):346–50.
28. van der Velde J, Serfontein L, Iohom G. Reducing the potential for tourniquet-associated reperfusion injury. Eur J Emerg Med 2013;20:391–6.
29. Drolet BC, Okhah Z, Phillips BZ, et al. Evidence for safe tourniquet use in 500 consecutive upper extremity procedures. Hand 2014;9(4):494–8.
30. Bogdan Y, Helfet D. Use of Tourniquets in limb trauma surgery. Orthop Clin North Am 2018;49: 157–65.
31. Chow JA, Bilos JZ, Chunprapaph B. Thirty thumb replantations: indications and results. Plast Reconstr Surg 1979;64(5):626e–30e.
32. Mahmoudi E, Huetteman HE, Chung KC. A population-based study of replantation after traumatic thumb

amputation, 2007-2012. J Hand Surg Am 2017;42(1): 25–33.
33. Goldner RD, Stevanovic MV, Nunley JA, et al. Digital replantation at the level of distal interphalangeal joint and the distal phalanx. J Hand Surg 1989;14A: 214–20.
34. Glickman LT, Mackinnon SE. Sensory recovery following digital replantation. Microsurgery 1990; 11(3):236–42.
35. Rondinelli R, editor. Guides to the evaluation of permanent impairment. 6th edition. Chicago: American Medical Association; 2008.
36. Harris AP, Goodman AD, Gil JA, et al. Incidence, timing, and risk factors for secondary revision after primary revision of traumatic digit amputations. J Hand Surg Am 2018;43(11):1040.e1-11.
37. Hattori Y, Doi K, Ikeda K, et al. A retrospective study of functional outcomes after successful replantation versus amputation closure for single fingertip amputations. J Hand Surg Am 2006;31A:811–8.
38. Drolet BG, Tandon VJ, Ha AY, et al. Unnecessary emergency transfers for evaluation by a Plastic Surgeon: A burden to patients and the health care system. Plast Reconstr Surg 2016;137:1927–33.
39. Drolet BC, Lifchez SD, Jacoby SM, et al. Perceptions of emergency medicine residency and hand surgery fellowship program directors in the appropriate disposition of upper extremity emergencies. J Hand Surg Am 2015;40(12):2435–9.
40. Thakur NA, Plante MJ, Kayiaros S, et al. Inappropriate transfer of patients with orthopaedic injuries to a level 1 trauma center: a prospective study. J Orthop Trauma 2010;24(6):336–9.
41. Wongworawat MD, Capistrant G, Stephenson JM. The opportunity awaits to lead orthopaedic telehealth innovation. J Bone Joint Surg Am 2017; 99(17):e93.
42. Bauer AS, Blazar PE, Earp BE, et al. Characteristics of emergency department transfers for hand surgery consultation. Hand (N Y) 2013;8(1):12–6.
43. Butala P, Fisher MD, Blueschke G, et al. Factors associated with transfer of hand injuries to a level 1 trauma center: a descriptive analysis of 1137 cases. Plast Reconstr Surg 2014;133:842–7.
44. Peterson BC, Mangiapani D, Kellogg R, et al. Hand and microvascular replantation call availability study: a national real-time survey of level-I and level-II trauma centers. J Bone Joint Surg Am 2012;94(24):e185.
45. Lynch KT, Essig RM, Long DM, et al. Nationwide secondary overtriage in level 3 and level 4 trauma centers: are these transfers necessary. J Surg Res 2016;204(2):460–6.
46. Hartzell TL, Kuo P, Eberlin KR, et al. The overutilization of resources in patients with acute upper extremity trauma and infection. J Hand Surg Am 2013;38(4):766–73.
47. Nolte MT, Shauver MJ, Chung KC, et al. Effect of policy change on the use of long-distance transport and follow-up care for patients with traumatic finger amputations. J Hand Surg Am 2017;42(8):610–7.
48. American College of Emergency Physicians and National Association of EMS Physicians. Guidelines for air medical dispatch: policy resource and education paper. Washington, DC: American College of Emergency Physicians; 2006.
49. Bastidas N, Cassidy L, Hoffman L, et al. A single-institution experience of hand surgery litigation in a major replantation center. Plast Reconstr Surg 2011;127(1):284–92.
50. Rodriguez L, Jung HS, Goulet JA, et al. Evidence-based protocol for prophylactic antibiotics in open fractures: Improved antibiotic stewardship with no increase in infection rates. J Trauma Acute Care Surg 2014;77:400–8.

Indications for Replantation and Revascularization in the Hand

Mitchell A. Pet, MD[a,*], Jason H. Ko, MD[b]

KEYWORDS

• Amputation • Finger replantation • Hand replantation • Indications

KEY POINTS

- The indications for upper extremity replantation are fluid, and it has long been appreciated that they change with time.
- Traditional strong indications for replantation include hand, thumb, or multiple digit amputation in adults, and almost any amputation in a child.
- Patients often desire replantation of single nonthumb digits based on aesthetic preference and personal/cultural values. Replantation in these situations is acceptable and rewarding, but individual consideration of patient, injury, and circumstantial factors is critical to avoid patient morbidity and unsatisfactory outcomes.

INTRODUCTION

As microsurgical capabilities have advanced, it is increasingly feasible to achieve revascularization or replantation of most amputations within the upper extremity. As a consequence, the focus of dialogue surrounding replantation has shifted from "can we replant this amputated part?" to "should we?" This is a much more difficult question to address because it requires reconciliation of multiple patient, injury, and circumstantial factors that often point the surgeon in opposite directions. This article provides a brief history of the development of traditional indications for upper extremity replantation/revascularization and explores the reasons why these indications remain fluid. Additionally, we offer our perspective on worthy considerations for the modern patient and surgeon when approaching this shared decision.

Traditional Indications for Replantation in the Upper Extremity

The development of indications for replantation in the upper extremity has been molded by parallel advancements in microsurgical capability and the understanding of surgical outcomes. In 1973, O'Brien and colleagues[1] published an early discussion of the indications for digital replantation. This group advocated replantation of multiple fingers and isolated amputations of the thumb or index finger. In 1974, Frykman and Wood recommended replantation/revascularization of any nonviable digit that remained partially attached, multiple digital amputations at or proximal to the proximal interphalangeal (PIP) joint, and amputations of the thumb or hand level.[2] In 1978, Manktelow offered a conservative perspective, arguing that replantation of one or two nonthumb digits may severely impair hand function. Manktelow's

Disclosures: The authors have no pertinent financial relationships to disclose.

[a] Washington University School of Medicine, 660 South Euclid Avenue, St Louis, MO 63110, USA; [b] Northwestern University School of Medicine, NMH/Galter Room 19-250, 675 North Saint Clair, Chicago, IL 60611, USA
* Corresponding author.
E-mail address: Mitchell.Pet@gmail.com

Hand Clin 35 (2019) 119–130
https://doi.org/10.1016/j.hcl.2018.12.003

hand.theclinics.com

indications for replantation were amputations of the hand, thumb, or greater than two nonthumb digits.[3]

Although these authors came to slightly different conclusions, their collective findings reflect early consensus supporting a strong indication to replant thumbs, multiple amputated digits, and extremities severed at the hand or wrist level. Essentially, this core triad of indications reflects that replantation is advisable when an amputation injury threatens a catastrophic functional deficit for which functional compensation is difficult.

As experience increased through the 1980s, replantation gained traction outside of devastating and functionally critical injuries. Replantation in the pediatric population is technically more challenging because of diminutive vessel size and the preponderance of crush/avulsion mechanisms. However, when microsurgical success is achieved, pediatric single-digit replantations generally achieve excellent functional outcomes attributable to superior regenerative capacity and cortical plasticity.[4,5] Because outcomes in this population are better than adults and a younger age warrants attempts at digital preservation, any amputation in the upper extremity of a pediatric patient is generally accepted as a strong indication for replantation.

Similarly, although replantation of single nonthumb digits was previously considered a functional detriment, evidence accumulated that in certain situations, excellent results could be obtained.[6] Several outcomes studies identified that replantations distal to the flexor digitorum superficialis (FDS) insertion achieved superior outcomes, especially with respect to range of motion (ROM).[7] For this reason, single digit amputation distal to the FDS insertion has been frequently cited as a relative indication for replantation.

Although no single source could be chosen to define the traditional indications for replantation, the fifth edition of *Green's Operative Hand Surgery* offers the following summary of indications and contraindications.[8] Indications for replantation include

- Thumb amputation
- Multiple digit amputation
- Partial or total hand through the palm, wrist, forearm, elbow, or above
- Almost any part in a child
- Single digit amputation distal to the FDS insertion

Contraindications to replantation include

- Severely crushed or mangled parts
- Amputations at multiple levels
- Amputations in patients with other serious injuries/diseases
- Severe atherosclerotic disease
- Prolonged warm ischemia
- Mentally unstable patient
- Individual finger amputation in an adult at a level proximal to the FDS insertion

Forces Driving the Modernization of Indications

Since the infancy of replantation surgery, authors experienced in the subject matter have recognized that surgical indications are flexible and likely to change with increasing experience and knowledge. In 1981, Zhong-Wei and colleagues[9] elegantly wrote the following: "Indications for upper limb reattachments at this time are neither absolute nor static. They are relative, dynamic, and surely will change as experience increases and techniques become even more refined. Success must not be equated with tissue survival but measured only in terms of what the effort has done for the patient in a global sense."

Among the most influential expansile forces influencing replantation surgery has been the vast improvement and proliferation of surgical instrumentation and magnification technology. Additionally, advanced techniques of bony fixation and tendon repair have facilitated earlier and more effective postoperative rehabilitation protocols. By increasing the frequency of microsurgical success and satisfactory functional rehabilitation, these advances have encouraged surgeons to be more aggressive in selecting patients for replantation/revascularization. Patient expectations are also influenced by the increasingly routine nature of replantation/revascularization, and many who present with amputations believe that microsurgical salvage can and should be performed.

Counteracting these expansile forces are some that exert a more conservative approach to patient selection. The increasing volume and influence of patient-reported outcomes data has highlighted that many patients who undergo revision amputation do well, and that not all who undergo replantation/revascularization are better off because of it. There has been an increasing consciousness among surgeons that the act of digital salvage can demonstrably impair long-term function. Even in situations where function is improved, growing concern exists surrounding excessive financial expenditure for sometimes marginal gains. Sears and colleagues[10] have demonstrated that the cost difference between replantation and revision amputation routinely exceeds $14,000, and that replantation of a single digit may cost in excess of $136,000 per quality-adjusted life-year. Although this cost should not be a primary driver of surgical decision-making, it does underscore that replantation requires a significant expenditure of health care resources, which should be carefully considered in the context of a larger system.

Updating the Indications for Upper Extremity Replantation and Revascularization

In general, we subscribe to the traditional strong indications for replantation: proximal thumb, multiple digit, or hand/arm amputations, and nearly all pediatric amputations. In these situations, replantation should be attempted if it can be safely done. However, most patients presenting with amputation/devascularization injuries are outside of these bounds. In modern practice, the decision to perform replantation/revascularization in cases of single nonthumb digital amputation is shared by the patient and surgeon. This decision process is complex and is influenced by numerous factors that must be weighed in each individual circumstance. We believe that formulation of an updated "indications list" that adequately respects these subtleties is not possible. Instead we offer a guide for rational consideration of the factors that should be weighed when navigating this situation (**Table 1**).

Patient factors

Medical comorbidity Chronic medical comorbidities negatively effects replantation success and postoperative complications. In perhaps the largest-scale examination of this relationship, Hustedt and colleagues[11] found in a cohort of 11,788 patients that the risk for replant failure is highest in patients with psychotic disorders, peripheral vascular disease, and electrolyte imbalances. Postoperative complications are most common among patients with electrolyte imbalances, drug abuse, or chronic obstructive pulmonary disease. Both replantation failure and risk of postoperative complications were all significantly elevated in patients with more than three comorbidities.

In noncritical amputations, even when the mechanism is favorable, a significant burden of chronic medical comorbidity is a relative contraindication for replantation. Good communication is critical in this situation, because patients with chronic medical conditions are at risk for feeling that revision amputation was recommended because they are in some way "not worth it." Careful and empathetic explanation of their risk profile for anesthetic and perioperative complications, coupled with the principle of "do no harm," is often helpful in reaching the understanding related to a thoughtful risk/benefit analysis.

In catastrophic amputation injuries (multiple fingers, thumb, hand) sustained by a patient with serious chronic medical comorbidity, decision-making is difficult. It is important to remember that no replantation is absolutely indicated, and that if the operative risk is overwhelmingly great, then replantation of even a hand or thumb can ethically be foregone. Prolonged anesthesia in multiply-comorbid patients is dangerous, and the extensive blood loss and reperfusion injury associated with major limb replantation has the potential to be life-threatening, especially in patients with cardiovascular or cerebrovascular disease.

In situations where replantation/revascularization in a comorbid patient is being considered, consultation with the on-call anesthesiologist may be advisable for risk stratification. During the process of informed consent, it is important to specifically discuss the negative implications of comorbidity on success and complication rates. During the operation, close communication with the anesthesiologist is critical, and the safety of continuing the replantation must be periodically reevaluated, even if the technical tasks are proceeding smoothly. Postoperative care requires vigilance, because many operative events, such as fluid administration, vascular stasis, and airway manipulation, have sequela that may occur in the days to follow.

Table 1
Factors for consideration when deciding whether replantation/revascularization should be offered

Patient Factors	Injury Factors	Circumstantial Factors
Medical comorbidity	Level of injury	Time to presentation
Age	Digits involved	Availability of post-replantation care
Physical and occupational demands	Mechanism	
Social factors	Injury to adjacent fingers	
Cultural and personal values	Incomplete or complete amputation	
Psychiatric disease		

Case 1

This 71-year-old female retiree and active gardener suffered an avulsion injury to the nondominant left ring finger (**Fig. 1**)*. Despite education regarding the poor functional prognosis for ring avulsion injuries, she was initially insistent on attempting replantation. Detailed history revealed that she had experienced cardiopulmonary complications necessitating intensive care unit care after her last two anesthetics. Replantation was not offered based on the unacceptable likelihood of serious postoperative complications. The noncritical nature of the amputation and unfavorable injury pattern were secondary factors in this case.*

Age Enthusiasm for replantation is appropriately high in pediatric and adult patients, but advanced age is often cited as a relative contraindication for replantation. However, in 2016 Hustedt and colleagues[11] demonstrated that the rate of microsurgical success in finger replantation varies independently from age after controlling for comorbidity. Kwon and colleagues[12] found that microsurgical success is unaffected by age up to a cutoff of 70 years, and that even in patients older than age 70 with a crushing mechanism of injury, successful replantation was achieved in excess of 70% of attempts. Although functional outcomes in the elderly are inferior to those in younger patients (mostly because of decreased sensory recovery),[13] 94% of elderly patients reported that they were completely or fairly satisfied with their replanted digits.[12]

Accepting that replantation in the elderly population can be accomplished, concern for the safety of this invasive intervention remains appropriate. In a study of more than 15,000 finger replantations, Barzin and colleagues[14] found that patients older than age 65 years had slightly higher rates of blood transfusion and disposition to a nursing home than those younger than 65. However, no intergroup difference was detected in such adverse events as deep venous thrombosis, pulmonary embolism, myocardial infarction, and sepsis.

Based on this information supporting the reliability and safety of this intervention, it is our opinion that advanced age alone should not be considered a contraindication for replantation. However, especially when considering replantation in patients exceeding 65, the absence of comorbidity should not be assumed and close attention to the patient's medical history is critical. This discovery process may include obtaining records, querying family members, and/or preoperative medical consultation. Furthermore, postoperative inpatient management must respect chronic conditions,

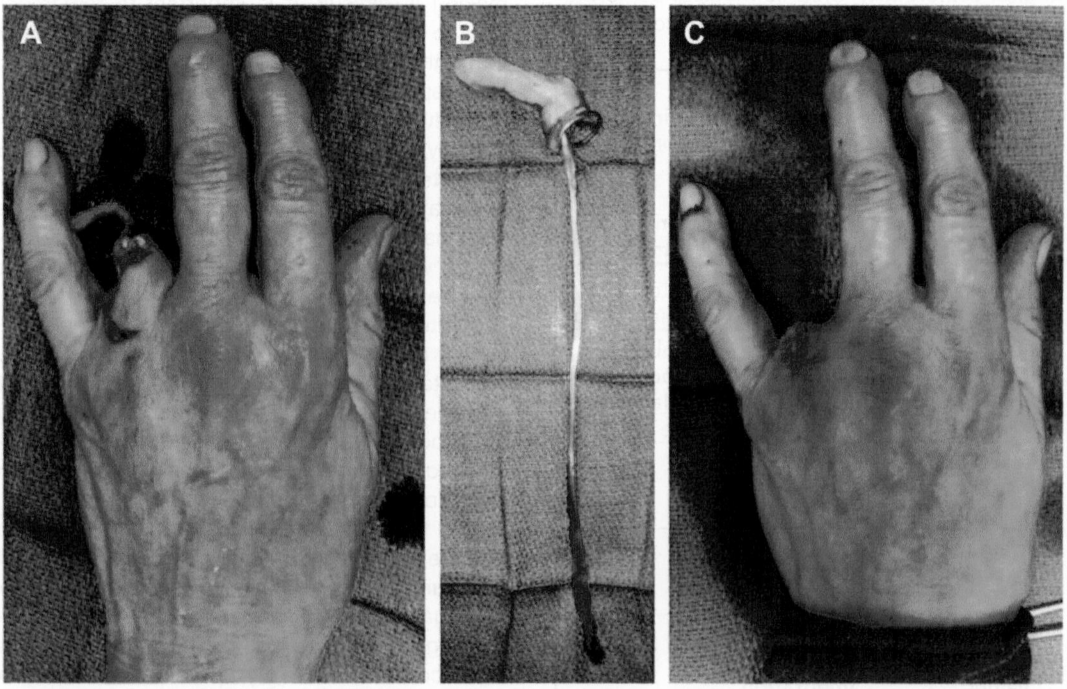

Fig. 1. (*A, B*) The patient from Case 1 presented with left ring finger avulsion. (*C*) Revision amputation was the chosen treatment primarily because of the patient's unacceptable operative risk profile, in addition to the avulsion mechanism and functionally noncritical nature of this single digit injury.

such a hypertension and diabetes, which can become dangerously destabilized if neglected.

Physical and occupational demands The first concern of many patients arriving with a partial or complete amputation is often the effect that this injury and its treatment will have on their ability to continue participation in their occupation or avocation. When considering replantation/revascularization of a single nonthumb digit, it is important to learn about the patient's occupational or avocational demands so that anticipated function after both replantation and revision amputation are discussed. Patients who perform manual labor often assume that because they are directly dependent on their hands to earn a wage, replantation is in their best interest when in fact, the opposite is often true. Return to a labor occupation may be faster and more complete with revision amputation, whereas replantation can delay or even prohibit achievement of this milestone. It is important that patients (especially manual laborers) understand that the benefits of replantation take many months to be realized, and require substantial postoperative therapy and often one to two additional procedures. For these reasons, a replanted finger may be burdensome for quite some time. Even after maximal recovery, these heavy outdoor laborers may find even moderate stiffness, numbness, and cold intolerance to be limiting. When provided with this information, laborers may lose interest in digital salvage.

On the other end of the spectrum are patients with particular occupational or other demands that depend on a full complement of fingers. These include, but are not limited to, persons who use sign language to communicate, musicians, and some athletes. In these patients, salvage of even an isolated index or small finger may provide great benefit and should be offered.

Most occupation classes and demand patterns neither strongly indicate nor contraindicate replantation of single nonthumb digits. With only modest accommodation, most patients can return to their previous activities after either revision amputation or replantation. In patients with low-demand jobs, return to work is often feasible even during postoperative immobilization and rehabilitation. It is in these situations that the patient and surgeon have the most latitude to consider other factors.

Social factors In addition to eliciting of the physical demands of a patient's occupation, careful consideration should be given to his or her social situation when deciding between revision amputation and replantation of a noncritical part. Social issues that might contraindicate replantation include, but are not limited to

- Unstable employment that would be lost during prolonged absence
- Financial unfeasibility of missing work while rehabilitating a replanted finger
- Lack of transportation to necessary postoperative hand therapy appointments

Especially in single nonthumb digital amputations, replantation results in a considerable delay in return to work.[15] In patients without a social support system and financial safety net, even temporary inability to earn a wage is catastrophic and results in extraordinary hardship. Failure to identify social barriers to successful replantation preoperatively can result in heartbreaking postdischarge digital necrosis caused by noncompliance, or serious social consequences for the patient. Just as one needs to be cognizant of causing systemic medical complications in comorbid patients, one must be aware of the social consequences that are incited by initiation of a prolonged hospitalization and convalescent period for a marginal indication.

Cultural and personal values Personal and cultural values have long been known to influence the shared decision to perform replantation of single nonthumb digits. A commonly cited example of this influence is the higher rate of replantation that occurs in Japan (29%) relative to the United States (12%).[16] This finding has long been attributed to a stronger preference for replantation among Japanese patients, which is presumably driven by Confucian values emphasizing body integrity and the stigma of finger amputation as a signal of gang affiliation in Japanese society.[16] Recently, this assumption has been called into question by evidence suggesting that most patients in the United States and Japan have a strong preference for replantation.[16] Instead, some suggest that cross-cultural difference in replantation rate may be caused by surgeon preference.[17]

This is in keeping with our experience that American patients generally desire replantation more often than surgeons recommend it. Although it is easy for the surgeon to assume that this represents a patient's unrealistically inflated estimation of their surgical outcome, this outlook was not supported by a recent survey study of patients and hand surgeons.[17] In fact, patients and surgeons had similar expectations for postreplantation outcomes and agreed that replantation would lead to better appearance. Instead, this discrepancy of patient and surgeon outlook is attributable to differing expectations for the post-revision amputation state. Patients expect significantly less functional recovery after a revision amputation than do surgeons, and patients exhibit increased association between revision amputation and social stigma.

The implication of these findings is that when deciding whether or not to pursue replantation, patients are much more concerned than surgeons about the social implications of living with a revision amputation. Whether or not this concern is rooted in some definable religious or moral values system is immaterial in our opinion, and attention to this issue is warranted in Eastern and Western cultures. Further study is needed to determine if the stigma and disability anticipated by lay survey-takers is actually experienced by patients who have undergone revision amputation.

Working with a patient who has a strong desire to pursue noncritical replantation for reasons of appearance is uncomfortable for the surgeon, especially when he/she expects that replantation may impair hand function. Although this may in fact be the case, the perceived positive impact of replantation on social function cannot be neglected. In some cases, the desire to reconstruct the most functional hand should yield to the obligation to reconstruct the most functional patient. In these difficult situations, there is no single correct course of action, although we argue that performing replantation is not necessarily contraindicated or unethical as long as the patient has been sufficiently apprised of the expected outcome. Importantly, this should not be interpreted as a universal mandate for replantation based on patient aesthetic preference, and surgeon judgment remains paramount.

Case 2

This 59-year-old male architect injured his nondominant left hand using a table saw **(Fig. 2)**. *He sustained amputation of the small finger through the PIP joint, in addition to distal phalanx fractures of the index, middle, and ring fingers. We initially advised against attempted replantation given the relatively poor functional prognosis of single nonthumb digits replanted within zone 2. However, the patient clearly communicated that maintaining a five-fingered aesthetic hand was a personal and cultural priority for him. Ultimately, replantation was performed, with consideration given to the fact that replantation would not hinder the rehabilitation of his adjacent finger injuries. The patient is extraordinarily pleased and appreciative, despite the fact that his small finger is fused at the PIP joint, and altogether stiff.*

Acute psychosis Although it is not a common occurrence, self-inflicted upper extremity amputations are so jarring and wrought with ethical challenges that they are deserving of individual attention. Psychological instability has been cited as a relative contraindication to replantation[8] and for this reason, it could be argued that self-inflicted amputations should be uniformly treated with revision amputation. This is a reasonable approach for amputations of noncritical parts, because replantation is unlikely to improve the overall prognosis and certainly will make emergent psychiatric treatment more complicated. However, in cases of multiple finger, thumb, or hand amputation, we believe that replantation should be at least considered.

In a thoughtful review of this topic, Schlozman[18] points out that most self-inflicted hand amputations in the literature are the result of nonsuicidal acute psychotic breaks, usually centered around some religious preoccupation or guilt over perceived transgressions. Although the patient may be psychotic and uncooperative at the time of presentation, this does not necessarily represent a permanent and unalterable psychological state. Immediate psychiatric consultation can rapidly determine if psychotic patients have capacity to refuse treatment. If a patient without capacity refuses treatment, it is ethically acceptable to perform replantation. Although the preoperative and immediate postoperative periods are routinely difficult, the collective published experience suggests that intense psychiatric care and antipsychotic medication usually stabilize a patient to the point that he/she cooperates with and appreciates treatment.

Injury factors

Level of injury and digits involved Amputations through the brachium, elbow, forearm, wrist, or palm should generally be replanted if the part and patient are in suitable condition. As myoelectric upper extremity prostheses have become increasingly advanced, it is sometimes suggested that major limb replantation could be foregone in favor of prosthetic rehabilitation. Although rehabilitation with an advanced prosthesis could feasibly offer function exceeding that of a replanted limb, it is important to remember that this type of prosthesis is not necessarily available to, or successfully integrated in, all patients. Furthermore, there is evidence to suggest that patients who have undergone hand/arm replantation regain better function and are more satisfied than patients who undergo prosthetic rehabilitation.[19,20]

Because thumb amputation represents such an enormous loss of hand function, great effort is

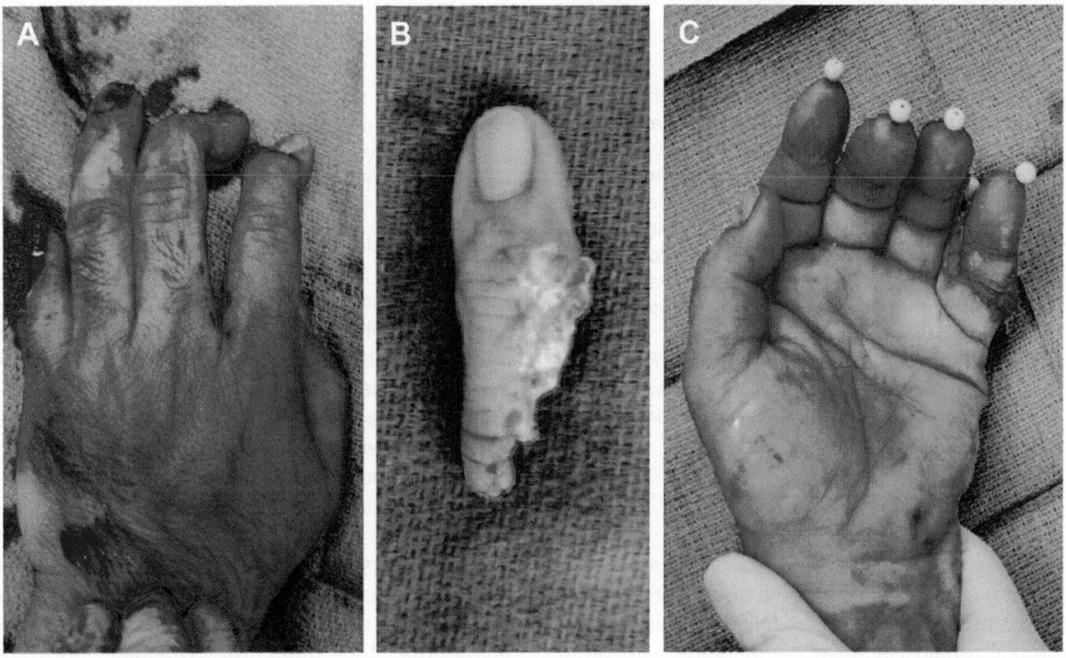

Fig. 2. (*A, B*) The patient from Case 2 presented with fractures of the distal phalanges of the index, middle, and ring fingers, and left small finger amputation. (*C*) Replantation was performed based on the patient's clear communication that maintenance of a five-fingered hand was a personal and cultural priority, even if it entailed some functional cost.

justified in performing replantation whenever possible. Nearly any thumb amputation occurring proximal to the interphalangeal joint (IPJ) should be replanted, including difficult cases of thumb crush or avulsion with tendons and nerves at the forearm level. Even if no motion or sensibility is restored, provision of a stable post of adequate length often represents a worthwhile salvage. Grasp and prehension are maintained even in the absence of IPJ and metacarpophalangeal joint motion, and sensation is restored secondarily using a variety of sensate flaps.

In cases of thumb amputation at or distal to the IPJ, replantation is only relatively indicated. This is because hand function is often acceptable after thumb tip amputation, as long as there is an intact proximal phalanx with adequate soft tissue coverage.[21] In our opinion, it is reasonable to recommend replantation of thumb injuries proximal to the nailfold. However, caution should be exercised if high-quality nerve repair is not possible, because a slightly shortened but fully sensate amputation stump is preferable to an insensate full-length thumb.

When replantation of a single nonthumb digit is strongly preferred by the patient, the primary surgical goal is preservation of a normal five-fingered aesthetic. When deciding whether or not to offer this intervention, the surgeon must consider how this aesthetically driven digit salvage could negatively impact hand function. Urbaniak and colleagues[7] found that single digits replanted at a level proximal to the insertion of the FDS tendon achieved only 35° of PIP joint ROM, whereas replantations occurring distal to the FDS insertion achieved 82°. In extremely distal replantations at or beyond distal IPJ, PIP motion may be even better at 94°.[15] Sensory recovery seems to follow the same trend, with better recovery expected in more distal injuries.[22] Although it is difficult to definitively quantify the functional impairment conferred by salvage of a stiff and minimally sensate finger, it is reasonable to suspect, based on these data, that replantation within flexor tendon zone 2 may decrease the overall utility of the hand. For this reason, many surgeons recommend against this and are more enthusiastic about distal injuries. This contrasts with the patient's perspective, where enthusiasm for single-digit replantation is generally proportional to the length of the amputated part. In our opinion, replantation of a single digit in zone 2 should be approached with caution and undertaken only if the patient's functional demands and priorities are truly compatible with accepting a potential functional deficit in favor of improved appearance of the hand.

> **Case 3**
>
> *This 19-year-old right-hand-dominant laborer sustained a sharp near-amputation of the small finger through the distal phalangeal shaft* (**Fig. 3**). *A 2-mm dorsal skin bridge remained intact, but the fingertip was dysvascular. Because of the distal level and sharp mechanism of this incomplete injury, the prognosis for functional recovery after replantation was believed to be excellent. The patient was counseled that either revision amputation or revascularization were options, and the patient strongly desired revascularization. Fracture pinning and repair of a single artery was performed without venous anastomosis, and venous drainage through the skin bridge proved to be adequate.*

Mechanism Sharp mechanisms, such as knives or metal machetes, produce a clean cut and narrow zone of injury, often allowing primary microsurgical repair. Because these injuries are often absent of bony comminution and tendon damage, rehabilitation is early and aggressive leading to favorable functional outcomes. Furthermore, primary coaptation of healthy nerve portends a good or excellent prognosis for sensory recovery. For these reasons, replantation/revascularization is favored for most injuries in this class.

Blunt (ie, table saw) lacerations and crush mechanisms are less favorable and considerably more common than sharp amputations. These injuries usually have an extended zone of injury that may necessitate considerable skeletal shortening and intercalary vein and/or nerve grafting. Functional recovery in these patients may be suboptimal, especially if rehabilitation is delayed by tenuous bony fixation or tendon repair. It is in this class of injury that one finds the most variability, and it is not unusual to proceed to the operating room for examination of the amputation stump and part before choosing a course of action. In our opinion, neither skeletal shortening nor the need for vascular graft to

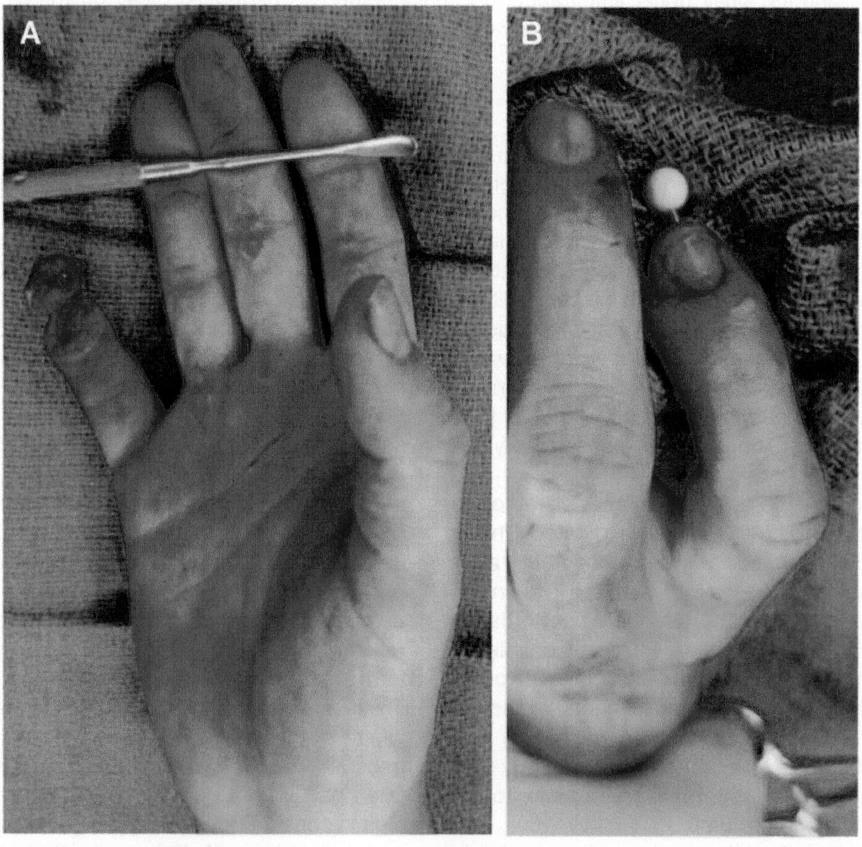

Fig. 3. (*A*) The patient in Case 3 presented with a dysvascular left small fingertip. Revascularization was believed to be a reasonable option based on the sharp and distal nature of the injury, in addition to the intact skin bridge obviating venous anastomosis. Both revascularization and revision amputation were offered, and (*B*) revascularization was performed.

reconstruct a digital artery are major barriers to replantation if other factors favor salvage. If reasonable skeletal shortening does not allow for primary nerve repair on the pinch surface of the finger (or ulnar border of the small finger), then strong consideration should be given to revision amputation. Nerve grafting is appropriate in some cases, especially when multiple fingers or a thumb are involved.

Avulsion by rope, ring, or other mechanism is a particularly difficult injury because of its large zone of vascular and nerve injury. Nerve and vessel repair of these injuries usually requires grafting or venous flow through flaps, and tendon repair is sometimes impossible because of avulsion at the musculotendinous junction. Skeletal repair often involves joint fusion because of transarticular amputation. A major problem with avulsion injuries is that a large area of skin becomes devitalized. Even if the distal segment is successfully revascularized, skin loss results in exposure of the neurovascular bundles and tendons, which can also be a difficult secondary problem to address.

Historically, replantation of avulsed digits was viewed with pessimism. However, in a recent review, Sears and Chung[23] found that replantation of an avulsed finger was successful between 66% and 78% of the time. ROM outcomes were also reasonable (total active motion 174°), although sensory outcomes were marginal (mean two-point discrimination, 13 mm). Given this evidence, we believe that replantation of many avulsed fingers is technically possible, and this should routinely be attempted in cases of hand, thumb, or multiple digital injury. In noncritical situations, reconstruction of an aesthetic five-fingered hand may be achievable, but consideration of replantation should take into account the poor sensory recovery that is expected and how this affects hand function.

Regardless of the mechanism, some zones of injury are too large to maintain any hope of replantation. Severe and diffuse crush, blast injury, or mangling of the amputated part is not uncommon and necessitates revision amputation. In cases where severe trauma makes the amputation stump unsuitable for replantation, revision amputation is generally recommended, but ectopic replantation should be considered for hands, thumbs, and three or more fingers.[24]

Injuries to adjacent fingers Injuries that devascularize or amputate a single nonthumb digit are often accompanied by lesser injury to adjacent fingers. In these cases, it is important to consider the trajectory of the whole hand before choosing a treatment of the amputated or dysvascular part. This includes the rehabilitation and anticipated pattern of hand use.

Replantation of a noncritical digit should not be offered if it significantly impairs rehabilitation of an adjacent finger with a better prognosis for long-term usefulness. This situation arises when adjacent injuries are at risk for severe stiffness and require immediate and aggressive ROM, which would be slowed by protection of an adjacent replanted digit. These injuries include, but are not limited to, soft tissue injuries, PIP articular injuries, and partial tendon injuries. In these cases, revision amputation should be strongly considered. One exception to this guideline is in children, where the indications for replantation are so broad in part because they are much less prone to this type of "collateral damage" stiffness.

The surgeon should try to anticipate the patterns of hand use that will emerge after recovery. For instance, in the case of an index finger amputation, the patient successfully substitutes an uninjured middle finger for pinch tasks, and index replantation may only get in the way.[25] However, if severe bony, tendon, or radial digital nerve injury impairs the utility of the middle finger for opposition against the thumb, salvage of the amputated index may eventually offer a functional benefit, because pinch bypass to the ring finger is less intuitive and useful. When multiple digits have sustained severe injuries and future functional use patterns are uncertain, replantation of a solitary amputated or dysvascular digit is encouraged.

Case 4

This 33-year-old right-hand-dominant male accountant sustained an injury to the right hand while using a table saw (**Fig. 4**). *The index finger was completely amputated through the PIP joint, and the middle finger common extensor tendon sustained a 60% laceration within zone 4. Given this injury pattern, our priority was to repair and rehabilitate the middle finger, which would undoubtedly serve as his best pinch surface in the future. Because we believed that index finger replantation would likely delay and impede rehabilitation of the middle finger extensor tendon injury, we recommended against this.*

Revascularization of an incomplete amputation Dysvascular fingers that are not completely

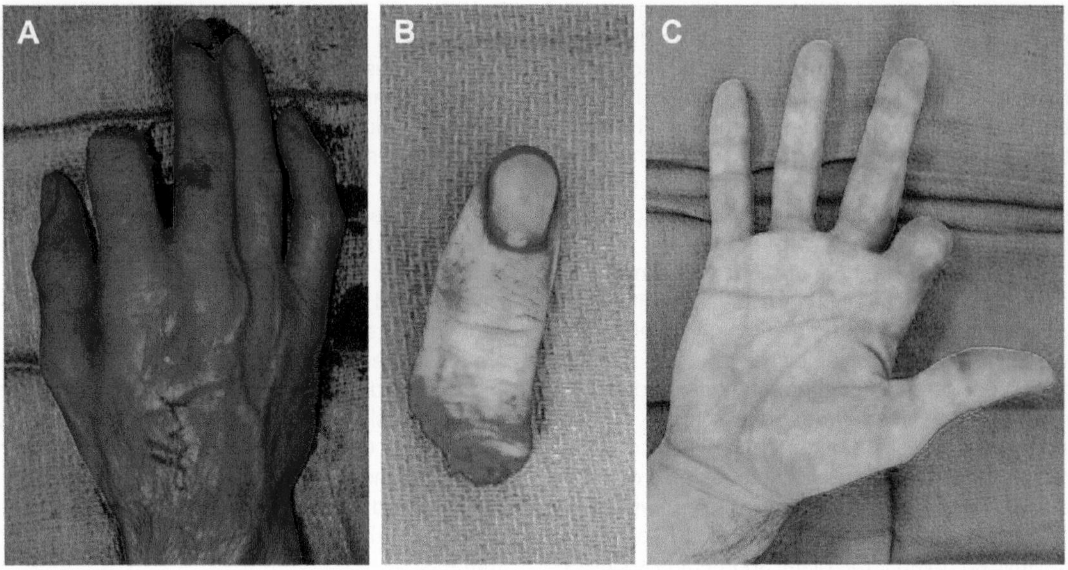

Fig. 4. (*A, B*) The patient from Case 4 presented with right middle finger extensor tendon laceration and index finger amputation. In this case, the middle finger will almost certainly become his preferred finger for pinch activities, and its repair and rehabilitation are the primary goals. (*C*) Revision amputation was the chosen treatment of the index, primarily because of concerns that replantation would interfere with rehabilitation of the middle finger.

amputated represent a gray area in the indications for digit salvage. Certainly, dysvascular hands, thumbs, and multiple fingers should be salvaged if there is an expectation of increased survival and potentially superior outcomes compared with corresponding complete amputations.[26] However, to our knowledge, no clear evidenced-based guidelines have been proposed guiding management of single dysvascular digits. One reason for this is that devascularizing injuries are heterogenous with respect to the remaining intact structures.

Logically, preservation of any viable tissue is advantageous. Even a small skin bridge can provide significant venous drainage and, in our experience, significantly improves survival of a revascularized digit. Intact tendon, bone, or nerve are unlikely to improve survival, but each enhances postoperative function. Although no study has specifically demonstrated the relative value of each preserved structure, there is evidence that as a whole, digits undergoing revascularization are more likely to be salvaged and achieve sensory outcomes superior to that seen with replantation.[13] For these reasons, in the absence of a social, occupational, or medical contraindication, we favor aggressive attempts to salvage dysvascular but incomplete single digit injuries.

Case 5

This 57-year-old right-hand-dominant artist sustained a crush injury to the nondominant left index finger at the level of the proximal phalanx (**Fig. 5**). *The proximal phalanx was fractured and the finger dysvascular, but a small skin bridge and several deep structures remained intact. The patient had no medical contraindications to digit salvage and desired revascularization. We proceeded to the operating room with consent for revascularization or revision amputation based on operative findings. On exploration, partial injuries of all flexor and extensor tendons were found. The radial digital artery was thrombosed, and the ulnar digital artery was transected. Both digital nerves were contused but in-continuity. Because of the improved prognosis conferred by intact tendons and nerves, we proceeded with digital salvage.*

Circumstantial factors

Time to presentation Acceptable ischemia time for consideration of replantation depends on the volume of muscle within the amputated part and the temperature of storage before reperfusion. Because muscle is the most ischemia-sensitive tissue in the upper extremity, proximal

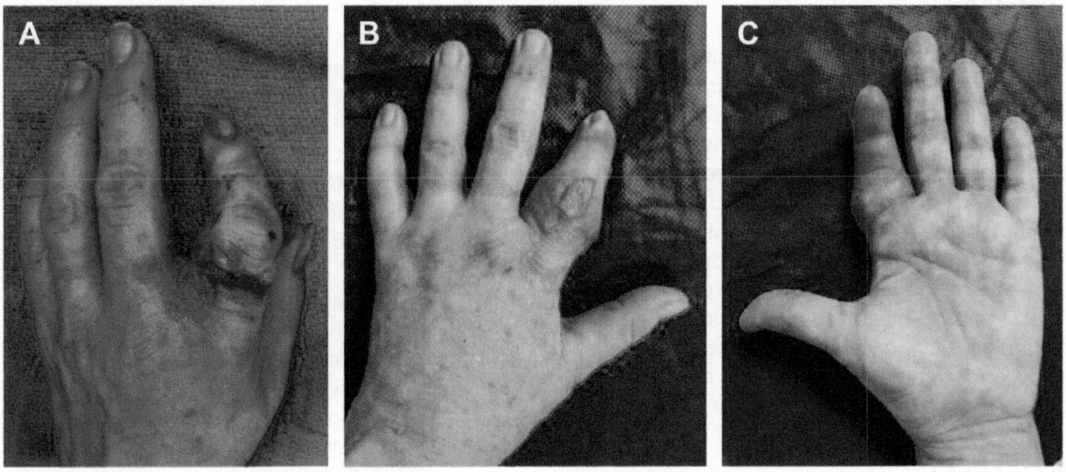

Fig. 5. (*A*) The patient in Case 5 presented with a dysvascular left index finger. After exploration of the injury, revascularization of the index finger was believed to be indicated given the good prognosis associated with intact tendons and digital nerves. (*B, C*) The appearance of the hand is shown 6 weeks postoperatively.

amputations are much more time-sensitive than digital amputations. Traditional limits of cold and warm ischemia are defined in **Table 2**.[27]

Beyond these limits, achievement of reperfusion may be impossible because of vascular thrombosis, and even if circulation is reestablished, considerable irreversible cellular damage has likely occurred. In major limb replantation, this can manifest as a fibrosis of the musculature, and in fingers sensory recovery is impaired.[28]

Despite these issues, numerous authors have documented successful replantation with acceptable results well beyond the traditional limits of ischemia time, including a digital replantation after 94 hours of cold ischemia.[27,29] Although delayed replantation is never desirable, we believe that it is indicated in certain uncommon clinical situations:

- Reversible critical illness (ie, hemorrhage) amenable to replantation after stabilization
- Prolonged travel time to a replantation center
- Concurrent microsurgical emergencies overwhelming a system's capacity for immediate care

Table 2
Traditional limits of cold and warm ischemia

	Warm Ischemia (h)	Cold Ischemia (h)
Major limb	2–4	6–8
Digit	6–12	12–24

Data from Lin CH, Aydyn N, Lin YT, et al. Hand and finger replantation after protracted ischemia (more than 24 hours). Ann Plast Surg 2010;64(3):286–90.

Based on their critical functional importance and low muscle content, ideal parts for delayed replantation are the thumb or multiple fingers. The hand is also deserving of consideration, with the expectation that intrinsic fibrosis is likely to impede the functional result. Although instances of significantly delayed major limb replantation have been reported,[30] this is not usually advisable because of the likelihood of systemic sequelae from reperfusion syndrome.

Availability of postreplantation care Although prompt and skilled microsurgical care is necessary to achieve successful replantation/revascularization of an amputated part, it is not sufficient to provide a maximally functional result. With the possible exception of the thumb, most replanted parts are minimally functional without considerable postreplantation care from a surgeon and occupational therapist. Important interventions may include wound care, splinting, ROM therapy, sensory reeducation, passive manipulation, and tenolysis.

Many regional medical systems have robust protocols for rapidly transporting patients over long distances for care of an amputated or dysvascular part. However, little infrastructure exists to help these patients receive follow-up care. When treating patients who have significant barriers to obtaining follow-up care, consideration should be given to revision amputation rather than salvage. These barriers may include a geographically remote residence, lack of transportation, or stated disinterest in ongoing care. This is especially pertinent in cases of single nonthumb digital amputation, where replantation is likely to impair function in the absence of considerable rehabilitative effort.

SUMMARY

The indications for upper extremity replantation are inherently relative, fluid over time, and require reconsideration on every patient encounter. Pediatric amputations and amputations of the hand, thumb, or multiple digits remain strong indications for replantation, and this should generally be attempted if deemed safe. Patients often desire replantation of single nonthumb digits based on aesthetic preference and personal/cultural values. Replantation in these situations is acceptable and rewarding, but individual consideration of patient, injury, and circumstantial factors is critical to avoid patient morbidity and unsatisfactory outcomes.

REFERENCES

1. O'Brien BM, MacLeod AM, Miller GD, et al. Clinical replantation of digits. Plast Reconstr Surg 1973; 52(5):490–502.
2. Frykman GK, Wood VE. Saving amputated digits. Current status of replantation of fingers and hands. West J Med 1974;121(4):265–9.
3. Manktelow RT. What are the indications for digital replantation? Ann Plast Surg 1978;1(3):336–7.
4. Ikeda K, Yamauchi S, Hashimoto F, et al. Digital replantation in children: a long-term follow-up study. Microsurgery 1990;11(4):261–4.
5. Mohan R, Panthaki Z, Armstrong MB. Replantation in the pediatric hand. J Craniofac Surg 2009;20(4):996–8.
6. Buntic RF, Brooks D, Buncke GM. Index finger salvage with replantation and revascularization: revisiting conventional wisdom. Microsurgery 2008;28(8):612–6.
7. Urbaniak JR, Roth JH, Nunley JA, et al. The results of replantation after amputation of a single finger. J Bone Joint Surg Am 1985;67(4):611–9.
8. Goldner RD, Urbaniak JR. Greens: operative hand surgery [Chapter 45]. In: Green's operative hand surgery. Philadelphia: Elsevier; 2005.
9. Zhong-Wei C, Meyer VE, Kleinert HE, et al. Present indications and contraindications for replantation as reflected by long-term functional results. Orthop Clin North Am 1981;12(4):849–70.
10. Sears ED, Shin R, Prosser LA, et al. Economic analysis of revision amputation and replantation treatment of finger amputation injuries. Plast Reconstr Surg 2014;133(4):827–40.
11. Hustedt JW, Chung A, Bohl DD, et al. Evaluating the effect of comorbidities on the success, risk, and cost of digital replantation. J Hand Surg Am 2016;41(12): 1145–52.e1.
12. Kwon G-D, Ahn B-M, Lee J-S, et al. The effect of patient age on the success rate of digital replantation. Plast Reconstr Surg 2017;139(2):420–6.
13. Chiu HY, Shieh SJ, Hsu HY. Multivariate analysis of factors influencing the functional recovery after finger replantation or revascularization. Microsurgery 1995;16(10):713–7.
14. Barzin A, Hernandez-Boussard T, Lee GK, et al. Adverse events following digital replantation in the elderly. J Hand Surg Am 2011;36(5):870–4.
15. Hattori Y, Doi K, Ikeda K, et al. A retrospective study of functional outcomes after successful replantation versus amputation closure for single fingertip amputations. J Hand Surg Am 2006;31(5):811–8.
16. Nishizuka T, Shauver MJ, Zhong L, et al. A comparative study of attitudes regarding digit replantation in the United States and Japan. J Hand Surg Am 2015;40(8):1646–56.e1–3.
17. Maroukis BL, Shauver MJ, Nishizuka T, et al. Cross-cultural variation in preference for replantation or revision amputation: societal and surgeon views. Injury 2016;47(4):818–23.
18. Schlozman SC. Upper-extremity self-amputation and replantation: 2 case reports and a review of the literature. J Clin Psychiatry 1998;59(12):681–6.
19. Otto IA, Kon M, Schuurman AH, et al. Replantation versus prosthetic fitting in traumatic arm amputations: a systematic review. PLoS One 2015;10(9):e0137729.
20. Pet MA, Morrison SD, Mack JS, et al. Comparison of patient-reported outcomes after traumatic upper extremity amputation: replantation versus prosthetic rehabilitation. Injury 2016;47(12):2783–8.
21. Lister G. The choice of procedure following thumb amputation. Clin Orthop Relat Res 1985;195:45–51.
22. Glickman LT, Mackinnon SE. Sensory recovery following digital replantation. Microsurgery 1990; 11(3):236–42.
23. Sears ED, Chung KC. Replantation of finger avulsion injuries: a systematic review of survival and functional outcomes. J Hand Surg Am 2011;36(4):686–94.
24. Higgins JP. Ectopic banking of amputated parts: a clinical review. J Hand Surg Am 2011;36(11):1868–76.
25. White WL. Why I hate the index finger. Hand (N Y) 2010;5(4):461–5.
26. Soucacos PN, Beris AE, Touliatos AS, et al. Complete versus incomplete nonviable amputations of the thumb. Comparison of the survival rate and functional results. Acta Orthop Scand Suppl 1995;264:16–8.
27. Lin C-H, Aydyn N, Lin Y-T, et al. Hand and finger replantation after protracted ischemia (more than 24 hours). Ann Plast Surg 2010;64(3):286–90.
28. Waikakul S, Sakkarnkosol S, Vanadurongwan V, et al. Results of 1018 digital replantations in 552 patients. Injury 2000;31(1):33–40.
29. Wei FC, Chang YL, Chen HC, et al. Three successful digital replantations in a patient after 84, 86, and 94 hours of cold ischemia time. Plast Reconstr Surg 1988;82(2):346–50.
30. Merican AM, Kwan MK, Cheok CY, et al. Successful revascularisation of near total amputation of the upper limb after ten hours of warm ischaemia. Med J Malaysia 2005;60(2):218–21.

Efficiency in Replantation/ Revascularization Surgery

Bauback Safa, MD, MBA[a,*], Mark A. Greyson, MD[b], Kyle R. Eberlin, MD[b]

KEYWORDS

• Replant • Digital • Efficiency • Revascularization • Microvascular • Technique • Reconstruction

KEY POINTS

- Replantation surgery is a technically demanding procedure that requires attention to efficiency to maximize outcomes and minimize surgeon fatigue.
- There are opportunities to streamline surgical work flow at every step, from the moment the patient enters the emergency department to the time of discharge.
- With a systematic plan in mind, a successful digital replantation can be performed under a single tourniquet run.

INTRODUCTION

Digital replantation and revascularization are triumphs of modern microvascular surgery. Since the first description of the use of the operating microscope in 1960,[1] to the first upper extremity revascularization by Malt and team in 1962 at Massachusetts General Hospital,[2] to the first complete digital replantation by Komatsu and Tamai in 1965,[3] surgeons have continued to pioneer microvascular techniques to optimize outcomes. Despite these key technological advancements, however, there has been a marked decline in the incidence of replant surgery in the United States, at a rate of 6% per year between 2000 and 2010. This represents more than a 50% decrease over this time period.[4]

To explain this trend, several possibilities have been suggested, including a decrease in reimbursement,[5] a decline in the incidence of work-related injuries,[4,6] questionable cost-effectiveness,[7] and the perception of poor functional outcomes. Although these factors may play a role, the impact of these issues alone seems to be overstated.[8,9] Collectively, they fail to account for the observed decrease in the incidence of replantation. Instead, clinical decision-making among hand surgeons and hospitals may be the driving force behind the changing practice patterns. This trend is concomitant with the decentralization of replantation surgery away from high volume centers, despite reports that hospitals with higher annual volume have greater success.[10,11] In addition, there has been decreasing individual experience with replantation, with most hand surgeons performing fewer than 5 per year.[12] In summary, clinical decision-making is rapidly changing along with regional practice patterns because greater numbers of surgeons are performing fewer replant cases.

For these reasons, replantation success rates in the United States may be decreasing.[13] This has a downstream effect on training programs: because individual centers perform fewer replants, there are fewer opportunities for residents and fellows to gain valuable experience to facilitate successful outcomes.

Disclosure Statement: The authors did not receive any funding for this study. Dr B. Safa is a consultant for AxoGen. Dr K.R. Eberlin is a consultant for AxoGen and Integra.
Level of Evidence: Expert Opinion V.
[a] The Buncke Clinic, 45 Castro Street, Suite 121, San Francisco, CA 94114, USA; [b] Division of Plastic and Reconstructive Surgery, Massachusetts General Hospital, Harvard Medical School, 55 Fruit Street, WAC 435, Boston, MA 02114, USA
* Corresponding author.
E-mail address: bauback@drsafa.com

Hand Clin 35 (2019) 131–141
https://doi.org/10.1016/j.hcl.2018.12.004
0749-0712/19/

It is therefore important to promote effective and reproducible techniques, so all qualified surgeons can reach a level of expertise in this demanding procedure. This article is therefore designed to provide an evidence-based and practical update to the practice of replantation, supplemented by expert opinion of the lead others.[14] It should serve as a succinct and high-yield reference for surgeons from the time the patient arrives in the emergency department (ED) until the day of discharge, with attention to minimizing tourniquet time and maximizing efficiency.

PREPARATION FOR REPLANTATION

Efficient replantation begins at the stage of triage and before patient arrival into the emergency room. Ideally, the patient will be brought to a specialized, regional center of expertise with qualified, experienced microsurgeons available.[15] As a first step, the operating room (OR) staff and anesthesia teams should be notified. The OR staff should prepare a back-table with ice, a second set of microsurgical instruments, heparinized saline, micro- and small vascular clip appliers, tenotomy scissors, Adson forceps, fine DeBakey forceps, and 4-0 and 5-0 nylon sutures (**Fig. 1**). Both the mini C-arm and microscope should be prepared, the former to confirm Kirschner wire (K-wire) placement in the amputated part and the latter for back-table dissection. A discussion with anesthesia should be held with specific reference to anticipated blood loss, potential need for heparin, likely operative time, and preference for regional anesthesia. The authors typically obtain an upper extremity block for the benefit of sympathetic blockade and subsequent vasodilation.[16,17]

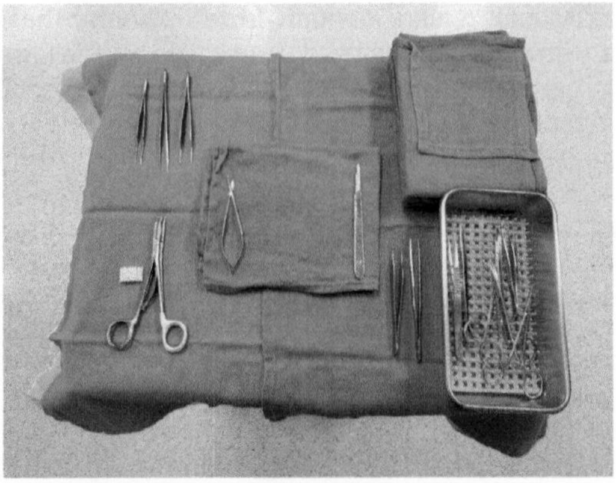

Fig. 1. The replant "tagging table" consisting of micro and macro instruments.

PATIENT ARRIVAL TO THE EMERGENCY DEPARTMENT

When the patient arrives in the ED and the decision to proceed with replantation has been made, informed consent is obtained. When the patient arrives in the ED, radiographs of the patient's hand and the amputated part(s) are obtained, with both the hand and the amputated part(s) together. Antibiotics are administered and tetanus vaccination given, if indicated, in addition to general resuscitative measures. The preoperative Buncke Clinic protocol consisting of a rectal aspirin, dry or slightly moistened gauze on the amputated part placed on indirect ice, and no digital block, was shown to significantly decrease complication rates during replantation.[18]

Next, the surgeon takes the amputated part to the OR. This is a critical time to maximize efficiency because a significant portion of the operation can be completed in a bloodless field before the patient enters the room and the block is complete.

The amputated part is first irrigated with betadine/saline and debrided on the back table, which has been set up before the induction of anesthesia (**Fig. 2**). Unless an assistant is available, the digit is secured to the towel covering the Mayo stand cover with a nylon suture, to prevent twisting and to secure it in place while structures are identified. Bruner incisions are made and the skin flaps are secured distally using 5-0 nylon sutures. Midlateral incisions may be used, but are often discouraged because they may leave the neurovascular bundle exposed and desiccated, or at risk for compression.[14,16]

Under the microscope, or using loupe magnification, arteries, veins, and nerves are tagged with small and micro clips on the back table. Clips are faster and less wieldy to use than micro sutures and also allow for more rapid identification of matched structures during replantation because different sizes are used for different structures: micro clips may be used on the vessels and small clips on the nerves (or vice versa), which may be labeled on the white board in the OR so that critical time is not lost for identification later in the operation. When anastomoses are performed, the small clips can be matched to the small clips, and the micro clips to the micro clips, to avoid confusion in a bloody field when the tourniquet is released.[19] Next, the distal half of a 4-strand core suture is placed into the flexor digitorum profundus (FDP) tendon. Some investigators advocate vein grafting on the back table[19]; we have not found this technique to be necessary. This is followed lastly by

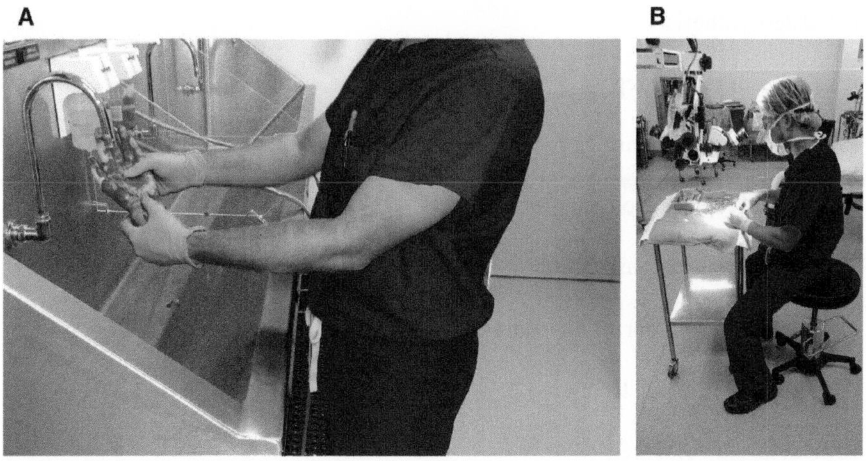

Fig. 2. (*A*) The part is washed in the sink, followed by betadine, and subsequently rinsed with sterile saline. (*B*) The structures are tagged on the back table. Loupe magnification may be used for preplacement of tendon sutures and K-wire placement. The microscope can be used for smaller structures such as vessel and nerve identification.

the insertion of K-wires, the placement of which is confirmed with the mini C-arm (**Fig. 3**).

The process of preparing the amputated part should occur while the patient is evaluated by the anesthesia team and prepared for surgery. The time frame required for regional anesthesia is an excellent opportunity for this stage of the operation.

OPERATIVE INTERVENTION

Although the exact sequence of operative repair in replantation may vary, the principles are immutable. Appropriate use of tourniquet time is paramount to efficient replantation; poor use of the tourniquet usually results in a painstaking, long operation that is universally disliked by all members of the team. If the surgeon is methodical and approaches the operation with a concrete, systematic plan in mind, it is possible to complete all essential components of the case in one tourniquet run. The following order of repair is advocated (after the amputated part has been prepared on the back table); there are 2 variations presented in the following section (**Figs. 4** and **5**), which can be used in individual situations.

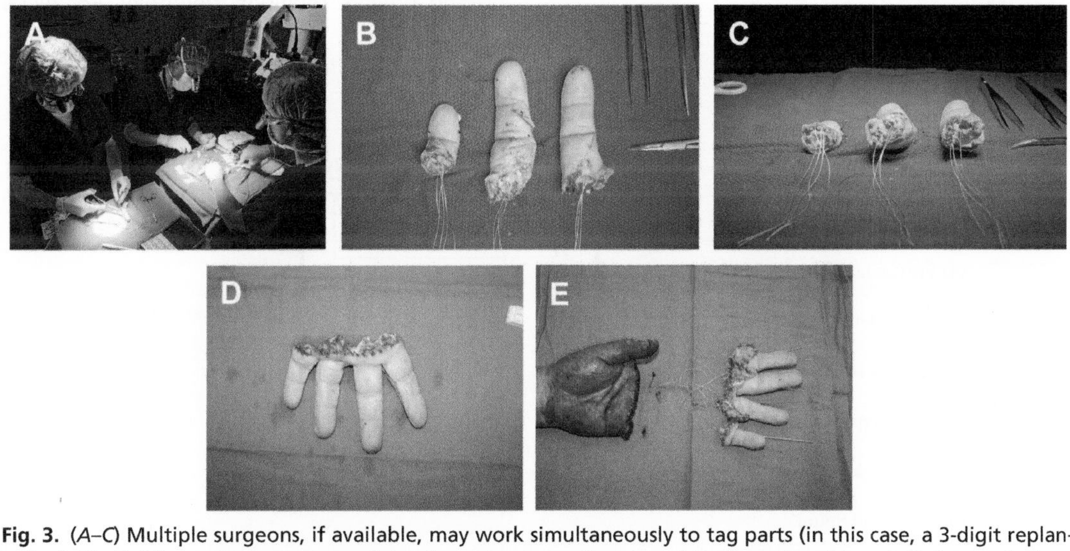

Fig. 3. (*A–C*) Multiple surgeons, if available, may work simultaneously to tag parts (in this case, a 3-digit replantation). (*D, E*) All structures are tagged, tendon sutures preplaced, and K-wires placed in a 4-digit amputation.

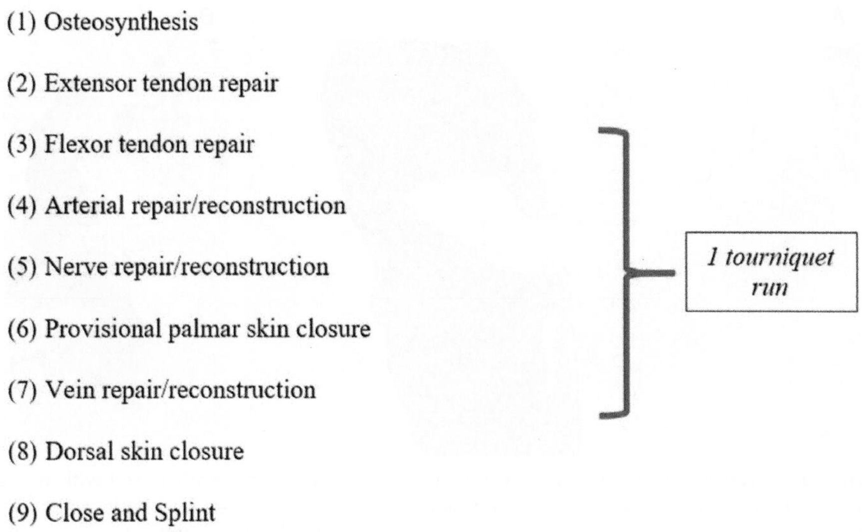

Fig. 4. Variation 1: Dorsal - > Volar - > Dorsal.

Osteosynthesis

In some cases, especially with multidigit replantation, it is preferred to perform osteosynthesis first and without the tourniquet. Skeletal shortening is a useful technique to bring the soft tissue structures into tension-free approximation. Shortening should be performed preferentially on the amputated part to preserve digital length in the case of replant failure. This can be done with a rongeur or with an oscillating saw. If a saw is used, extreme care must be taken to avoid injury to the soft tissues; the soft tissues are typically mobilized off the bone and a piece of Esmarch bandage or a glove with a small perforation is slid over the bone to protect adjacent structures.[19]

To the inexperienced surgeon, osteosynthesis can be a time-consuming part of the operation. It is tempting to aspire to perfect skeletal fixation, with bony compression and rigid fixation. This can be done using plate and screw constructs or alternatively 90-90 wiring.[20] In the authors' experience, using K-wires is most often sufficient and provides a technically simple, streamlined way to move the operation forward in order to execute the other necessary steps. Also, in their experience, rigid fixation with plates or 90-90 wires increases operative time but does not decrease rates of revision operations such as tenolysis and capsulotomy. The authors typically use two 0.035 or 0.045 K-wires to achieve fixation and prevent rotational deformity. For distal

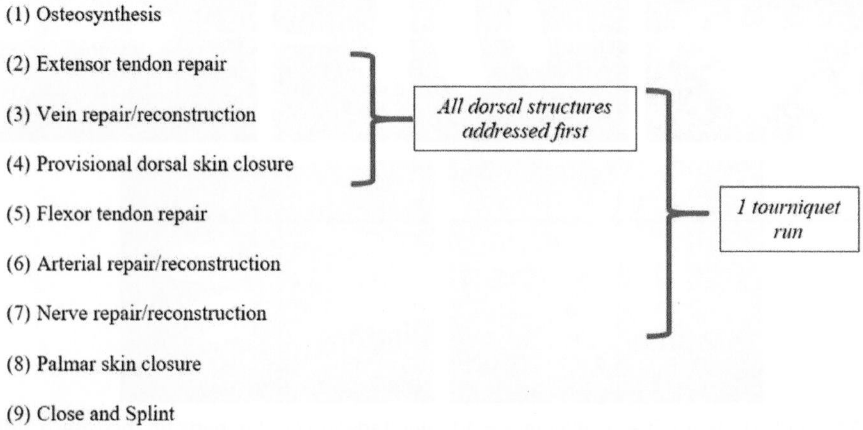

Fig. 5. Variation 2: Dorsal - > Volar.

(or pediatric) replants, 0.035 or 0.028 K-wires may be used. An initial attempt at crossing, periarticular K-wires is reasonable, but if this proves difficult they are converted expeditiously to transarticular K-wires.

For amputations through the carpus, 0.062 Steinman pins are typically used. In appropriate candidates, a proximal row carpectomy may also be performed in order to achieve appropriate shortening. For amputations through the distal forearm, the pronator quadratus muscle is removed and a distal radius plate (and a distal ulna plate if necessary) is applied on the back table. For amputations through the diaphyseal radius and ulna, 3.5 mm plates (from the "small frag" set) or a metadiaphyseal distal radius plate are applied on the back table. Bone shortening on the amputated part is performed with an oscillating saw before placement of the plates on the back table. The proximal bone is then shortened before placement of the proximal screws. Amputations through the elbow, or highly contaminated injuries, typically require external fixation.

Extensor Tendon Repair

Following bony stabilization, the extensor tendons are repaired. In order to preserve tourniquet time, this may be done without the use of tourniquet, especially in the setting of a multidigit replant. Figure of 8 sutures are used; 1 to 2 sutures are usually sufficient for this repair. During this portion of the procedure, care is taken to preserve the dorsal veins and these are identified during the extensor tendon repair.

Flexor Tendon Repair

After the extensor mechanism is repaired, the hand is placed in supination with the palm facing upwards. Most commonly, the tourniquet is inflated at this time for subsequent portions of the operation. The tendon coaptation is performed next to set the appropriate tension and posture of the digit before repairing the microvascular structures. After wide proximal exposure with the tourniquet inflated, the FDP is repaired. Modest improvement in postoperative function may be seen with the additional repair of flexor digitorum superficialis (FDS),[21] but this repair takes additional precious time and the authors often forego repair of the FDS in the interest of expediency in digit replantation. In addition, they have found that it often does not add digital excursion to the final outcome, and it greatly complicates future flexor tenolysis (particularly in Zone II), which is often necessary to maximize function in digit replants.

Arterial Repair/Reconstruction

Following flexor tendon repair, the microsurgical portion of the operation begins. Although a vein first approach was originally described, the authors often begin with the arterial anastomoses.[17] The vein-first approach is reserved for proximal digit replants (eg, through the metacarpals) where the veins are large and readily visible. In these cases, the veins may be repaired after extensor repair and the dorsal skin can be provisionally closed to protect the anastomoses on supination.

The sequence of arterial repair or reconstruction proceeds with a goal of efficiency, as the hand is in a position to perform the arterial anastomoses following flexor tendon repair. At this juncture, it is important to consider thorough debridement of injured segments of the vessels. After an avulsion injury, intimal damage can extend 3 cm or more beyond the point of vessel rupture, which is often underappreciated.[22] The "ribbon" sign, the "red line" sign, and intraluminal white clots are all indications of extensive vessel injury.[23]

To the inexperienced surgeon, the decision about the extent of vessel debridement is challenging. It is preferable to trim vessels under the microscope with the tourniquet inflated and to make an expeditious decision about the length of resection and potential need for vein grafts. If there is an avulsion injury, and it seems that the vessel ends are inherently damaged, the authors resect aggressively and perform vein graft reconstruction without hesitation. It should be noted that significant mobilization of the arteries may be achieved proximally by clipping side branches. Mobilization of the digital arteries may obviate a vein graft. This contrasts significantly with digital nerves, which exhibit little stretch even with significant mobilization. Should a vein graft be necessary, the authors prefer distal volar forearm veins for digital arteries. They typically use dorsal foot veins or the saphenous vein for more proximal injuries.

Although the tourniquet may be deflated to check for inflow, this step is often unnecessary in experienced hands because the morphologic appearance of the vessel and its lumen can be used to determine adequacy of arterial debridement. If any doubt exists, the tourniquet may be deflated to ensure adequate flow, then reinflated to assist with the arterial anastomosis. The anastomosis is performed most commonly under tourniquet using interrupted 9-0 or 10-0 nylon sutures (11-0 nylon sutures may be needed for very distal replants). One option is to use double-opposing clamps to facilitate back wall repair, whereas another technique uses Serafin clamps proximally and distally while performing a free-hand anastomosis.

In proximal replantations, vascular shunts can be used to minimize ischemia time while the osteosynthesis is performed, although this is uncommon (**Fig. 6**). In these cases, distal fasciotomies are typically performed on the back table. Blood products should be readily available because the use of vascular shunts can result in significant blood loss. Early transfusion is preferable to avoid use of vasopressors and should be communicated to the anesthesiology team at the beginning of the operation.

Nerve Repair/Reconstruction

Following the arterial anastomosis, attention is turned to the digital nerve repair, which is most commonly performed under tourniquet control. The digital nerve repairs should not be an afterthought for surgeons performing replantation or revascularization; they are a critical component of the procedure, the success of which may portend long-term functionality of the digit. Most replanted digits develop some stiffness, but an insensate, stiff digit, especially in the index or long finger, is functionally useless and is a relative indication for amputation.

The extent of injury to the digital nerves often parallels the injury to the vessels. If aggressive resection and debridement is required to achieve adequate anterograde flow to reperfuse the digit, it is expected that nerve debridement will be required, which most often results in a nerve gap. Both autograft and allograft nerve reconstruction are appropriate and can be used for this purpose. More proximal amputations typically involve wider zones of injury. In these cases, the surgeon may elect to repair the nerves in a delayed fashion, allowing time for the zone of injury to fully demarcate. If the surgeon foresees the use of nerve conduits or allografts, the products should be called for before beginning the arterial anastomoses, because obtaining these products may take precious time in the OR.

Critical features of digital nerve reconstruction include sufficient debridement to healthy nerve endings and the provision of a tension-free neurorrhaphy through digital range of motion. To achieve this, nerve grafts are often required. Options include nerve conduits for short gaps (<6 mm), as well as autograft and allograft for longer gaps. There is currently one commercially available processed nerve allograft option for use in the hand. In recent years, the use of nerve allografts in the authors' practice has greatly supplanted the use of autografts in digit replantation.[24–26] Autograft options include the sural nerve, medial or lateral antebrachial cutaneous nerve, superficial peroneal nerve, posterior interosseous nerve, or nerves harvested from spare parts.[27,28] However, size mismatch and donor site morbidity are important considerations.

Despite the historical assertion that nerve repair is not an essential maneuver during replantation or revascularization surgery,[8,29,30] it is thought that contemporary techniques for nerve repair typically allow for a single-stage approach to nerve repair in the dysvascular digit.

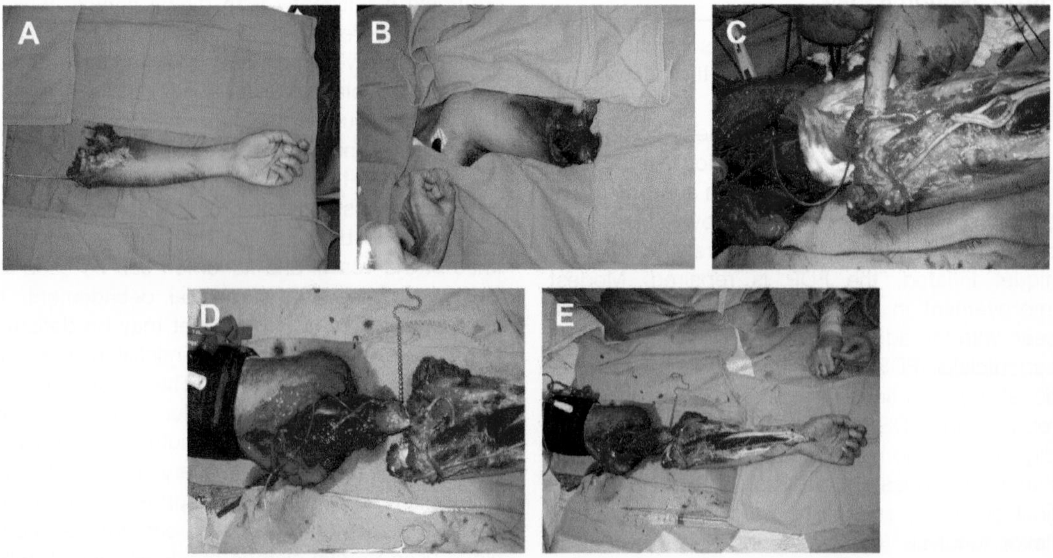

Fig. 6. (*A–E*) An amputation through the elbow with 6 hours of ischemia time. A vascular shunt is used immediately after fasciotomies are performed. Once the part is perfused, bony fixation is obtained.

Palmar Skin Closure

Following arterial and nerve repair, skin closure is performed. Tension is to be strictly avoided with closure, because it may compromise patency of the anastomoses performed. Liberal use of split-thickness and full-thickness grafts from spare parts can be used for resurfacing to avoid tension on the volar closure. Once the volar structures are repaired, the tourniquet may be kept inflated or taken down depending on the amount of time elapsed. The authors prefer to keep the tourniquet insufflated for as long as possible and will extend the tourniquet time up to 150 minutes, if necessary.

Venous Repair/Reconstruction

The hand is then pronated and as many venous anastomoses are performed as possible while the tourniquet remains inflated. Additional anastomoses may be performed once the tourniquet is released. This provides the added benefit of vein distension after arterial inflow is reestablished. However, deflating the tourniquet comes at the expense of visualization, because the amount of bleeding from the dorsal veins following tourniquet deflation can be challenging. Consideration should be given to multiple venous anastomoses, especially in zone 3, and the authors prefer to repair as many veins as is technically feasible.[31] If vein grafts are used for venous drainage, precise attention should be paid to vein length to avoid kinking during closure as they dilate and distend significantly.[14] Volar veins are commonly used for venous grafting, particularly in distal replants (eg, Tamai zone I). In these cases, all the microsurgery (artery, nerve, and vein) may be done in the same field. The dorsal skin is closed loosely (**Fig. 7**).

SPECIAL CIRCUMSTANCES

Vein First Replantation/Revascularization

The vein first approach is reserved for proximal digital replantation (eg, through the metacarpals) where the veins are large and readily visible. In these cases, the veins may be repaired after extensor tendon repair and the dorsal skin can be provisionally closed to protect the anastomoses on supination.

Distal Replantation

Distal replantation is deserving of separate discussion. Once regarded as superfluous, with the advancement of microsurgical technique and recognition of more optimal aesthetic and functional outcomes, zone I amputations are now considered a good indication for replantation.[32,33] Several excellent classification schemata have been described for distal digital replantation. The system proposed by Tamai divides zone 1 and 2 at the base of the nail and DIPJ, respectively.[34] Further refinements have been made by Allen, Hirase, and Sebastin, among others.[8,35,36] Regardless of the exact level, these distal replants are often more technically straightforward (although they require “supermicrosurgery” techniques), and alternatives including local flaps that pilfer from an already injured hand bestow not inconsequential morbidity. A key technique to employ in distal replantation is the use of volar veins for venous anastomoses.

Unique to the case of very distal replantation, especially zone 1, is the flexibility to forego a venous anastomosis because this is sometimes not possible.[37,38] The authors prefer to create a fish mouth incision in the distal pulp to provide for venous egress until formal intrinsic outflow is reestablished. Systemic heparin is administered, and the rate of infusion is titrated to a slow ooze from the fish mouth opening. Heparin scrubs with heparin-soaked sponges are performed at the bedside every hour. In case of venous congestion, leech therapy can be initiated. Although effective, these artery-only techniques come with the added cost of requiring an average of 1 week in the hospital to bleed the part and months of recovery before anticipated return to work.[33,39] These

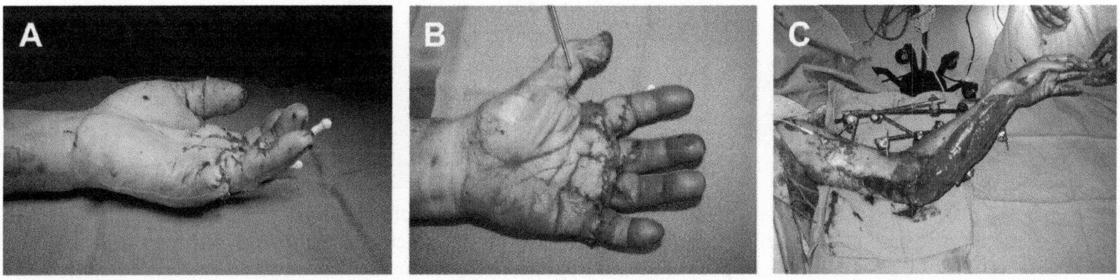

Fig. 7. (*A*) Immediate postoperative result of 3-finger replant (see **Figs.** 3A–C). (*B*) Immediate postoperative result of 4-finger replant (see **Figs.** 3D, E). (*C*) Immediate postoperative result of elbow replant (see **Fig.** 4A–E).

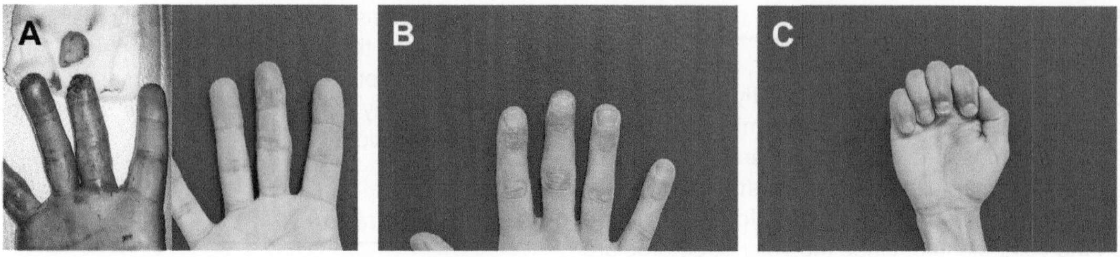

Fig. 8. (*A–C*) Distal replant with postoperative results.

patients may occasionally need blood transfusions. However, with increased experience, transfusions have become rare in our experience (**Fig. 8**).

EFFICIENCY IN POSTOPERATIVE REHABILITATION

Attention to efficiency should not end when the tourniquet is deflated. Perhaps the most important principle is to maintain excellent communication between the surgeon, hand therapist, and patient in order to lay the groundwork for meaningful functional recovery after these life-altering and unexpected events.[19]

The postoperative rehabilitation should be tailored to the patient, injury, operation, and level of patient compliance. The postoperative course should remain streamlined and efficient for the patient, hand therapist, and surgeon alike.

TOP 10 REPLANTATION PEARLS AND PITFALLS

1. High-power loupes (4X or above)
2. Microscope capable of minimum 20X magnification

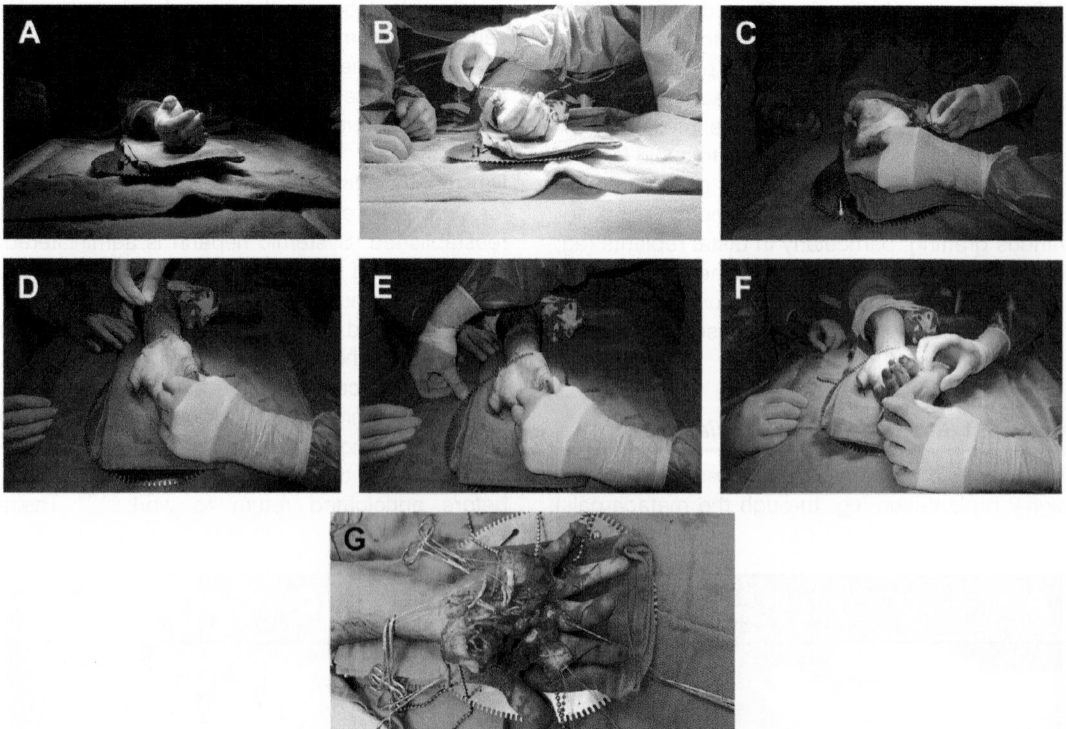

Fig. 9. (*A*) The use of the Tupper hand table to achieve hypersupination: resting hand position. (*B, C*) A hook-chain is placed in the thenar eminence, wrapped under the hand, retracted ulnarly, and attached to the Tupper hand table. (*D–F*) A hook-chain is then placed in the hypothenar eminence and retracted radially to assist in hypersupination. (*G*) The Tupper hand is used to quickly and easily retract skin flaps in a 4-finger revascularization. The hook-chains can be easily and quickly adjusted during the case.

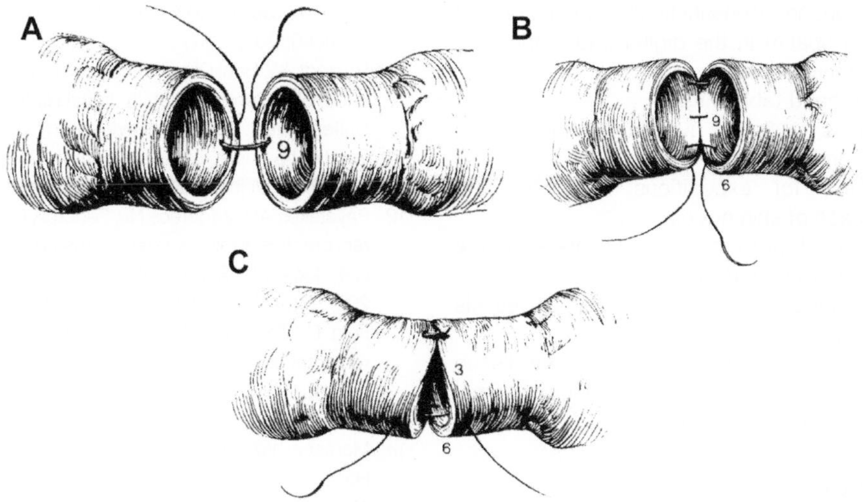

Fig. 10. (*A–C*) The "posterior wall technique" of vascular anastomosis. The back wall is sutured first and sutures are subsequently placed from the back to front, with the final suture placed in the front wall. The lumen is easily visible during the entire anastomosis. This technique is especially useful in very small vessels where 0-180 retraction tends to collapse the lumen. (*From* Hou SM, Seaber AV, Urbaniak JR. An alternative technique of microvascular anastomosis. Microsurgery 1987;8(1):23; with permission.)

3. Expeditious dissection of the amputated part on the back table with careful tagging of injured structures with differential size clips for the different neurovascular structures
4. Efficient use of tourniquet time: optimize tourniquet usage for arterial and nerve repair/reconstruction
5. 30-gauge 30-degree anterior-chamber cannula for heparin irrigation; connected via intravenous tubing to a syringe controlled by the scrub tech. "On" and "Off" commands are used for the scrub tech to initiate irrigation. This puts the surgeon's hand directly in the field near the vessel instead of having to hold a syringe outside the field, which is cumbersome
6. Liberal use of Papaverine for vasodilation
7. Meticulous clipping of all side branches of digital arteries during mobilization. Any unclipped

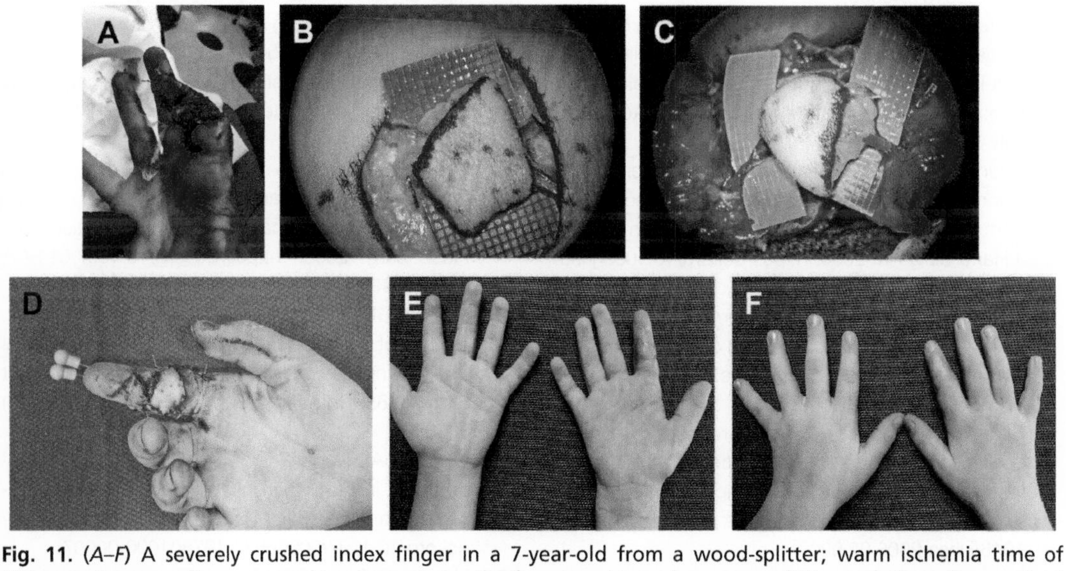

Fig. 11. (*A–F*) A severely crushed index finger in a 7-year-old from a wood-splitter; warm ischemia time of 13 hours. A venous flap was used to revascularize the finger and introduce new soft tissue to the volar proximal phalanx.

side branches ("unsatisfied" branches) result in focal spasm in the digital artery and may lead to thrombosis

8. Tupper hand table (**Fig. 9**)
   a. Allows for hypersupination and hyperpronation
   b. Allows for expeditious retraction and release of skin edges
   c. No need for retractors to be placed in the hand or finger (frees up space)
9. The posterior wall technique for small vessels (**Fig. 10**)[40]
10. Liberal use of venous flaps for soft tissue coverage over the volar aspect of the proximal interphalangeal joint (**Fig. 11**)

REFERENCES

1. Doft MA, Widmann WD, Hardy MA. Under a microscope: Julius H. Jacobson, MD (1927-). J Surg Educ 2008. https://doi.org/10.1016/j.jsurg.2008.01.004.
2. Malt RA, Mckhann CF. Replantation of severed arms. JAMA 1964. https://doi.org/10.1001/jama.1964.03070100010002.
3. Masuhara K, Tamai S, Fukunishi H, et al. Experience with reanastomosis of the amputated thumb. Seikei Geka 1967;18(4):403–4.
4. Reavey PL, Stranix JT, Muresan H, et al. Disappearing digits: analysis of National trends in amputation and replantation in the United States. Plast Reconstr Surg 2018;141(6):857–67.
5. Chen MW, Narayan D. Economics of upper extremity replantation: National and local trends. Plast Reconstr Surg 2009. https://doi.org/10.1097/PRS.0b013e3181bf8008.
6. United States Department of Labor, Bureau of Labor Statistics. Occupational injuries and illnesses: employment statistics and projections. Available at: http://www.bls.gov/data/#employment. Accessed July 7, 2018.
7. Chung KC, Kowalski CP, Walters MR. Finger replantation in the United States: rates and resource use from the 1996 healthcare cost and utilization project. J Hand Surg Am 2000. https://doi.org/10.1053/jhsu.2000.16356.
8. Sebastin SJ, Chung KC. A systematic review of the outcomes of replantation of distal digital amputation. Plast Reconstr Surg 2011. https://doi.org/10.1097/PRS.0b013e318221dc83.
9. Hattori Y, Doi K, Ikeda K, et al. A retrospective study of functional outcomes after successful replantation versus amputation closure for single fingertip amputations. J Hand Surg Am 2006. https://doi.org/10.1016/j.jhsa.2006.02.020.
10. Brown M, Lu Y, Chung KC, et al. Annual hospital volume and success of digital replantation. Plast Reconstr Surg 2017. https://doi.org/10.1097/PRS.0000000000003087.
11. Hustedt JW, Bohl DD, Champagne L. The detrimental effect of decentralization in digital replantation in the United States: 15 years of evidence from the National Inpatient Sample. J Hand Surg Am 2016. https://doi.org/10.1016/j.jhsa.2016.02.011.
12. Payatakes AH, Zagoreos NP, Fedorcik GG, et al. Current practice of microsurgery by members of the American Society for Surgery of the hand. J Hand Surg Am 2007. https://doi.org/10.1016/j.jhsa.2006.12.006.
13. Fufa D, Zeng W, Wall L, et al. Success of digital replantation: experience of two U.S. level-I trauma centers: level 4 evidence. J Hand Surg Am 2012. https://doi.org/10.1016/S0363-5023(12)60050-1.
14. Morrison WA, McCombe D. Digital replantation. Hand Clin 2007. https://doi.org/10.1016/j.hcl.2006.12.001.
15. Misra S, Wilkens SC, Chen NC, et al. Patients transferred for upper extremity amputation: participation of regional trauma centers. J Hand Surg Am 2017. https://doi.org/10.1016/j.jhsa.2017.08.006.
16. Maricevich M, Carlsen B, Mardini S, et al. Upper extremity and digital replantation. Hand 2011. https://doi.org/10.1007/s11552-011-9353-5.
17. Weiland AJ, Villarreal-Rios A, Kleinert HE, et al. Replantation of digits and hands: analysis of surgical techniques and functional results in 71 patients with 86 replantations. J Hand Surg Am 1977. https://doi.org/10.1016/S0363-5023(77)80002-6.
18. Ngaage LM, Oni G, Buntic R, et al. Initial management of traumatic digit amputations: a retrospective study of functional outcomes. J Reconstr Microsurg 2018;34:250–7.
19. Chang J, Jones N. Twelve simple maneuvers to optimize digital replantation and revascularization. Tech Hand Up Extrem Surg 2004. https://doi.org/10.1097/01.bth.0000134711.75677.3b.
20. Nash J. Digital replantation. Using the ninety-ninety intraosseous wiring technique. Todays OR Nurse 1990;12(3):22–7.
21. Ross DC, Manktelow RT, Wells MT, et al. Tendon function after replantation: prognostic factors and strategies to enhance total active motion. Ann Plast Surg 2003. https://doi.org/10.1097/01.SAP.0000058499.74279.D8.
22. Mitchell GM, Morrison WA, Papadopoulos O, et al. A study of the extent and pathology of experimental avulsion injury in rabbit arteries and veins. Br J Plast Surg 1985. https://doi.org/10.1016/0007-1226(85)90064-5.
23. Van Beek AL, Kutz JE, Zook EG. Importance of the ribbon sign, indicating unsuitability of the vessel, in replanting a finger. Plast Reconstr Surg 1978. https://doi.org/10.1097/00006534-197801000-00007.
24. Means KR, Rinker BD, Higgins JP, et al. A multicenter, prospective, randomized, pilot study of outcomes for

digital nerve repair in the hand using hollow conduit compared with processed allograft nerve. Hand 2016. https://doi.org/10.1177/1558944715627233.
25. Rinker B, Zoldos J, Weber RV, et al. Use of processed nerve allografts to repair nerve injuries greater than 25 mm in the hand. Ann Plast Surg 2017. https://doi.org/10.1097/SAP.0000000000001037.
26. Cho MS, Rinker BD, Weber RV, et al. Functional outcome following nerve repair in the upper extremity using processed nerve allograft. J Hand Surg Am 2012. https://doi.org/10.1016/j.jhsa.2012.08.028.
27. Paprottka FJ, Wolf P, Harder Y, et al. Sensory recovery outcome after digital nerve repair in relation to different reconstructive techniques: meta-analysis and systematic review. Plast Surg Int 2013. https://doi.org/10.1155/2013/704589.
28. Higgins JP, Fisher S, Serletti JM, et al. Assessment of nerve graft donor sites used for reconstruction of traumatic digital nerve defects. J Hand Surg Am 2002. https://doi.org/10.1053/jhsu.2002.31154.
29. Ozcelik IB, Tuncer S, Purisa H, et al. Sensory outcome of fingertip replantations without nerve repair. Microsurgery 2008. https://doi.org/10.1002/micr.20543.
30. Wong C, Cheong Ho P, Tse WL, et al. Do we need to repair the nerves when replanting distal finger amputations? J Reconstr Microsurg 2010. https://doi.org/10.1055/s-0030-1249320.
31. Matsuda M, Chikamatsu E, Shimizu Y. Correlation between number of anastomosed vessels and survival rate in finger replantation. J Reconstr Microsurg 1993;9(1):1–4.
32. Foucher G, Norris RW. Distal and very distal digital replantations. Br J Plast Surg 1992. https://doi.org/10.1016/0007-1226(92)90076-A.
33. Jazayeri L, Klausner JQ, Chang J. Distal digital replantation. Plast Reconstr Surg 2013. https://doi.org/10.1097/PRS.0b013e3182a3c0e7.
34. Tamai S. Twenty years' experience of limb replantation—Review of 293 upper extremity replants. J Hand Surg Am 1982. https://doi.org/10.1016/S0363-5023(82)80100-7.
35. Hirase Y. Salvage of fingertip amputated at nail level: new surgical principles and treatments. Ann Plast Surg 1997. https://doi.org/10.1097/00000637-199702000-00009.
36. Allen MJ. Conservative management of finger tip injuries in adults. Hand 1980. https://doi.org/10.1016/S0072-968X(80)80049-0.
37. Buntic RF, Brooks D. Standardized protocol for artery-only fingertip replantation. J Hand Surg Am 2010. https://doi.org/10.1016/j.jhsa.2010.06.004.
38. Erken HY, Takka S, Akmaz I. Artery-only fingertip replantations using a controlled nailbed bleeding protocol. J Hand Surg Am 2013. https://doi.org/10.1016/j.jhsa.2013.08.110.
39. Chen YC, Chan FC, Hsu CC, et al. Fingertip replantation without venous anastomosis. Ann Plast Surg 2013. https://doi.org/10.1097/SAP.0b013e3182321b81.
40. Harris GD, Finseth F, Buncke HJ. Posterior-wall-first microvascular anastomotic technique. Br J Plast Surg 1981. https://doi.org/10.1016/0007-1226(81)90096-5.

Hand, Wrist, Forearm, and Arm Replantation

Matthew L. Iorio, MD[a,b,*]

KEYWORDS

• Hand • Wrist • Forearm • Arm • Replantation

KEY POINTS

- Antibiotics should be given within 3 hours of major amputation and include a first generation cephalosporin, whereas the addition of a third-generation cephalosporin, aminoglycoside, and/or penicillin remains controversial.
- The level of injury plays a significant role in the decision to perform replantation, with improved function, nerve regeneration, and reperfusion.
- The principles of a functional and sensate outcome dictate replantable parts, whereas patient comorbidity, expectations, and safety dictate patient candidacy.
- Vascular grafts are an expected part of the operation, and the contralateral arm or a lower extremity should be prepped into the surgical field.
- Despite diminished function, patient satisfaction and independence remain high after a major upper extremity replantation.

INTRODUCTION

The goals of upper extremity major replantation are the preservation of function, independence, and prevention of chronic pain. Admittedly, the replanted part may not have the same function as the contralateral limb, but by providing a sensate extremity that can be utilized as a helper hand, some function may be maintained. In a review of 26 patients with wrist and wrist-proximal replantations, protective sensation was recovered in 20 patients and the overall grip strength was 32% of the contralateral, which the investigators and patients cited as functional with regard to assistance with daily activities and independence.[1]

Accurately predicting postoperative chronic pain and dysfunction can be difficult in the acute setting, where a majority of patients may be overcome by a sense of loss or despair, and most request replantation at any cost. Sometimes—despite patient preferences—there are intercalary defects of tendon nerve and bone that may be insurmountable for providing a replant that will be a useful extremity. From a technical standpoint, these instances may be difficult, although possible, and it is the guiding principle of a functional, sensate, and pain-free outcome that dictates operative candidates for replantation.

The motivation and occupation of the patient should be considered in conjunction with medical comorbidities. A well-cited article that reviewed the functional outcomes of 183 surgeons with amputated digits, including loss of the thumb in 29 patients, found that only 3 noted a significant

Disclosures: The author has no financial relationships to disclose. This work was not supported by any sources of external funding.

[a] Department of Surgery, Division of Plastic and Reconstructive Surgery, University of Colorado, Anschutz Medical Center, 12631 East 17th Avenue, C309 (Room 6414), Aurora, CO 80045, USA; [b] Department of Orthopedics, University of Colorado, Anschutz Medical Center, 12631 East 17th Avenue, C309 (Room 6414), Aurora, CO 80045, USA

* Department of Orthopedics, University of Colorado, Anschutz Medical Center, 12631 East 17th Avenue, C309 (Room 6414), Aurora, CO 80045.

E-mail address: mattiorio@gmail.com

Hand Clin 35 (2019) 143–154
https://doi.org/10.1016/j.hcl.2018.12.005
0749-0712/19/

professional disability, demonstrating the strong association of patient motivation and acceptance having an impact on the final outcome.[2] Because the return to work or gainful employment after a major upper extremity replantation is usually greater than 24 months, this should be discussed with the patient, because time to recovery may be unacceptable to many self-employed laborers.[3]

This article reviews techniques for upper extremity amputation, patient-based outcomes, and potential alternatives or revisions to improve patient function.

GENERAL PRINCIPLES AND INITIAL MANAGEMENT

The initial management of an upper extremity amputation is similar to the triage of any major trauma, using the advanced trauma and life support (ATLS) survey. Management includes evaluation of concomitant injuries, medical comorbidities, and patient hemodynamic stability owing to the frequently high blood loss at the time of injury (**Box 1**). For patients with severe medical comorbidities, prolonged ischemia time, or mangling/contamination of the amputated part, a revision amputation may be advisable (**Fig. 1**).

Box 1
Consensus guidelines for the initial assessment and management of traumatic amputation injuries

- ATLS assessment of patient and coexisting injuries.
- Control active bleeding with direct pressure.
- Intravenous access and intravenous fluid or blood, depending on hemodynamic status.
- Blood samples for hematology, biochemistry, coagulation studies, and cross-match blood.
- Broad-spectrum intravenous antibiotics.
- Radiography of both the stump and amputated part.
- Determine and update tetanus status.
- Place part in saline-soaked gauze and seal in a plastic bag. Immerse the bag in icy water, and ensure patient information on bag. Never use dry ice.
- Cover the stump with a moist, nonadherent sterile dressing, covered by a dry dressing.
- Early and effective analgesia.
- Early referral to a specialist microsurgical center.

Adapted from Win TS, Henderson J. Management of traumatic amputations of the upper limb. BMJ 2014;348:g255; with permission.

Initial hematologic and metabolic laboratory tests should be obtained expeditiously, and used in consideration of proceeding with a lengthy operation. Additionally, due to the high risk of exsanguination, packed red blood cells should be cross-matched and readily available.

Despite the high rate of blood loss, prolonged tourniquet use is discouraged owing to the possibility of local tissue ischemia and compression as well as potential for metabolic acidosis during incomplete injuries with intact venous return, which explains the typically cited durations of permissible ischemia time, as dictated by the presence of skeletal muscle (eg, warm ischemia of the arm up to 6 hours versus 12 hours in digits).[3] If bleeding cannot be controlled by local pressure, the tourniquet should be cycled to prevent lactic acid build-up and systemic distribution. Additionally, the random or poorly visualized application of hemostats or other tools may cause unnecessary vascular injury and nerve damage.

For patients who are hemodynamically stable, the initial evaluation also should include radiographs of both the extremity and amputated part to aide in surgical planning of osteosynthesis, including direct plating or external fixation. Otherwise, a detailed examination should be completed for both the amputation site and part, evaluating for multilevel injuries, timing, mechanism, contamination, general medical status, and patient goals.

The mechanism of amputation seems to have the greatest predictive effect on the success of the replantation. In a study of 1018 replantations, sharp amputations had the highest survival rate, followed by avulsion, degloving, and, finally, crush injuries with the lowest success.[4] Medical comorbidity, smoking status, patient age, and ischemia are additional considerations, but, given the complexity of microvascular reconstruction, injuries with a wide zone of crush, intimal damage, and vascular thrombosis are frequently not replantable. From an operative standpoint, the microvascular circulation can be protected by keeping the patient normothermic and well hydrated, with avoidance of hypotension or vasopressor use and the potential addition of a regional nerve block for additional vasospastic control through sympathetic blockade.[5]

TECHNIQUE

The amputated part should be brought immediately to the operating room while the patient

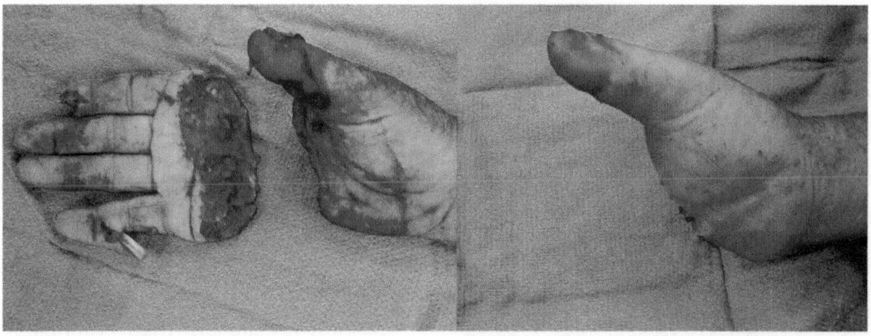

Fig. 1. (*Left*) Multilevel hand amputation in an 80-year-old patient with a recent history of myocardial infarction, multiple cerebrovascular accidents, and leukemia. (*Right*) He was not hemodynamically stable for replantation and underwent a revision amputation with regional anesthesia.

completes preoperative clearance and examination by the anesthesia and nursing teams. The surgeon can then proceed with the initial washout, removal of all foreign debris and either preparation of the part for replantation or, in severe mangling injuries, a determination of the overall viability of the part. Foreign debris should be meticulously removed, and intraoperative fluoroscopy can helpful in cases of radiopaque material, such as shrapnel or road debris. Depending on the mechanism, the part may be heavily contaminated and require extensive débridement of any devitalized structures, even if they pose a functional consequence, in lieu of allowing necrotic or nonviable tissue to remain a potential infectious burden.

Vascular tissue should be cut back to an area without concern for crush, stretch, or accumulated clot. Arterial and venous tissue free from vascular injury should demonstrate soft, pliable vessels, without a hemorrhagic adventitia and with no intimal clot or stippling, and should flush freely with heparinized saline. As a simple rule, an artery or vein with accumulated intraluminal clot should be cut back to an area proximal to the clot, based on the reactive changes of the intima to clot and injury. Vascular damage may dictate whether a part is replantable: if the vessels are damaged with multiple areas of crush, adventitial stippling, or stretch-rupture, the débridement can at times proceed from the level of the forearm and into the hand and fingers, potentially indicating a devastating vascular injury that may not be replantable.

Considerable time should be spent on the appropriate identification and débridement of neurovascular structures, because failed neural regeneration tends to favor a late revision amputation, given the lack of function and sensibility (**Figs. 2** and **3**). Similar to vascular débridement, the nerve should be cut back to an area of healthy-appearing epineurium, without signs of hemorrhage, stretch, or crush. The individual fascicular groups should be visible at the end of the cut nerve.

In patients with prolonged ischemia in the setting of a proximal amputation, vascular shunting should proceed immediately to stop any ongoing muscle necrosis. The initial surgical approach should then involve a meticulous débridement of any nonviable tissue or foreign debris, bony shortening and stabilization to aid in vascular and nerve repair, and distal fasciotomies.[6] Full compartment releases and fasciotomies are standard in major upper extremity

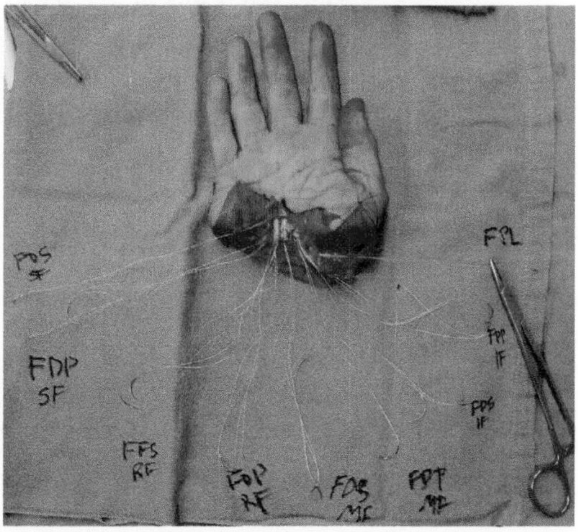

Fig. 2. The amputated part is brought to the back table and prepared and assessed for replantation. Lateral incisions are made for exposure, and the skin is tied back with nylon sutures. Double, modified Tsuge-type core stitches are placed and tagged in the individual flexor tendons to facilitate rapid repair.

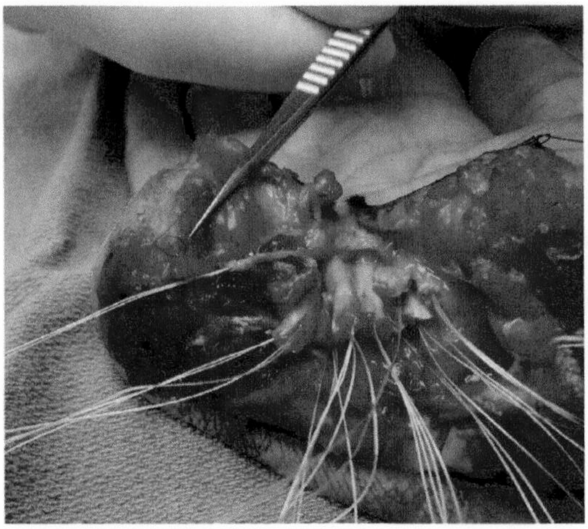

Fig. 3. The nerves are tagged with a blue stitch to aid identification once the tourniquet is released.

replantation, depending on the level of the injury, ischemia time, and whether the soft tissue in various compartments has remained intact. Fasciotomies are especially important for forearm-level and proximal injuries.

After this, bony shortening is then completed both to remove fragmented or nonviable bone and to potentially decrease the length of vein and nerve grafting. At the wrist, shortening can be readily completed through a proximal row carpectomy, whereas several centimeters of shortening can be readily tolerated in the forearm and upper arm.[7] When choosing an internal implant, a guideline may be for at least a 3.5-mm compression plate in the forearm and 4.5-mm compression plate in the upper arm, depending on a patient's body habitus.[3]

Tendon repairs are then completed with core sutures when possible, or, in instances of musculotendinous disruption, the proximal tendon can be woven into the muscle belly. Additionally, tissue grafts can be used to create a scar bridge within the injured muscle belly if a gap remains after definitive fixation (**Fig. 4**).

The vascular anastomoses are then completed, first through the arterial system, with efflux allowed through the venous channels. Once this is completed, the venous channels can be anastomosed, but the anesthesia team should be notified prior to removing the vascular clamps in the event that some lactic acid or reperfusion products are still present, given the risk for cardiovascular collapse.

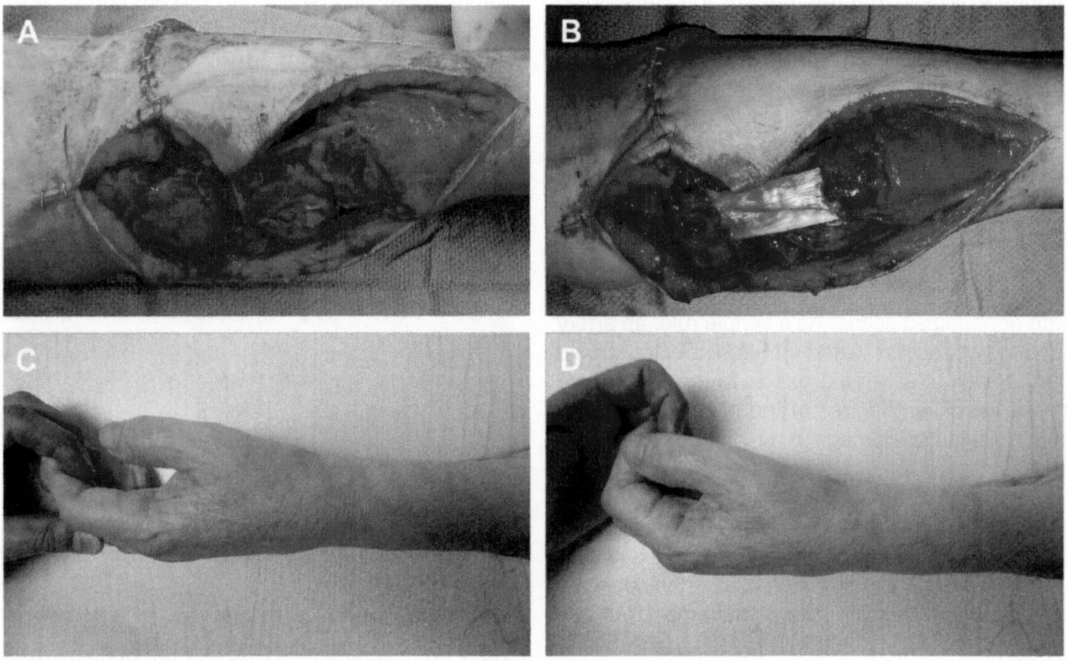

Fig. 4. (*A*) A forearm-level replantation with a significant defect in the superficial and deep flexor muscle bellies. (*B*) The patient was brought back to the operating room 48 hours following replantation to ensure viability and no ongoing signs of necrosis or infection, and an Achilles tendon allograft was woven into the proximal and distal muscle bellies to transmit longitudinal pull. Postoperatively, (*C*) the hand in repose and (*D*) with good resisted finger flexion.

Great attention should be given to the nerve coaptations. Frequently, as nerve repairs occur at the end of the case, it may be seen as a lesser part of the procedure, but a nonsensate or painful replantation is not necessarily a successful replantation (**Figs. 5** and **6**). And, in cases of significant loss of nerve tissue after a crush or intercalary injury, the proximal and distal nerve stumps can be tagged with suture or surgical clips to facilitate a repair through nerve grafting once the soft tissue bed has stabilized.

After reperfusion of the distal limb, the muscle in the zone of injury should be re-examined to see what is perfused and not perfused. Any nonperfused muscle is then débrided to avoid contracture and help limit postoperative infection. The carpal tunnel is generally released and distal fasciotomies are considered if not already performed. Particular attention should be placed on the metacarpophalangeal joint position and the first webspace. Some surgeons recommend pinning the metacarpophalangeal joints at maximum flexion and pinning the first webspace in maximal abduction to help preserve later function and reconstruction.

If possible, the surgical management also should be proactive about preventing infection, with cultures taken at the time of the replantation. If the cultures are positive or there was severe soft tissue injury or contamination, the patient should be taken back to the operating room at 48 hours for a secondary washout and débridement to prevent active infection, osteomyelitis, or microvascular collapse.

Vascular Shunts and Grafts

A vascular shunt can be placed in the distal radial, ulnar, or brachial artery to facilitate immediate reperfusion once the patient and stump are prepared in the operating room. Several shunts are commercially available; however, in the setting of forearm or wrist-level injuries, these products can be difficult to locate within the hospital or can be too large in caliber, and a pediatric feeding tube or high-gauge Foley catheter can be supplemented. The French gauge system describes the outer diameter of the tubbing, in distinction from the inner, or luminal, diameter. As a point of reference, a 3-French feeding tube is equivalent to an outer diameter of 1 mm, with each increase in French gauge of 0.33 mm. If possible, a 3-French to 6-French tube should be selected to allow adequate flow without clotting at the ostium. The shunt should be secured with a tie very close to the ostium of the vessel or with a vessel loop to

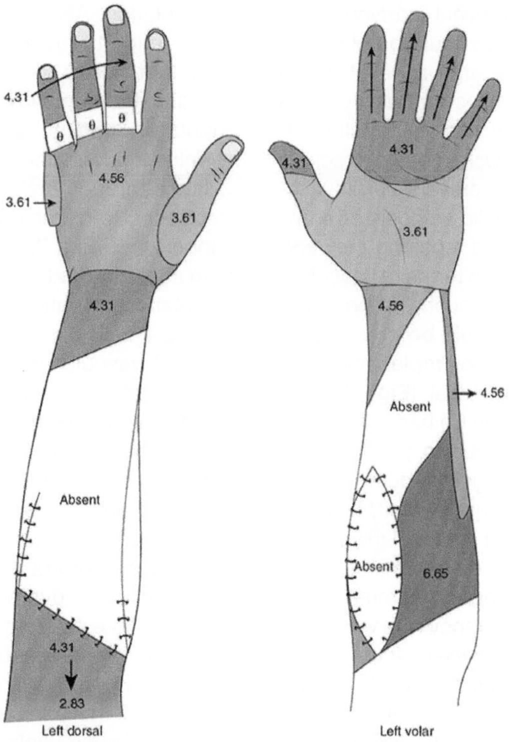

Fig. 6. Sensory recovery 15 months after a transforearm-level replantation in a 74-year-old patient. Evaluator monofilament sizes listed on image of 2.83, 3.61, 4.31, 4.56, and 6.65 correspond to target forces of 0.07 g, 0.4 g, 2.0 g, 4.0 g, and 300 g, respectively. Colors correspond to threshold of sensation: blue, diminished light touch; purple, diminished protective sensation; red, loss of protective sensation; and red lined, tested with no response. (*Adapted from* Taylor EM, Iorio ML. Lateral femoral circumflex arterial system as donor vessels for extremity replantation. J Reconstr Microsurg Open 2016;1(2):88–91; with permission.)

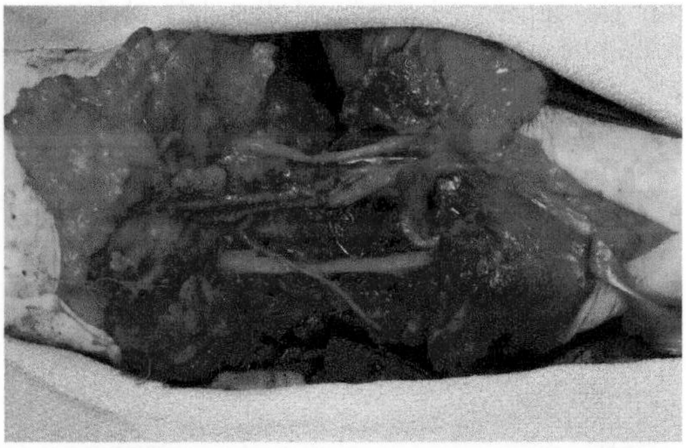

Fig. 5. A forearm-level replantation where the bone has been shortened to allow primary coaptation of the nerves without tension. Additionally, several vein and artery grafts are seen crossing the wound to re-establish arterial and venous flow to the replanted part.

prevent inadvertent loss of cannulation. Also, the tie should be placed close to the edge to prevent a large zone of vascular injury that needs to be resected prior to the anastomosis. It also may be advisable to allow the amputated part to be flushed of lactic acid with the veins freely draining, to prevent cardiovascular collapse through metabolic acidosis or emboli, as opposed to clamping and repairing the venous channels first (**Fig. 7**).

In terms of vascular grafts, an additional extremity, such as the leg or contralateral arm, always should be prepped into the surgical field during a major replantation as a source of vascular graft material (**Fig. 8**). Typically, the saphenous vein can be harvested from anterior to the medial malleolus to the level of the thigh to create multiple, large-diameter grafts (**Fig. 9**). There may be a slight benefit, however, to arterial grafts as used for revascularization compared with venous grafts.

In a review of 152 arterial and venous grafts for upper extremity revascularization, an overall patency rate was found of 87%. The investigators, however, found a narrow margin of increased patency in the arterial grafts compared with venous grafts, with patency rates of the arterial grafts at 18 months of 100% and a slightly diminished patency, albeit at a longer time point, of 85% at 37 months in venous grafts.[8]

When determining the proper source for vascular graft, a few things should be considered, including the state of the donor extremity with any baseline venous insufficiency or arterial atherosclerosis. At all costs, the surgeon should avoid creating a second site of surgical morbidity whenever possible. Additionally, if there are significant soft tissue deficits at the amputated site that may require free tissue transfers, the decision of donor graft should be carefully considered to not preclude a viable flap option. If that risk remains low, however, common arterial donor vessels include the thoracodorsal, inferior epigastric, and the descending branch of the lateral femoral circumflex arteries (LFCA).[9] The LFCA may be especially suitable because the artery as well as the venae comitantes can be taken from the leg with the patient in supine position and within

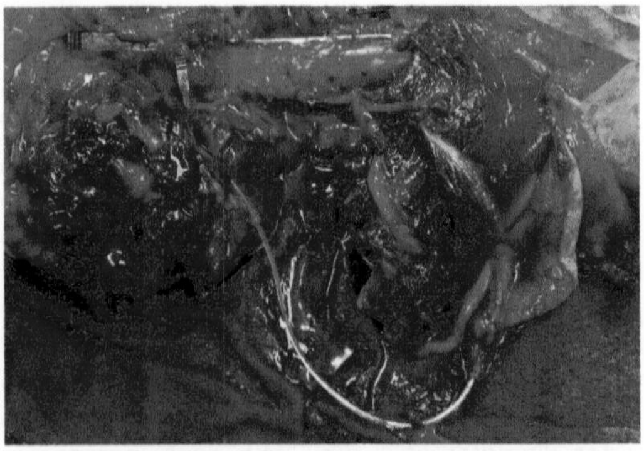

Fig. 7. A shunt is placed in a forearm-level replantation to bridge the defect in the ulnar artery and to allow immediate perfusion to the distal part. In this case, a pediatric feeding tube was utilized. It is securely tied to allow bony stabilization to proceed without accidental dislodgement of the shunt.

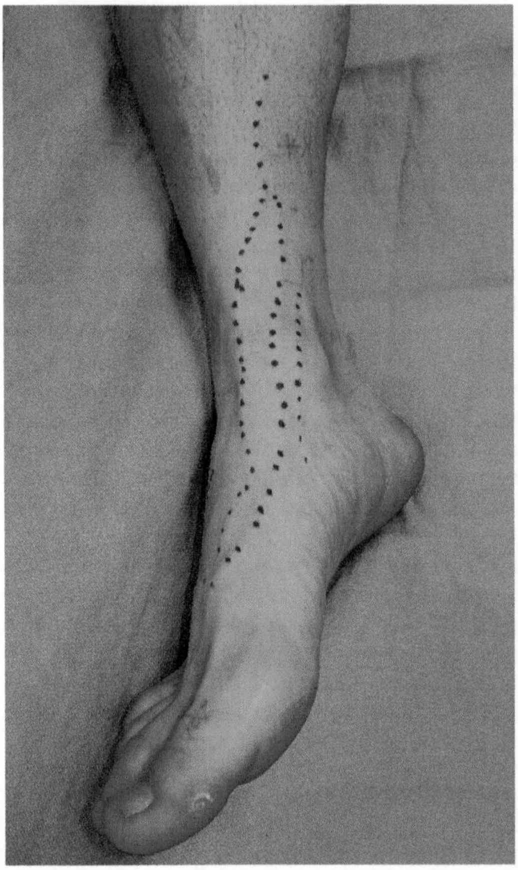

Fig. 8. An additional extremity should always be prepped in for potential vein graft material, and the superficial system can be marked at the start of the case so that a graft can later be easily chosen to fit the appropriate defect.

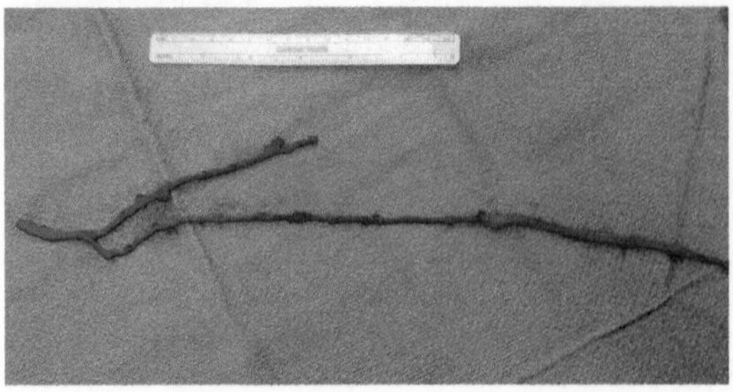

Fig. 9. The saphenous vein can be utilized for multiple, high-caliber vein grafts.

what is most likely a familiar surgical anatomy. The descending branch of the lateral circumflex femoral arterial system often is spared from peripheral vascular disease. In a retrospective review examining angiograms of patients with peripheral vascular disease, the investigators found that the descending branch of the lateral circumflex femoral artery was spared from atherosclerosis in 87% of patients.[10]

Timing of Internal Fixation

The timing of definitive fixation remains a point of surgeon preference, to some degree based on the level and contamination of the injury as well as the overall status or expectation for the replanted part.

At the level of the forearm, several studies have evaluated outcomes after fixation for either complete amputation or incomplete injuries with open fractures. Amongst these studies, immediate or early techniques of plate fixation or wiring are favored, with little evidence for an increased rate of surgical site or hardware-associated infections. Despite the timing of the fixation, however, the rate of nonunion typically is higher than that associated with a closed fracture, at approximately one-third, most likely due to the additional periosteal devitalization and soft tissue stripping.

Based on few existing data, basic principles of operative fixation should prevail in either closed or open injuries, with the type of fixation chosen based strongly on the fracture pattern as opposed to a scoring system. In instances of heavy contamination, however, verification of débridement of devitalized tissue and foreign material is mandatory prior to proceeding with any method of fixation. Additionally, in those circumstances where the fixation technique may interfere with soft tissue management or would be at high risk for subsequent erosion or exposure, alternate techniques should be considered.[11]

Supplementary Techniques

Several techniques may aid in the operation or overall rate of a successful replantation. Vein grafting onto the amputated part can be performed on the back table, so that teams can work simultaneously on both the injury site and the amputated part. This also may make the microsurgery more feasible, by allowing the part to be rotated in 3-D space prior to osteosynthesis.

Additionally, there should be a strict avoidance of pressure or tension on the wound closure, and, as such, split-thickness skin grafts should be liberally used[12] (**Fig. 10**). If needed, coverage of a portion of the vascular reconstruction with a skin graft may be preferred compared with tightly closing the tissue envelope and causing a point of constriction or vascular compromise. If the exposed area is extensive, or if it is unclear as to whether the replanted part will survive and donor sites are to be conserved, temporary coverage may be obtained by several different xenograft and allograft skin substitutes.[13] In cases of flap coverage or secondary skin grafting planned, a xenograft, such as porcine skin, may function as an excellent choice by both covering tissue and preventing desiccation, in addition to indicating the suitability of final coverage or grafting, such that, if the initial xenograft is destroyed by bacterial lysis or demonstrates nonadherence, the wound bed is unsuitable for definitive grafting and may instead require repeat débridement. Several other acellular dermal matrices are commercially available, but, if they are to be used as a temporary dressing for only a few days and then removed, this technique may be economically prohibitive.

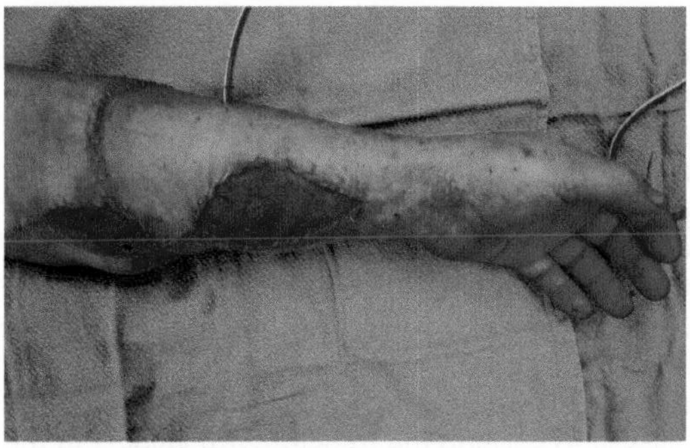

Fig. 10. Skin grafts should be used to prevent tension on the closure or vascular repair.

In terms of the postoperative monitoring of the replantation, pulse oximetry may provide an objective tool in lieu of subjective techniques, such as capillary refill or skin turgor. In a study of lacerating trauma to the hand, pulse oximetry was used to record data from the injured side as well as the contralateral limb to normalize for patient temperature, hemodynamic status, and environmental factors, with a measure of digital hypoxia followed by surgical exploration and correlation with vascular injury. The investigators found that a pulse oximetry value below 84% indicated a positive predictive value of arterial insufficiency and injury at 100%, whereas above an oximetry value of 95%, the negative predictive value of arterial insufficiency was 100%.[14]

Soft Tissue Reconstruction

When attempting to salvage an amputation with inadequate soft tissue coverage, the surgical algorithm should consider use of the amputated part when possible as a filet flap.[15] This spare-part strategy offers the potential for an immediate and robust reconstruction without the expenditure of a donor site. Alternatively, free tissue transfer can offer several different types of tissue coverage, including neurotized muscle and innervated skin (**Fig. 11**). In a report of 13 cases of residual limb coverage through microsurgical transfer done for length preservation, 3 of these flaps (2 latissimus dorsi and 1 anterolateral thigh) were specifically to salvage the transforearm level.[16] In the report, elbow preservation was cited as a major indication for microsurgical coverage of a residual limb, along with shoulder preservation, preservation of pinch function, and preservation of skeletal length greater than 7 cm below the shoulder or elbow joint (**Fig. 12**).

Volitional control of elbow flexion followed by elbow extension allows the patient to position the hand or prosthetic to the mouth for feeding or to assist with daily hygiene and activities. In cases of muscle in the upper arm, the pectoralis major muscle or latissimus dorsi muscle can be pedicled on their blood supply and reoriented for restoration of function. A pedicled flap obviates additional microsurgery and potentially comes with little surgical morbidity.[17] In a report of 5 patients who underwent latissimus transfer after upper arm replantation, 3 patients demonstrated M4 function and 2 patients demonstrated M3 function at an average follow-up of 43 months. In the procedure, the entire latissimus dorsi muscle can be harvested and released from the lesser tuberosity and iliac crest, brought anteriorly, and anchored to the coracoid or clavipectoral fascia to create a linear line of pull. Distally, the muscle can be tubularized to prevent lateral tissue adhesion and woven into the remnant of the coracobrachialis or biceps tendon and insertion.

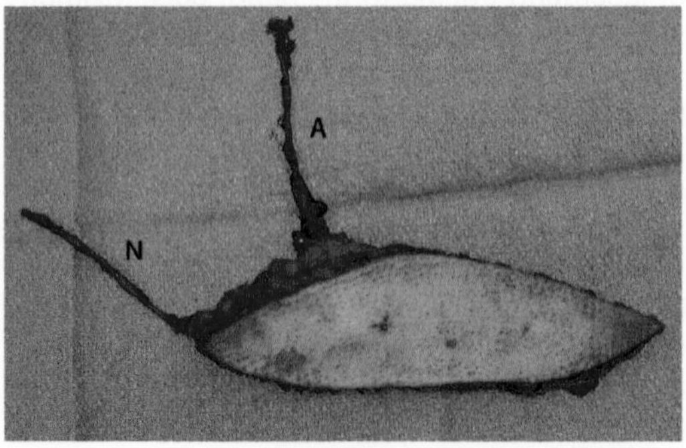

Fig. 11. The anterolateral thigh flap is based on irrigating perforators from the descending branch of the lateral femoral circumflex artery (A). The flap can be taken with skin and subcutaneous tissue, fascia, muscle, or a branch of the lateral femoral cutaneous nerve for a sensate reconstruction (N).

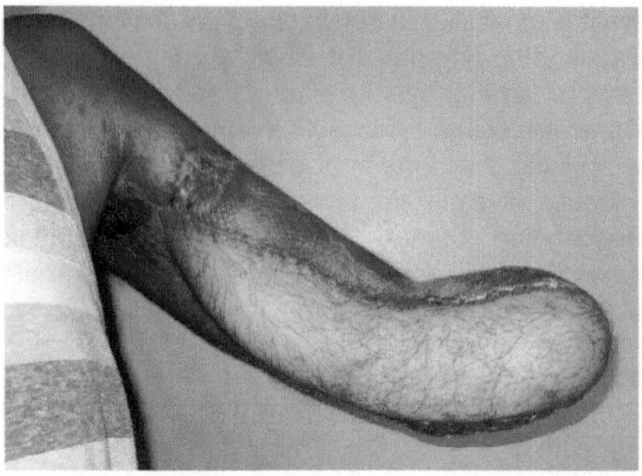

Fig. 12. Proximal forearm-level revision amputation with salvage of the elbow joint using an anterolateral thigh flap for coverage.

In cases of local pedicled flaps not available outside of the zone of injury or extensive soft tissue defects and exposed bone, tendon, hardware, or nerve tissue, free tissue transfers should be considered.[18] The choice to proceed with an immediate tissue transfer at the time of replantation, as opposed to delayed coverage within the acute postoperative period, is based on the hemodynamic stability of the patient, the likelihood of replant viability, infection, the risk of flap loss, and a prediction of secondary procedures or revisions that would benefit from a vascularized soft tissue envelope.

COMPLICATIONS

Early complications are typically related to microvascular collapse or infection, based on the degree of contamination, débridement, and tissue quality of the injury. In open fractures, the Gustilo classification typically is used to dictate general outcomes and principles of antibiotic management.[11] A greater emphasis on the severity of the tissue injury, however, with full-thickness defects, skin and muscle loss, and gross contamination can be used in the Tscherne-Oestern system to help guide antibiotic use based on the severity of the tissue trauma.[19] In a review of open fractures of the forearm and distal radius, the highest risks for postoperative infection were based on severity of tissue trauma and type of contamination, with road/soil and sewage/fecal contamination relating to the highest risks of infection.

The initial antibiotic management of a major amputation should be based on the type of injury as well as the overall medical status of the patient (immunocompromised, chronic injury, and smoking status), with the optimal timing of antibiotic administration within the first 3 hours. This recommendation is based on outcomes that demonstrated a 4.7% infection rate versus 7.4%, when antibiotics were given either within 3 hours or more, respectively.[11,20] There are few data, however, to support prolonged antibiotic administration beyond 24 hours. The choice of antibiotic has been demonstrated in level I studies to include a first-generation cephalosporin, given the broad coverage and activity against a majority of gram-positive cocci, gram-negative rods, *Escherichia coli* and *Klebsiella pneumoniae*.

Late complications after replantation may include nerve pain, cold intolerance, joint ankylosis, tendon adhesions, or bony malunion and nonunions.[21] In the pediatric population, however, it is possible to find ongoing longitudinal bone growth. In a series of 162 digital replants, the digits averaged 81% of normal length at the time of skeletal maturity, although it is difficult to determine if this discrepancy is secondary to physis arrest versus primary bone shortening at the time of replantation.[22]

OUTCOMES

The rate of successful replantation varies widely, with reported rates from the thirtieth to the midninetieth percentiles, largely due to the variability in injury level, mechanism, and surgeon experience. What seems to remain consistent, however, is a relatively high rate of patient satisfaction. A multicenter study evaluated transforearm-level amputees with patients who had a successful replantation at the same level to determine intergroup comparisons with the Disabilities of the Arm, Shoulder and Hand (DASH) and Michigan Hand Questionnaire (MHQ) instruments. The investigators found that within the replantation group, there was a significantly higher aggregate MHQ score as well the domains of overall function (41.1 vs 19.7; $P = .03$), activities of daily living (28.3 vs 6.0; $P = .03$), and patient satisfaction (24.6 vs 39.8; $P = .08$).[23] This satisfaction occurs, however, despite a marked reduction in function. In a review of 11 patients who underwent forearm replantation, there was a demonstrated an average grip strength of 39.4% and pinch strength of 36.2% of the contralateral side.[24] Based on these and similar outcomes, functional evaluations may be less important than a patient's individual perception of function, again highlighting the importance of adequate patient understanding and shared decision making in the treatment plan.

The replanted limb does not, however, seem to diminish in function over time and may instead accrue improvements in function, range of motion, and sensibility.[25] In a review of long-term outcomes after replantation, 16 patients at an average follow-up of 13.5 years demonstrated a mean DASH of 41 and reported good functional independence, which may explain why, despite a frequent rate of postoperative pain, commonly quoted between 39% and 79%, a majority of patients note that they are happy with their replantation and would undergo the procedure again if placed in the same situation.

The overall psychological health of the patient should be carefully considered, because a review of 22 upper extremity amputees found that 5 required treatment of acute stress disorder and 17 required treatment of posttraumatic stress disorder beyond 6 months after the initial injury. In the circumstance of major upper extremity amputation, psychiatric or psychological referrals should be part of the standard postoperative counseling.[26]

UPPER EXTREMITY PROSTHETIC USE WITHOUT REPLANTATION

Unfortunately, despite the high functional challenges of a major upper extremity amputation without replantation, a large portion of patients are unable to either accommodate or tolerate a prosthesis. In several reviews, the rate of prosthesis rejection for proximal amputations is at least 23% to 38%, which is substantially different from the low rates of prosthetic rejection in the lower extremity.[27,28] In a comparison of replantation and revision amputation outcomes, 20 patients underwent successful upper extremity major replantation and 22 were treated with a revision amputation and fitted with a body-powered prosthetic. The investigators found that even with a low satisfaction in the replantation group (37%), the prosthetic group fared far worse with a satisfaction rate of 0% ($P < .006$), although the results favored a younger patient age and more distal injury. With the advent of myoelectric prostheses, prosthetic function is a relative outcome that is best determined by the surgeon and patient.

An additional consideration, especially in cases of severe mangling or avulsion injuries with soft tissue loss, is that the distal-most part of the exposed bone may be considerably longer than the available tissue coverage. In these circumstances, and when replantation is not feasible or advisable, the surgeon must decide on the level of the proximal revision amputation. In the forearm, this may mean bony shortening of a few centimeters, but in the proximal forearm, efforts should be made to maintain elbow flexion and the insertion of the biceps onto the radial tuberosity, whenever possible. Some studies have shown little difference in DASH scores or activities of daily living for a transhumeral-level versus transforearm-level amputation; however, functional tasks may be more limited with a proximal amputation.[29,30] A performance-based outcome measure, called the Activities Measure for Upper Extremity Amputees, was developed to evaluate functional outcomes after amputation and found significantly better scores with prosthesis use for transradial amputees compared with transhumeral amputees.[31] When evaluating return to work, 66% (20/30) of transradial amputees but only 18% of transhumeral amputees had success reintegrating

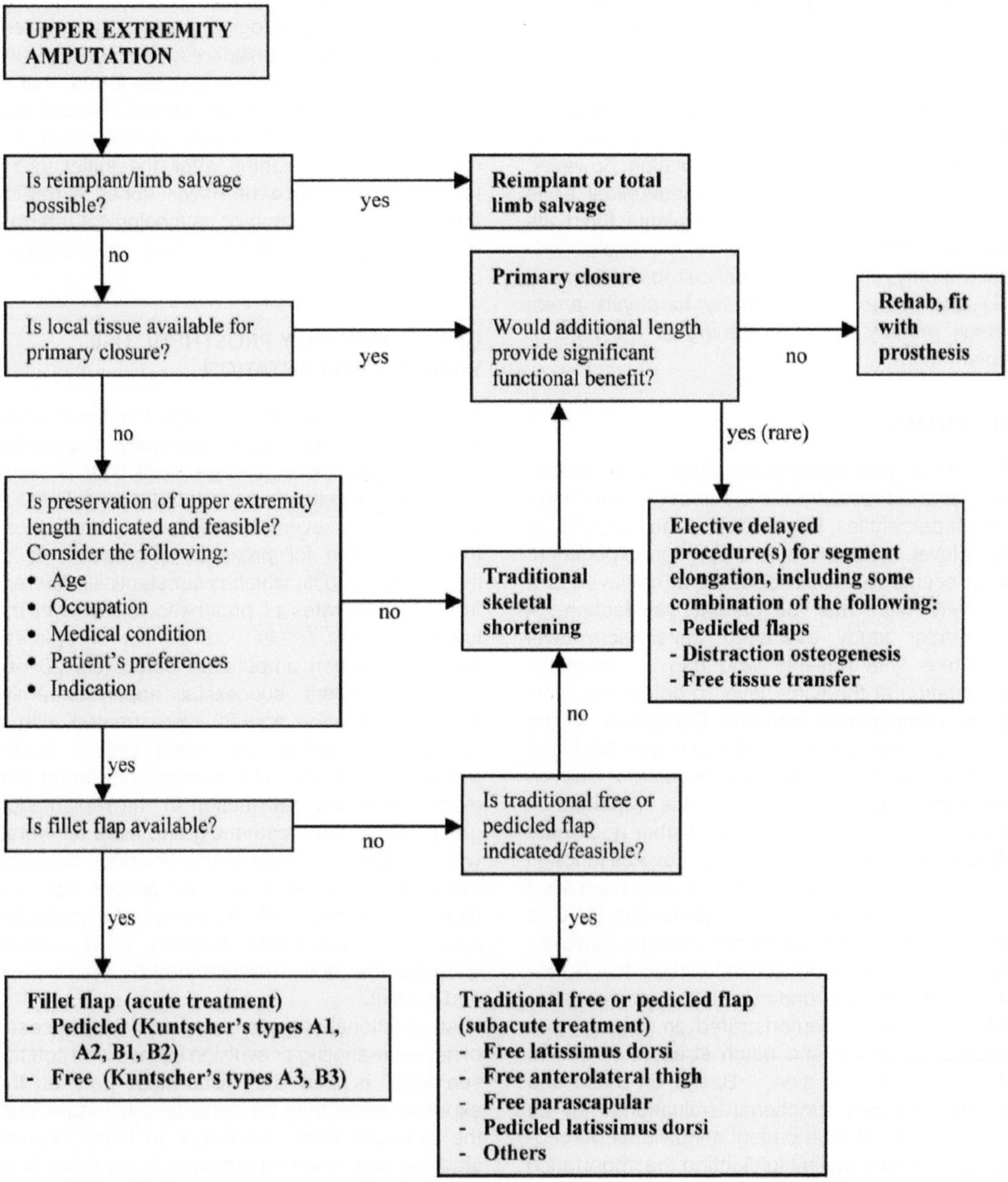

Fig. 13. Treatment algorithm for management of the amputated upper extremity. Therapeutic actions are in bold; questions that determine the path along the decision tree are in plain text. (*From* Baccarani A, Follmar KE, De Santis G, et al. Free vascularized tissue transfer to preserve upper extremity amputation levels. Plast Reconstr Surg 2007;120(4):971–81; with permission.)

into the workplace, a finding confirmed by other groups.[30,32]

Elbow joint preservation facilitates myoelectric prosthesis use by simplifying the control algorithms and requiring fewer distinct electromyographic signals. With the myoelectric device, a below-elbow amputee can initiate palmar tip grasp or other types of grip by contracting residual forearm flexors and can release by contracting residual extensors.[16] In contrast, transhumeral amputees often lack adequate electromyographic signals, and myoelectric prosthesis fitting requires complex control algorithms and/or including targeted muscle reinnervation.[26]

SUMMARY

Major upper extremity replantation is dependent on adequate consideration of patient goals, motivation, and functional needs (**Fig. 13**). Above all, patient safety should be prioritized, and medical comorbidities and hemodynamic instability should be considered in the decision of replantation versus revision amputation.

REFERENCES

1. Sugun TS, Ozaksar K, Ada S, et al. Long-term results of major upper extremity replantations. Acta Orthop Traumatol Turc 2009;43(3):206–13.
2. Brown PW. Less than ten-surgeons with amputated fingers. J Hand Surg Am 1982;7(1):31–7.
3. Hanel DP, Chin SH. Wrist level and proximal-upper extremity replantation. Hand Clin 2007;23(1):13–21.
4. Waikakul S, Sakkarnkosol S, Vanadurongwan V, et al. Results of 1018 digital replantations in 552 patients. Injury 2000;31(1):33–40.
5. Sammer DM. Management of complications with flap procedures and replantation. Hand Clin 2015;31(2):339–44.
6. Yaffe B, Hutt D, Yaniv Y, et al. Major upper extremity replantations. J Hand Microsurg 2009;1(2):63–7.
7. Sabapathy SR, Venkatramani H, Bharathi RR, et al. Replantation surgery. J Hand Surg Am 2011;36(6):1104–10.
8. Masden DL, Seruya M, Higgins JP. A systematic review of the outcomes of distal upper extremity bypass surgery with arterial and venous conduits. J Hand Surg Am 2012;37(11):2362–7.
9. Taylor E, Iorio ML. Lateral femoral circumflex arterial system as donor vessels for extremity replantation. J Reconstr Microsurg Open 2016;1:88–91.
10. Halvorson EG, Taylor HO, Orgill DP. Patency of the descending branch of the lateral circumflex femoral artery in patients with vascular disease. Plast Reconstr Surg 2008;121(1):121–9.
11. Iorio ML, Harper CM, Rozental TD. Open distal radius fractures: timing and strategies for surgical management. Hand Clin 2018;34(1):33–40.
12. Chang J, Jones N. Twelve simple maneuvers to optimize digital replantation and revascularization. Tech Hand Up Extrem Surg 2004;8(3):161–6.
13. Iorio ML, Shuck J, Attinger CE. Wound healing in the upper and lower extremities: a systematic review on the use of acellular dermal matrices. Plast Reconstr Surg 2012;130(5 Suppl 2):232S–41S.
14. Tarabadkar N, Iorio ML, Gundle K, et al. The use of pulse oximetry for objective quantification of vascular injuries in the hand. Plast Reconstr Surg 2015;136(6):1227–33.
15. Flurry M, Melissinos EG, Livingston CK. Composite forearm free fillet flaps to preserve stump length following traumatic amputations of the upper extremity. Ann Plast Surg 2008;60(4):391–4.
16. Baccarani A, Follmar KE, De Santis G, et al. Free vascularized tissue transfer to preserve upper extremity amputation levels. Plast Reconstr Surg 2007;120(4):971–81.
17. Schoeller T, Wechselberger G, Hussl H, et al. Functional transposition of the latissimus dorsi muscle for biceps reconstruction after upper arm replantation. J Plast Reconstr Aesthet Surg 2007;60(7):755–9.
18. Saint-Cyr M, Wong C, Buchel EW, et al. Free tissue transfers and replantation. Plast Reconstr Surg 2012;130(6):858e–78e.
19. Valderrama-Molina CO, Estrada-Castrillón M, Hincapie JA, et al. Intra- and interobserver agreement on the Oestern and Tscherne classification of soft tissue injury in periarticular lower-limb closed fractures. Colomb Med (Cali) 2014;45(4):173–8.
20. Patzakis MJ, Wilkins J. Factors influencing infection rate in open fracture wounds. Clin Orthop Relat Res 1989;243:36–40.
21. Win TS, Henderson J. Management of traumatic amputations of the upper limb. BMJ 2014;348:g255.
22. Taras JS, Nunley JA, Urbaniak JR, et al. Replantation in children. Microsurgery 1991;12:216–20.
23. Pet MA, Morrison SD, Mack JS, et al. Comparison of patient-reported outcomes after traumatic upper extremity amputation: replantation versus prosthetic rehabilitation. Injury 2016;47(12):2783–8.
24. Assouline U, Feuvrier D, Lepage D, et al. Functional assessment and quality of life in patients following replantation of the distal half of the forearm (except fingers): a review of 11 cases. Hand Surg Rehabil 2017;36(4):261–7.
25. Mattiassich G, Rittenschober F, Dorninger L, et al. Long-term outcome following upper extremity replantation after major traumatic amputation. BMC Musculoskelet Disord 2017;18(1):77.
26. Solarz MK, Thoder JJ, Rehman S. Management of major traumatic upper extremity amputations. Orthop Clin North Am 2016;47(1):127–36.

27. Wright TW, Hagen AD, Wood MB. Prosthetic usage in major upper extremity amputations. J Hand Surg Am 1995;20(4):619–22.
28. Biddiss EA, Chau TT. Upper limb prosthesis use and abandonment: a survey of the last 25 years. Prosthet Orthot Int 2007;31(3):236–57.
29. Ostlie K, Franklin RJ, Skjeldal OH, et al. Assessing physical function in adult acquired major upper-limb amputees by combining the Disabilities of the Arm, Shoulder and Hand (DASH) Outcome Questionnaire and clinical examination. Arch Phys Med Rehabil 2011;92(10):1636–45.
30. Fernández A, Isusi I, Gómez M. Factors conditioning the return to work of upper limb amputees in Asturias, Spain. Prosthet Orthot Int 2000;24(2):143–7.
31. Resnik L, Adams L, Borgia M, et al. Development and evaluation of the activities measure for upper limb amputees. Arch Phys Med Rehabil 2013;94(3):488–94.
32. Pinzur MS, Angelats J, Light TR, et al. Functional outcome following traumatic upper limb amputation and prosthetic limb fitting. J Hand Surg Am 1994;19(5):836–9.

Pediatric Replantation and Revascularization

Amir H. Taghinia, MD, MPH, MBA

KEYWORDS

• Replantation • Revascularization • Pediatric • Children • Amputation

KEY POINTS

- In children, successful replantation and revascularization promises good functional outcomes, thus the indications for attempting these procedures are broad.
- Children differ from adults in multiple facets: technical execution, healing, functional outcomes, and complications.
- In children these procedures are necessary mainly after trauma, but can also be required after extirpation of lesions such as vascular malformations and malignant tumors, or for treatment of vascular disease.
- Probability of functional success can be improved with experience in pediatric microsurgery, understanding of the technical challenges in children, and adequate protection after repair.

INTRODUCTION

The adage that children are not small adults rings ever true in pediatric upper extremity replantation and revascularization. Although many principles and technical points are shared between adults and children, there are distinct differences that make pediatric replantation and revascularization easier and more challenging simultaneously. It may not be simple coincidence that the first reported functionally successful replantation in humans was performed in a child.[1,2] Children heal better than adults: soft and hard tissues heal faster and nerves regenerate more rapidly and robustly. The major determinant of long-term functional outcome after extremity injury is nerve recovery, an area where children dramatically excel compared with adults. Children are also less affected by stiffness, joint contractures, and pain syndromes. They adapt faster to functional deficits and display remarkable long-term resiliency when coping with loss. The psychosocial care of children and their families, especially those subjected to significant trauma, requires specialized expertise and should not be neglected. Microsurgical treatment of children can be technically challenging and requires meticulous technique and attention to detail. This article reviews basic principles of pediatric microsurgery, replantation, and revascularization. In addition, it outlines specific technical considerations and maneuvers to optimize success. A review of literature-reported outcomes and considerations is provided. Although the broad subjects of replantation and revascularization apply to all end appendages in the body (eg, ears, lips, scalp), the discussions in this article focus solely on the extremities.

MICROSURGICAL PRINCIPLES

Pediatric replantation and revascularization procedures represent a subset of reconstructive operations under the discipline of pediatric microsurgery. As such, the principles of microsurgery, especially as applied in children,[3] should be followed carefully to better understand disease pathophysiology and optimize treatment.

Disclosure: No disclosures.

Department of Plastic and Oral Surgery, Boston Children's Hospital, Harvard Medical School, 300 Longwood Avenue, Enders 1, Boston, MA 02115, USA
E-mail address: amir.taghinia@childrens.harvard.edu

Hand Clin 35 (2019) 155–178
https://doi.org/10.1016/j.hcl.2018.12.006

General Considerations

It is preferable to perform direct, end-to-end vascular and neural coaptation without grafts when feasible. Direct repair avoids the extra time and morbidity of harvesting grafts, and ensures higher vascular patency rates and better nerve recovery. However, graftless repairs should never be done under tension. Undue tension undoes microsurgery: vascular and nerve repairs under tension are much more likely to fail.

Repositioning of joints may help avoid tension in vascular and neural repair. However, this option should be exercised cautiously and conservatively. Extreme joint positioning to avoid tension may be effective initially, but the repair is prone to disruption if the patient moves in the early period. In children, this is especially problematic if they slip out of casts or splints. Nerve grafts survive by inosculation from the surrounding soft tissues. A nerve graft sutured under tension is likely to have its blood supply sheared once motion starts. Surgical judgment plays an important role in balancing the degree of tension versus the degree of joint repositioning. It is usually best to repair without having to reposition the joint to reduce tension. The surgeon should put the involved adjacent joints through their full range of motion before making final decisions about the length of vascular and/or nerve grafts.

In the case of a gap or undue tension, the first option is shortening of the bone at the site of injury. This option is almost always best (if possible) because bone shortening helps gaps/tension on multiple structures simultaneously. However, the downsides of bone shortening should be counterbalanced against the need for grafting. In general, bone shortening is better tolerated distally than proximally, and better tolerated in the upper extremity than the lower extremity. Bone transport and distraction lengthening techniques can be used later to remedy any functional deficits.

One of the most difficult decisions in acute or subacute nerve repair is determining the zone of injury. In acute sharp lacerations, the zone of injury is likely small; minimal debridement and end-to-end repair is usually sufficient and provides the best outcome. In delayed cases where the nerves have been crushed and/or the ends have retracted, the zone of injury is more obvious and the resultant gap almost always needs a graft. However, in acute crush or avulsion injuries it is very difficult to determine how much of the nerve needs debridement acutely. In these cases, it may be best to do the bone shortening as needed, tag the ends of the nerves, and return in 10 to 14 days for reconstruction with a nerve graft.

Grafts

If bone shortening is not possible or only a few structures are gapped, grafting may become a necessity. Options for vascular grafts include arterial or venous grafts. In young children, it is best to avoid synthetic vascular conduits because they do not grow and in theory would need to be replaced in the future. Spare structures from nonreplantable parts are a readily available source of graft material.

For arterial gaps, arterial grafts are the ideal. However, these grafts are usually not easily expendable and are rarely used. One exception is when an arterial graft becomes available in a spare part (**Fig. 1**). Vein grafts are usually available in all sizes and lengths, but not necessarily in children with medical problems requiring previous vascular access. In nonacute cases, vein mapping can be invaluable to avoid wasting time and unnecessary incisions.

The choice and location of vein graft are dictated by the reconstructive need. Ideal vein grafts mimic the reconstructive deficit in terms of lumen diameter and wall thickness. In digital replants, arterial gaps are best repaired with dorsal veins from the foot, which are thicker walled than veins from the hand. However, digital vein gaps are best treated with similar veins from adjacent digits (**Fig. 2**). The walls of foot veins are too thick and muscular; they collapse readily and diminish flow in the low-pressure venous system of the fingers. The saphenous vein is ideal for brachial artery reconstruction because it closely mimics its lumen diameter and wall thickness.

The types of nerve grafts and indications for nerve grafting continue to be debated in the literature, especially given the additional choices in synthetic and cadaveric conduits introduced in the past several decades. The first decision is whether to graft or not based on the principles outlined earlier (bone shortening, minimal joint repositioning, injury type, and timing of repair). The main goal is a tension-free repair with the digit/extremity in extension.[4] If a graft is needed, the ideal reconstruction remains autologous nerve. However, this decision needs to be balanced with the requirements of the deficit. Newer modalities of nerve grafting with conduit or processed nerve allograft are gaining popularity and are reasonable options for small gaps.[4–7] For longer gaps, and perhaps for deficits that would pose a greater functional loss (eg, thumb ulnar digital nerve), autologous grafts are likely superior theoretically because of the presence of progenitor cells. There are limited data supporting the use of cadaveric or synthetic grafts for reconstruction of motor or combined

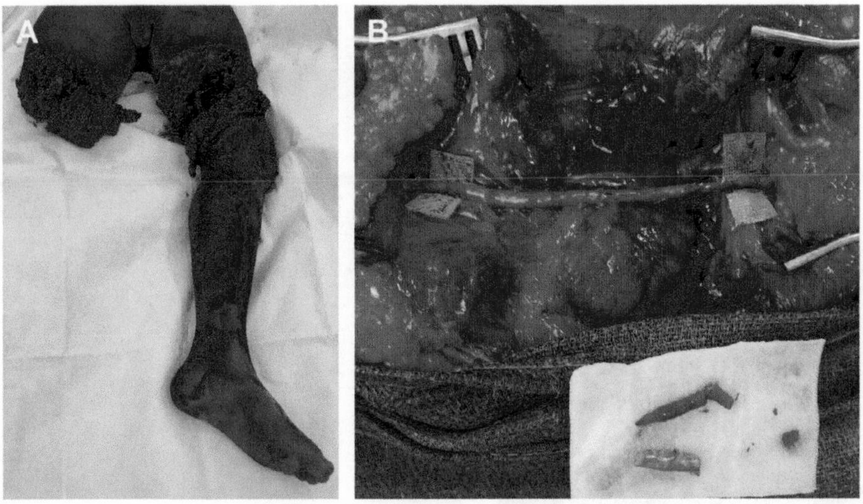

Fig. 1. A 3-year-old boy sustained midthigh crush injuries from an industrial backhoe. (*A*) The left lower limb was partially amputated, held on by a small skin and muscle bridge anterolaterally. The femoral artery was lacerated; the sciatic nerve was intact but bruised. (*B*) An 11-cm arterial graft was harvested from the nonreplantable right leg and used to revascularize the left leg. Note the nearly 4 cm of (definite and presumed) injured artery excised before reconstruction (on white pad). The left leg survived.

sensory/motor nerves. Nevertheless, there are situations in which long-segment, large-diameter cadaveric nerve grafts are necessary. For example, in proximal avulsion or crush injuries, large nerve gaps may require more dispensable autologous nerve than is available. In these situations, the entire nerve may need reconstruction with cadaveric graft; alternatively, if the motor and sensory bundles can be separated, autologous nerve may be used for the functionally more important bundles and cadaveric for the less important ones. To date, there are no studies documenting long-term results of conduit or cadaveric nerve grafts in children.

Pediatric Considerations

Children show faster and more vigorous healing than adults. This aspect of pediatric recovery is best manifested after major extremity injury, for which the biggest obstacle in functional improvement is nerve regeneration. Sensory and motor recovery in pediatric extremity injuries is excellent.[8–10] Great recovery can be expected even without nerve repair in amputations at or distal to the distal interphalangeal joint. This conclusion has been reached by multiple studies[11–15] and is consistent with the clinical observations of the author. Nevertheless, recovery from peripheral nerve injury encompasses not only restoration of sensory and motor function but also avoidance of motor dysfunction (eg, synkinesia or dyskinesia), chronic pain, and pain syndromes. The pediatric brain shows remarkable plasticity and adapts well to crisscrossed neural pathways after reinnervation. Children rarely develop painful neuromas[16] or other long-term problems of peripheral nerve injury. For these reasons, every attempt should be made to salvage amputated structures in this patient population.

In addition to healing differences, there are certain other technical elements that differentiate pediatric microsurgery from adult microsurgery. Most children do not have long-term sequelae from vascular disease induced by smoking, diabetes, or atherosclerosis. Pediatric arteries are soft and elastic; hence they are more tolerant to stretching but also retract more when lacerated. In children, digital vessels are smaller and technically more difficult to repair, requiring superfine instruments and high magnification. Nevertheless, technically well-repaired, nondiseased vessels are much less likely to fail in children.

One concern about pediatric vessels is their tendency to vasospasm, an issue that has been debated in the literature.[17–20] It is the author's experience that vasospasm in pediatric microsurgery does occur but is no more frequent than in adults. Vasospasm can be either seen directly or inferred. When seen directly, vasospasm describes the phenomenon of a vessel shrinking to a smaller diameter, usually during manipulation. When inferred, vasospasm describes sluggish flow across a technically patent anastomosis. Both these scenarios usually respond to a

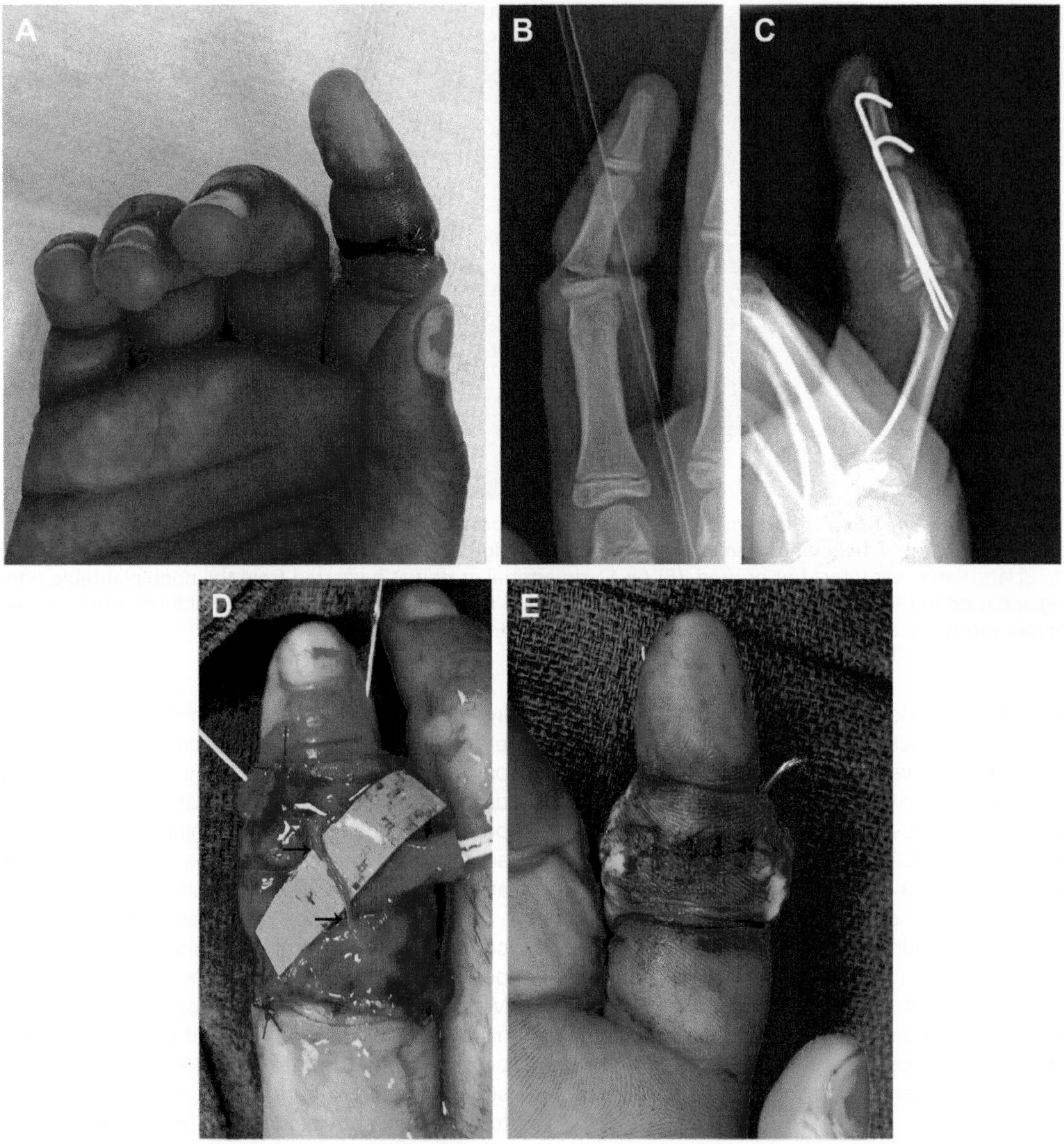

Fig. 2. An 8-year-old girl had a near-complete amputation with circumferential skin and soft tissue injury after the edge of a television crushed her index finger. (*A*) The flexor tendon was intact and the finger was ischemic. (*B*) The juxtaphyseal middle phalangeal fracture was (*C*) cross-pinned. (*D*) After aggressive debridement, an 8-mm digital vein graft provided the ideal reconstructive vessel to bridge the venous gap; arrows indicate proximal and distal anastomoses using 11-0 suture. (*E*) One-week postoperative clinical view (before casting) shows good tip vascularity.

combination of warm irrigation, vasodilating agents, and (most importantly) time and patience. When vasospasm is encountered, ensure that the patient is well hydrated and warm, that the blood pressure is normal, and that vasopressors have been held. A smaller blood volume and greater surface area/mass ratio means that children have higher insensible losses. Dehydration and hypothermia both lead to vasoconstriction and should be strictly avoided.

Another concern in pediatric arterial repairs is the long-term fate of vein grafts, especially in proximal extremity reconstructions. Early reports documented aneurysmal changes of vein grafts used for nonextremity (aortorenal) vascular reconstructions in children.[21–24] Few long-term reports (>10 years) address this concern in the extremities. Cardneau and colleagues[25] reported on 14 patients who underwent 16 revascularization procedures with greater saphenous vein in the lower extremity. After an average of 11 years postoperatively, 50% developed nonaneurysmal dilatation and 14% showed nonprogressive aneurysmal expansion. In another study of brachial artery reconstruction after supracondylar humeral fracture, Konstantiniuk and colleagues[26] noted that all 6 greater saphenous vein grafts had developed dilatation (ectasia) without aneurysms after an average follow-up of 14 years. It is not clear whether these dilatory changes will ultimately lead to extremity ischemia or thrombosis. Nevertheless, given the absence of other options, vein grafts still represent the best reconstruction for proximal extremity arterial gaps in children. While surgeons await additional data, patients should continue to be periodically monitored for development of vascular problems.

In addition, pediatric microsurgical patients should be protected postoperatively. Nowhere is this more important than the extremities, which children use directly for environmental interaction. When the initial pain subsides, children are very likely to use the extremity and can potentially jeopardize the reconstruction. A minimum of a cast is required in the early postoperative period. Smaller children require long arm/leg casts. If swelling is a concern, the cast can be bivalved or a temporary splint placed several days before definitive casting.

SPECIFIC CONDITIONS IN REPLANTATION AND REVASCULARIZATION

The most common indication for replantation and revascularization in children is trauma. Trauma can include complete or partial amputations, or injuries that damage end blood vessels in the extremities. A less common indication is the need for revascularization (or replantation) after extirpation of masses such as tumors or vascular anomalies. The least common indication for revascularization in children is vascular disease. Each of these indications is reviewed herein.

Trauma

Traumatic amputations or injuries with a dysvascular part in the pediatric extremity are rare. The most common mechanism of injury in the digits is sharp lacerations with saws or machinery. Young children sustain more amputations from a caught-between-object mechanism, resulting in crush or avulsion injuries.[27,28] These injuries can occur with bicycle chains, doors, adjustable car seats, home exercise equipment,[29] fishing line, sailing rope, cords of window blinds, fireworks, and animal bites. Every imaginable digital amputation mechanism has likely occurred at some point owing to the curiosity of young children and their tendency to use their hands for exploring the environment. Adolescents digital amputations are usually caused by heavy machinery, motor vehicle crashes, or firearm accidents.[28]

More proximal (partial or complete) amputations are usually caused by motor vehicle collisions, train accidents, or power tools.[27] Common reasons for revascularization occur in adolescents who get piercing or cutting injuries from knives or glass. These injuries occur because of sports (hockey); altercations with others; suicide attempts; or, more commonly, punching glass in a fit of rage (**Fig. 3**). There is a distinct population of younger children who may require proximal-level revascularization not because of a partial amputation but because of a displaced supracondylar humeral fracture.[30,31] In addition, an even smaller group of young patients may require revascularization because of iatrogenic arterial injury from misplaced access catheters. However, many of these patients tend to be small, very ill infants who cannot tolerate surgical operations with potential blood loss, and are thus mainly treated with anticoagulation.[32,33]

Indications: replantation

The indications for replantation in children are more liberal than in adults[34] because children have better functional and sensory outcomes and fewer complications,[17,35–37] but the psychological and functional impairments for children last a lifetime. Children are also less likely to develop pain syndromes, and gain greater psychosocial benefits over the long term. As a result, replantation should be attempted in almost any part in a child. Sharp amputations in flexor zone I are ideal candidates (**Fig. 4**). For very distal amputations, success is possible with artery-only replantations[38] (with leeching for venous outflow) or palmar venous anastomoses.[13,15] Contraindications are similar to adult scenarios and include severely crushed or mangled parts; multilevel injury; serious illness or injury; proximal amputations with prolonged warm ischemia time; and amputations in mentally impaired patients,[39] particularly those who self-mutilate, such as in Lesch-Nyhan syndrome. In contrast with adults, individual finger amputations in children proximal to the flexor digitorum superficialis insertion, even for the index or small finger, can be replanted with good functional outcomes.

Indications: revascularization

The indications for extremity revascularization after trauma have been less developed than those for replantation. Revascularization is needed in

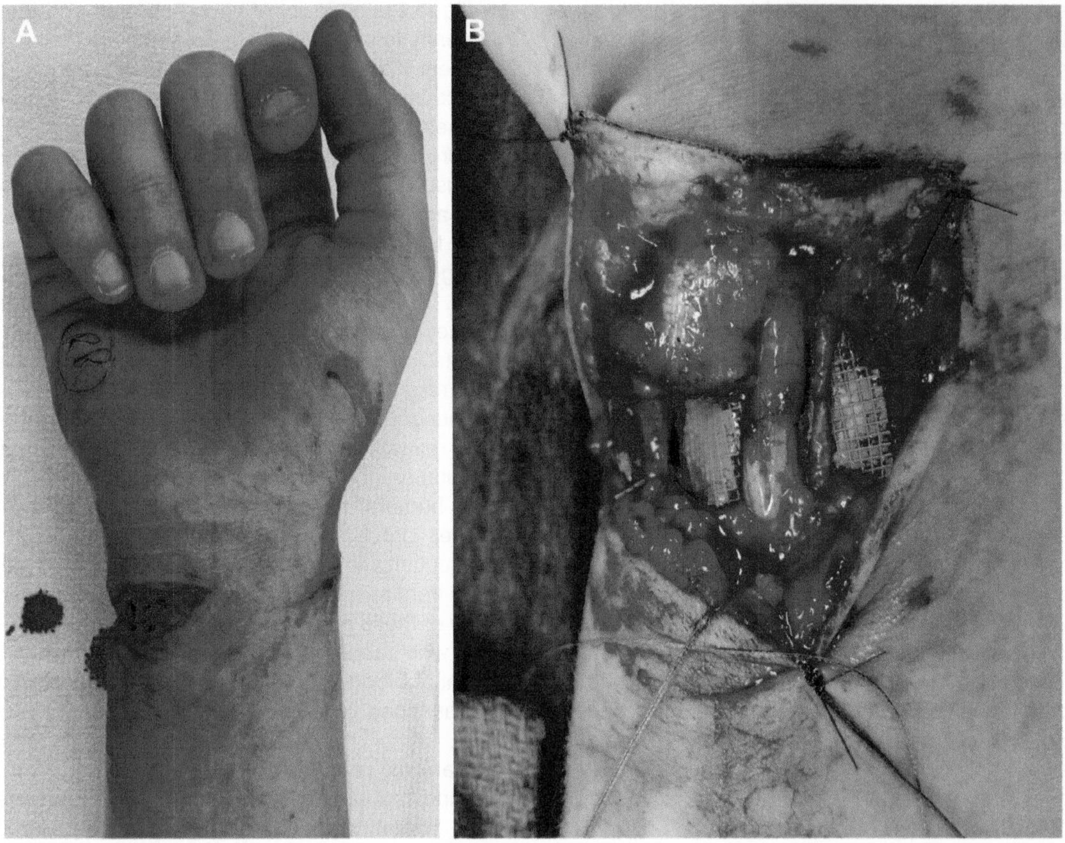

Fig. 3. (*A*) This 15-year-old boy lacerated his dominant ulnar artery and ulnar nerve in the distal forearm after punching a glass window in a fit of rage. (*B*) Clinical view after repair of the injured artery and nerve. Ethilon braided suture loaded in proximal edge of lacerated flexor carpi ulnaris tendon before repair.

cases of partial amputation or arterial injury. Venous reconstruction is rarely needed in these cases because a skin or soft tissue bridge usually provides enough outflow. In cases in which the distal limb is ischemic, the need for revascularization is obvious. However, controversy exists in cases in which an artery has been (possibly) injured but the distal extremity is pink and well perfused. In children, this situation occurs in isolated radial, ulnar, and even brachial artery lacerations, or in displaced supracondylar humeral fractures with vascular injury.

There is no concrete evidence to recommend for or against repair of isolated radial or ulnar artery injuries in the pediatric population. Most of the research on consequences of radial artery harvest (from the cardiac surgery literature) suggest no significant problems with vascularity.[40] Long term, the ulnar artery lumen enlarges to accommodate greater flow after radial artery harvesting. Although some have suggested that this enlargement would predispose to early vascular disease, recent evidence refutes this supposition.[41] The long-term consequences of ulnar artery harvest/ligation are less clear. Furthermore, there are no data about the long-term effects of radial or ulnar artery harvest/ligation in children. It is not clear whether repairing a radial or ulnar artery in a pink, well-perfused extremity of a child may predispose to cold intolerance and growth problems. Accordingly, without any evidence to guide treatment, the more conservative option is to attempt restoration of the patient's premorbid state by repairing the injured vessels, especially if the patient is otherwise healthy. Although propagation of clot has been touted as a potential risk in these cases, it is unlikely to occur if the vessel ends are adequately prepped, flashed (clamps removed to assess flow), and flushed (irrigated with heparinized saline) before microanastomosis. Little is known about the long-term patency of these repairs in young patients.

Controversy exists in the vascular treatment of displaced supracondylar humeral fractures that present with a pink, pulseless hand. These fractures are the most common pediatric elbow injury,

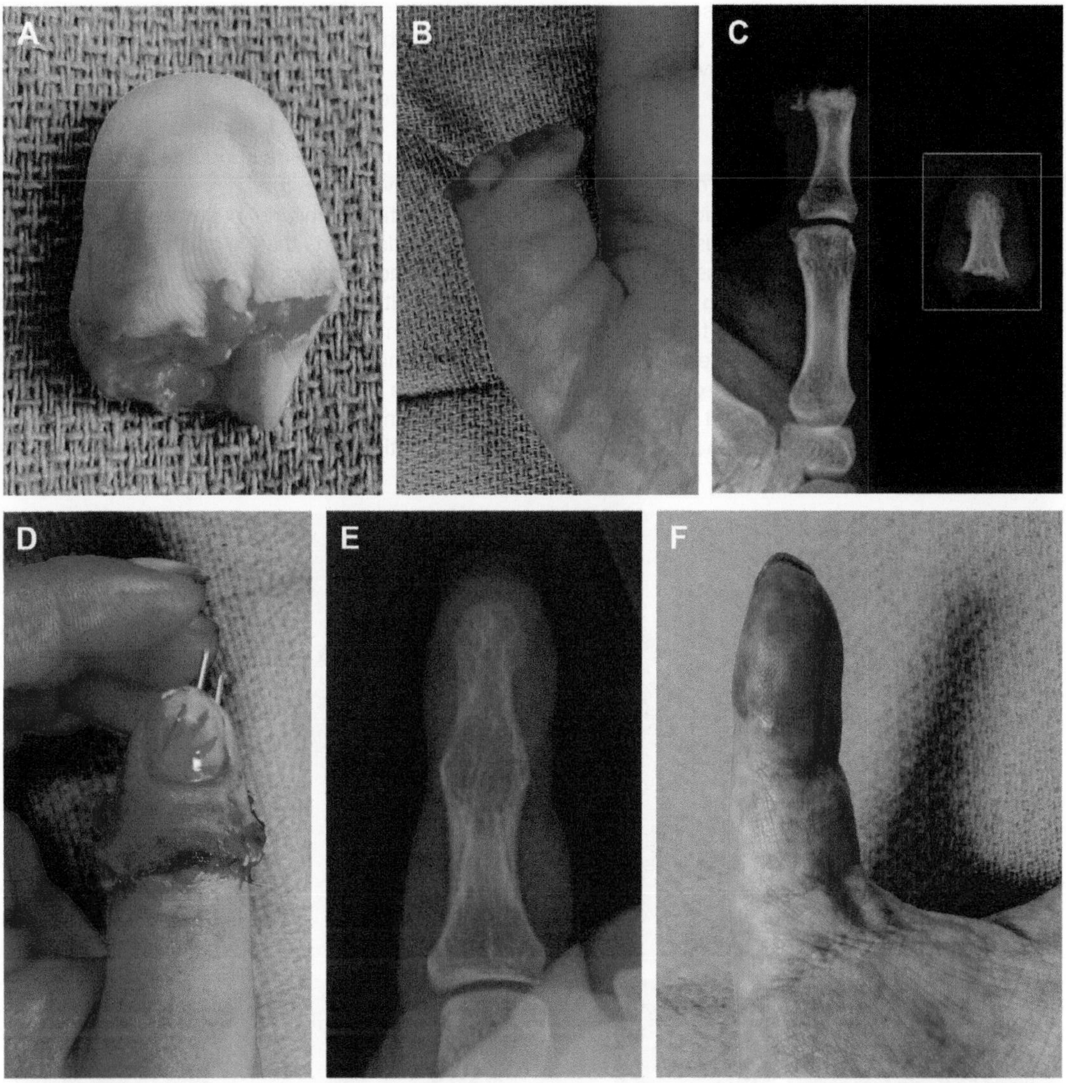

Fig. 4. A 15-year-old girl amputated her nondominant thumb with a saw in woodshop class. (*A*) The volar injury was just proximal to the palmar whorl and (*B*) the dorsal injury was distal to the interphalangeal joint. (*C*) The proximal aspect of the distal phalanx was lost so the joint was fused (the distal phalangeal physis had already closed). (*D*) One artery distal to the trifurcation and 2 dorsal veins were coapted and the skin was closed loosely. Nerve repair was not done given the distal nature of the palmar injury. (*E*) One year after the injury, the fusion was fully healed. (*F*) The thumb tip had 2-point discrimination of 5 mm and was used normally but displayed mild soft tissue atrophy.

with vascular compromise occurring in up to 20% of patients with displaced fractures.[31,42–44] The proximal humeral fracture fragment (spike) usually displaces anteriorly and can stretch, kink, compress, or lacerate the brachial artery. Initial treatment is to reduce and stabilize the fracture and reassess vascularity. Most often reduction of the fracture restores distal pulses. If the distal extremity is poorly perfused, then the artery should be explored, tethering or kinking should be addressed, antispasm agent administered, and vascular repair performed if needed. If the hand is pink but pulseless (a more common scenario), the patient should either be observed closely for 24 to 48 hours or immediate exploration should be undertaken. The merits of both approaches are debated without strong evidence to shift the balance either way.[30,31] If there is no distal Doppler signal, this usually indicates substantial arterial trouble. In these cases, the potential for dire consequences, such as ischemia, cold intolerance, compartment syndrome, intermittent claudication, and poor growth,[45–48] tilts the scales toward exploration and repair, especially in centers where microvascular expertise is readily available.

Techniques of replantation and revascularization

The author advocates assessment of all pediatric replantation/revascularization candidates/parts in the operating room, and ideally using a microscope.[11] Not only does this increase the chances of accurate assessment but it also reinforces to the patient and family that the most thorough evaluation for salvage is being undertaken. The history and early assessment allow the surgeon to delineate the most important aspect of deciding whether a part can be salvaged: the zone of injury. Amputations with a sharp mechanism have a higher chance of success and better function than those with avulsion or crushing mechanisms.[49] Avoid turning a near-complete amputation into a complete amputation; even a small skin bridge may provide adequate venous outflow postoperatively (**Fig. 5**).

Replantation in children has a few different technical considerations than in adults. The sequence of repair should be no different than recommended in adults: structure-by-structure replantation is more time-efficient, but this is not a rigid rule and the thumb should be given priority if many digits are involved.[17] The author prefers to take the amputated parts to the operating room as the patient is being transported from the

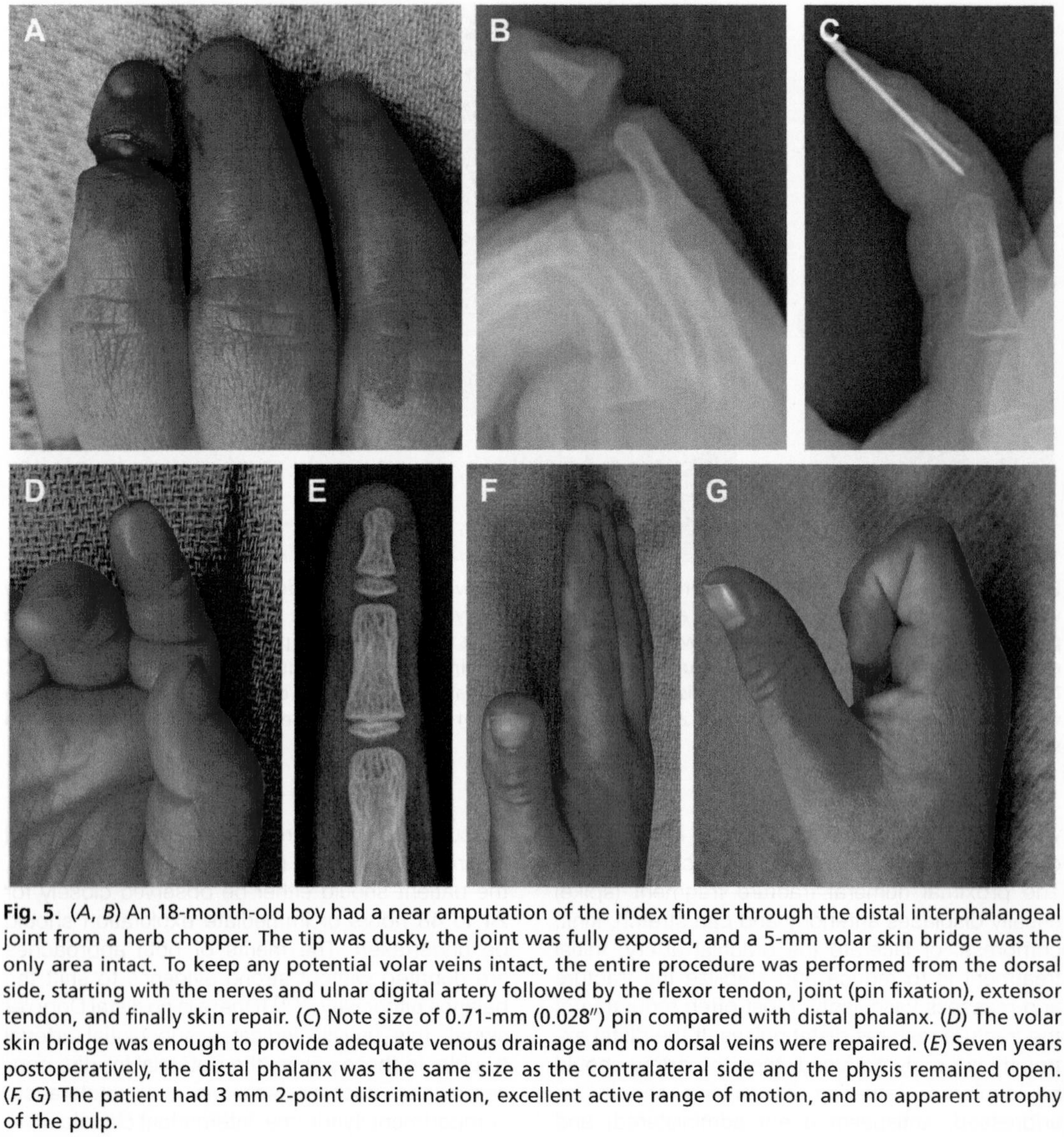

Fig. 5. (*A*, *B*) An 18-month-old boy had a near amputation of the index finger through the distal interphalangeal joint from a herb chopper. The tip was dusky, the joint was fully exposed, and a 5-mm volar skin bridge was the only area intact. To keep any potential volar veins intact, the entire procedure was performed from the dorsal side, starting with the nerves and ulnar digital artery followed by the flexor tendon, joint (pin fixation), extensor tendon, and finally skin repair. (*C*) Note size of 0.71-mm (0.028″) pin compared with distal phalanx. (*D*) The volar skin bridge was enough to provide adequate venous drainage and no dorsal veins were repaired. (*E*) Seven years postoperatively, the distal phalanx was the same size as the contralateral side and the physis remained open. (*F*, *G*) The patient had 3 mm 2-point discrimination, excellent active range of motion, and no apparent atrophy of the pulp.

emergency room. The parts are explored, all relevant structures tagged, pins driven, and tenorrhaphy sutures placed. Midlateral incisions are preferred. Dissection of the arteries and nerves is easier in children because the subcutaneous digital fat has smaller globules and is a different color than the nerves. Once the patient is asleep, under tourniquet control, the proximal part of the amputation is explored and relevant structures are tagged. The amputated parts are then secured with pins and the extensor tenorrhaphy is performed. Venous anastomoses are then performed, the dorsal skin is closed, and the hand is turned over to complete the flexor tenorrhaphies followed by artery and nerve repairs. The author prefers extensor tenorrhaphy with absorbable, figure-of-eight sutures for digital replants. Flexor tenorrhaphy is done using any standard technique, although a multicore repair is not necessary because the replant is usually protected for several weeks before starting motion.

Arteries are more elastic in small children and tolerate a fair bit of stretch; small sections of artery can be removed and successful primary anastomosis is still possible. As many veins as possible should be done, because patency of outflow is one of the most critical factors in survival.[50] Some surgeons suggest doing the veins last, once they become engorged after arterial repair. The author has found that there is usually too much bleeding with this approach, resulting in poor visualization and unnecessary blood loss.

The other consideration in children is regarding future growth. Growth is maintained after replantation[51]; thus, every attempt should be made to preserve the growth plates, especially in young children. The physis is radiolucent, so it is easy to miss it on plain radiographs, especially when the anatomy is disarranged. If fusion of a joint is needed, an epiphyseal arthrodesis provides more predictable healing than a chondrodesis (**Fig. 6**). If shortening of the bone is required, it should be done away from the physis. Patients should be followed long term to assess growth.

Revascularization of a distal extremity requires the same attention to detail, and similar sequencing, as replantation. The most common indications for revascularization in the pediatric extremity is partial amputation of a digit, vascular injury from laceration of a major artery, or a supracondylar humeral fracture. In revascularization of digits, clinicians should bear in mind similar technical considerations as for replantation (outlined earlier). When a major extremity artery is lacerated, the injury can be complete or partial. A complete arterial laceration rarely shows up with bleeding (**Fig. 7**). The elastic arterial ends retract and the muscular media of the artery undergo spasm to completely occlude the ends, especially in healthy pediatric vessels. However, partial lacerations present with profuse bleeding that is difficult to control (**Fig. 8**). In these cases, the intact wall prevents full obliteration of the lumen, and thus retraction of the lacerated edges keeps the defect open. Emergent exploration and repair is necessary.

As mentioned previously, displaced supracondylar humeral fractures in children can stretch, kink, trap, tether, compress, or lacerate the brachial artery (**Fig. 9**). Several important pearls are outlined in **Table 1** for undertaking revascularization after supracondylar humeral fracture.

Nonreplantable amputations

If careful intraoperative assessment reveals that the digits are not replantable or if vascular flow cannot be established, there are 2 options: a primary amputation or reattachment followed by burial in a vascularized pocket. Primary amputation can be done directly if there is adequate skin or if the bone is trimmed back. An amputation should be considered a reconstructive opportunity rather than a failure.[52] In children, especially, the goal is to maximize length and growth. As such, the surgeon should make liberal use of the spare part as skin or composite graft. Composite grafts of the fingertip have not been as reliable as previously thought, even in small children.[53,54] Skin grafting is likely more reliable and provides a higher likelihood of take.[55] Skin grafting directly over bone, even without the presence of periosteum, yields better healing in children than in adults.

Burial in a subcutaneous pocket is also a possible strategy.[56–59] The digit is pinned, tendons and skin lacerations are repaired, and the outside skin of the amputated part is deepithelialized. A subcutaneous pocket is created in the abdomen[58,59] or the chest[56] and the finger is buried within this pocket and sutured into place. Theoretically, vascular ingrowth from the pocket will allow the amputated portion to live temporarily while it develops blood supply from the attached proximal digit. The part must be small for it to have a chance (eg, distal interphalangeal joint level or beyond). The finger can be exteriorized in 2 to 3 weeks. Long-term outcomes using this technique have not been reported in children, but it is likely that growth will be impaired even if vascularity is established. Keeping a young child's finger attached to the trunk for several weeks is challenging; some investigators have

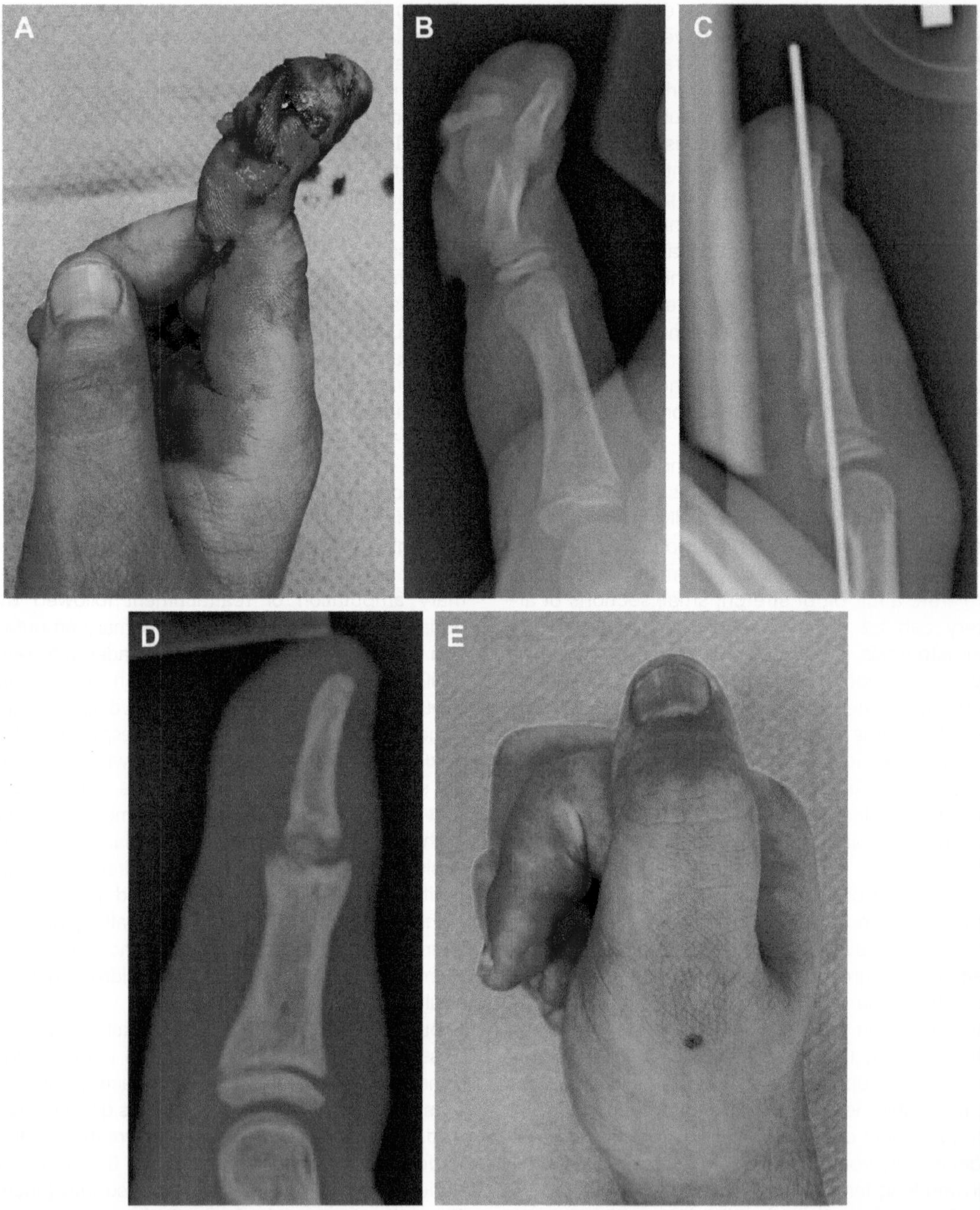

Fig. 6. (*A*) A 12-year-old boy injured his dominant index finger in a bicycle chain. (*B*) Part of the distal phalangeal epiphysis had detached and extruded. (*C*) The articular surface of the distal interphalangeal joint was destroyed so an epiphyseal arthrodesis was performed, fusing the remaining attached epiphysis to the middle phalanx and securing the middle phalangeal fracture. (*D*) A year later, part of the distal phalangeal physis remains open and (*E*) the joint is fused, stable, and pain free.

recommended using palmar pockets.[57] The pocket principle can only be applied to small amputated parts, which typically would not cause significant functional loss regardless, and thus its merits are questionable.

Impending failure

The best opportunity for success is the first opportunity, so surgeons should do a meticulous assessment of the injured structures, debride all tissues in the zone of injury, and perform grafting

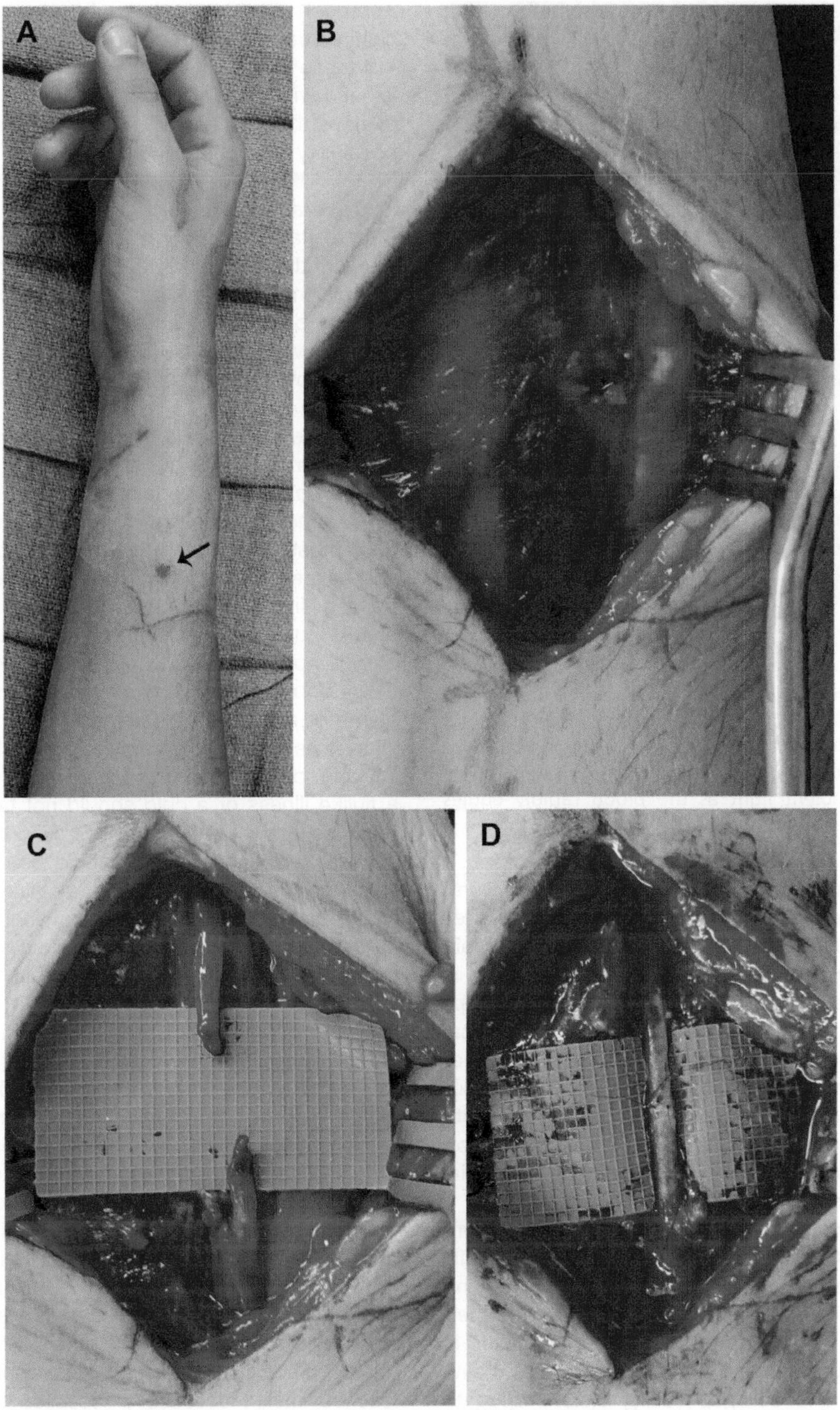

Fig. 7. (*A*) A seemingly innocuous puncture wound is seen in this 14-year-old boy who punched a glass window (*black arrow*). The hand was well perfused and there was no active bleeding. Allen test suggested discontinuity of the radial artery. Exploration revealed (*B*) a small hole in the superficial fascia, and (*C*) complete laceration of the radial artery, which was (*D*) repaired directly.

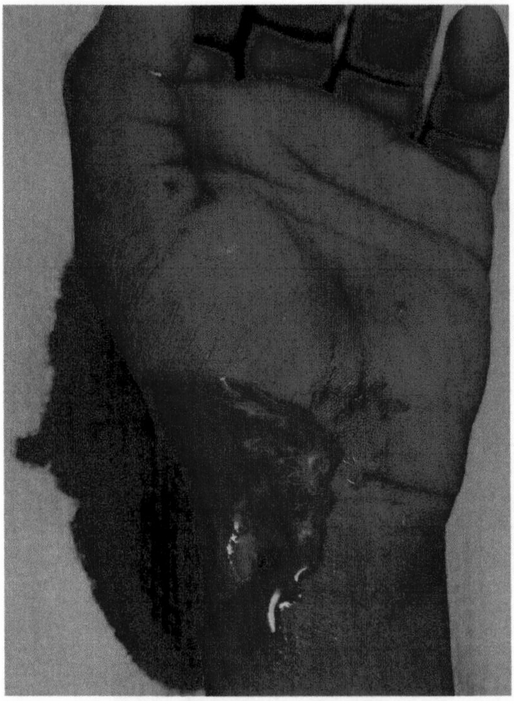

Fig. 8. Partial laceration of the distal radial artery in this 7-year-old boy resulted in hemorrhage that was difficult to control with pressure dressings. The white swirls in the blood represent dissipation plume of reflecting ambient light as the blood rapidly eddies about the exit wound.

liberally. In the case of impending vascular failure, the reason should be determined: venous or arterial. Sometimes the reason is not clear. The main reason for arterial failure in a healthy child is inadequate bypass of the zone of injury. If this happens after meticulous assessment and technical execution, then the zone of injury is much larger than evident. Exploration should be considered, although the rate of salvage in pediatric reports is less than 10%.[60] Systemic anticoagulation should also be considered in the case of arterial compromise.

The reasons for venous congestion are more extensive (kinking, swelling, low flow) and usually manifest at the end of the operation (when the bleeding has stopped) or soon thereafter. Salvaging compromised venous anastomoses is even more challenging than for arterial ones. Veins are small and collapse easily, clots propagate more quickly in the low-flow system, and congestion causes bleeding that impairs visualization. As such, venous congestion is often best treated with leeching and/or local application of anticoagulants to open wounds. A well-opposed skin closure is necessary to promote growth of venous channels while the leeches are applied over several days. Approach leeching with caution because small children can lose a lot of blood quickly.[61]

If these treatments fail, then the part is likely to fail and will need to be amputated. It is important to have the patient and family prepared for this possibility beforehand.

Postoperative care

After digital replants or revascularizations, children are admitted to a high-acuity care ward for close vascular monitoring. Color, turgor, capillary refill, and temperature[62] can be monitored. A warm room prevents cold-induced vasoconstriction but should not be prioritized over the comfort of the child.

The role of routine anticoagulation in replantation continues to be debated,[63,64] and its role in children is even less certain. At present, there is little evidence to guide postoperative anticoagulation; most of the literature consists of surveys and expert opinion.[64] Thus, experience and training in reconstructive free tissue transfer should guide the decision making in this realm. The author has had success with using only so-called baby aspirin (81 mg or weight-based equivalent) for a month in cases in which the zone of injury was clear and was successfully bypassed. Children or adolescents who are recovering from a flulike illness or a cold should not take aspirin because it may precipitate Reye syndrome.

Heparin anticoagulation should be considered in injuries in which the zone of injury is wider (eg, crushing mechanism). Intravenous heparin is the best initial choice because it can be titrated. However, partial thromboplastin time is notoriously unreliable as a measure of therapeutic anticoagulation in children, so anti-Xa levels should be followed instead.[65,66] Early transition to low-molecular-weight heparin provides more stable levels of anticoagulation while minimizing blood draws. Dextran is difficult to dose in children and can cause allergic reactions and pulmonary edema, so its use is mostly abandoned.

One of the most important aspects of caring for children with injuries of the extremities is immobilization, especially in younger children. After replantation, patients are placed in a sugar-tong splint and monitored in the hospital for several days. Immobilization also makes application of leeches easier, because a recessed tunnel can be created in the splint where leeches are placed. When close to discharge, the splint is changed to a cast. In younger children, this change should be done in the operating room under light inhalational anesthesia to avoid disturbing the suture line where some vessel ingrowth and inosculation has likely taken place. The cast is removed after

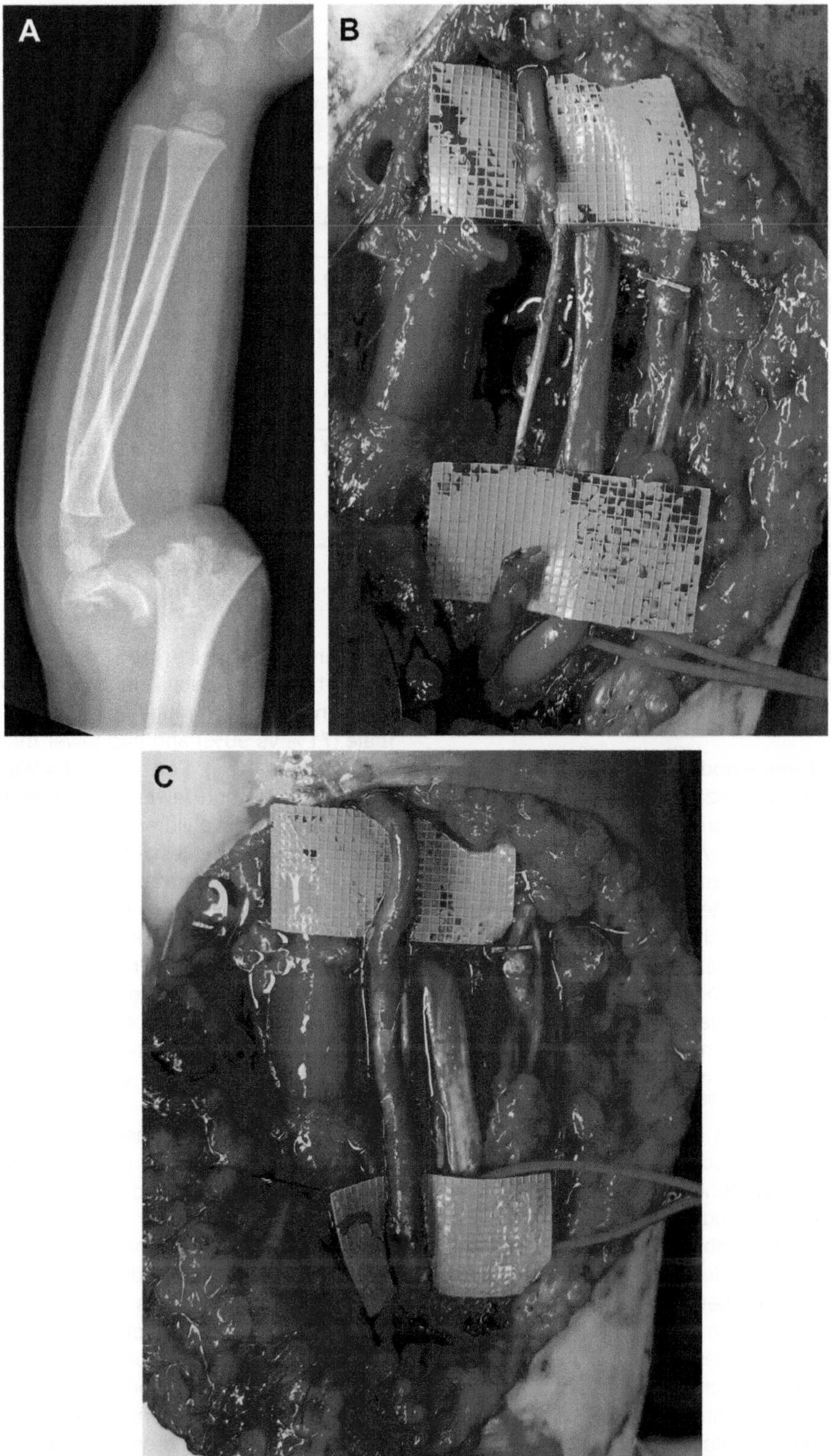

Fig. 9. (*A*) A 5-year-old boy fell and developed a Gartland IIIb supracondylar humeral fracture with loss of distal pulses. After fracture reduction and pinning, arterial pulses did not return. (*B*) Exploration revealed complete laceration of the brachial artery (figure bottom is proximal). (*C*) After debridement of the injured ends, an 8-cm reverse saphenous vein graft was used to reconstruct the defect, with subsequent restoration of palpable distal pulses (figure bottom is proximal). Note slight redundancy of vein graft caused by flexion of the elbow. One year after the injury, the pulses remain palpable; ultrasonography of the graft showed good patency and normal contour.

Table 1
Pearls for successful revascularization after brachial artery injury

Pearl	Explanation
Use reverse SVG	Reverse SVG from the distal leg usually provides matching vessel diameter and thickness to the brachial artery, and it is out of the zone of injury
Brachial artery in children has high elasticity	It can retract significantly so needs a large wound and good exposure
Release the antebrachial fascia	This structure can kink the brachial artery and impede flow, especially once swelling occurs
Consider elbow motion	Assess length of needed vein graft based on elbow extension, knowing that flexion creates laxity
Excise any injured segment of vessel and flash each end before committing to repair	Often more of a segment of brachial artery is traumatized than is initially apparent

Abbreviation: SVG, saphenous vein graft.

3 weeks, bony healing is checked, the pins are removed, and therapy is commenced.

Outcomes

Reporting of series dedicated to pediatric replantation and revascularization started in the 1980s with a few articles focusing on survival and technical feasibility.[27,67] As techniques improved and survival became more predictable, clinicians became more interested in functional outcomes. Several reports published in the 1990s showed favorable outcomes,[36,37,51,60,68,69] whereas others continued to focus on survival and feasibility.[70–72] Additional dedicated studies published since then have been sparse,[73,74] and mainly address the results of technically challenging distal replants.[12,13,15,38]

Table 2 provides a list of dedicated pediatric replantation and revascularization articles with reported survival and functional outcomes. Survival rates between 43% and 100% have been reported in digital and major limb replants. In contrast, large revascularization series have reported higher mean survival rates between 80% and 95%. The most consistent theme is that survival after sharp or guillotine-type injuries is much higher than after crush or avulsion injuries. There has been less consistency in reporting of functional measures such as range of motion, strength, sensibility, and self-reported outcomes. The functional measures that have been reported are excellent, especially in sensory recovery.

In a large nationwide analysis of digital replants using the Nationwide Inpatient Sample from 1999 to 2011, Berlin and colleagues[35] identified 455 children who underwent digital replants, and compared outcomes and complications with more than 2500 adults. In contrast with adults, children who had replantation were less often male (71% vs 90%) and had fewer medical problems (6% vs 10%). Fewer thumbs were involved (23% vs 40%) and fewer multiple-digit replantations were seen in children (8% vs 13%). For all replantations, children less often had a complication (13% vs 20%), underwent microvascular revision (16% vs 20%), or required an amputation (19% vs 29%). Similar results were noted when comparing single-finger replantation in children and adults. A cursory review of the functional outcomes reported in adults compared with children shows that pediatric function is better than adults, but there have not been any direct comparative studies.

Outcomes of arterial vascular extremity trauma in pediatric patients are also favorable. Kirkilas and colleagues[75] reviewed 23 children who underwent repair of vascular injury after extremity trauma and found a survival rate of 87% after repair.[75] The study included various indications, multiple different vessels proximal to the hand and foot, and repair of other injured structures. The most common short-term and long-term complication was functional impairment but this was not fully characterized. Another study of vascular trauma in children showed 100% patency of the vascular reconstruction (median follow-up, 52 months) and transient functional impairment that was mainly related to nerve or muscle injury.[76] Schoenecker and colleagues[77] reported on 7 patients who underwent brachial artery detethering or vascular reconstruction after supracondylar humeral fractures. At a mean follow-up of 30 months,

Table 2
Summary of dedicated pediatric replantation series

Author, Year	Description	Patients	Ages	Replantations	Revasc (n)	Replant Survival (%)	Revasc Survival (%)	Active Motion	Sensation	Grip and Pinch	Bone Growth	Comments
Zhu et al,[13] 2017	Fingertips only	8	2–18 y, avg 6.8 y	9	—	100	—	—	Avg s2PD 6.8 mm; SW normal in 50% and reduced tactile sensation in 50%	—	—	—
Wen et al,[15] 2017	Fingertips only	16	3–12 y, avg 6.6 y	21	—	95	—	DIP mean ROM 89.3°	Avg s2PD 3.8 mm	—	—	—
Linnaus et al,[74] 2016	Digital artery revasc	25	Median 6.8 y	—	25	—	92	—	—	—	—	Graded functional outcome as favorable. Self-reported impaired function was most common long-term complaint in 9% of patients
Lindfors & Marttila,[73] 2012	Digits	26	<16 y	14	15	43	87	Avg TAM 70% of normal for fingers, 39% of normal for thumb	Normal SW in most patients	—	—	Only 65% of patients had functional measures checked
Shi et al,[38] 2010	Fingertips only	12	4–10 y, avg 6 y	12	—	91	—	DIP mean ROM 89°	Avg s2PD 4.2 mm: 3.8 mm in neurorrhaphy cases and 4.4 mm in non–nerve repair cases	—	—	No venous anastomoses

(*continued on next page*)

Table 2
(*continued*)

Author, Year	Description	Patients	Ages	Replantations	Revasc (n)	Replant Survival (%)	Revasc Survival (%)	Active Motion	Sensation	Grip and Pinch	Bone Growth	Comments
Dautel & Barbary,[12] 2007	Fingertips only	18	<16 y	—	—	67	—	—	8 patients available, none with any neural repair: avg 2PD 4.6 mm	—	—	Children tolerated replantations without venous anastomoses better
Cheng et al,[36] 1998	Digits	26	14 mo–12 y, avg 4 y	44	Anastomoses	98	—	Avg TAM thumb 130°, fingers 151°	Normal 2PD in 88% of cases	Grip 79% and pinch 88% of normal side	Mean relative length of 93% of normal in digits without joint involvement and 88% in those with joint involvement	—
Yildiz et al,[69] 1998	Digits	25	2–15 y, avg 6.4 y	13	12	85	95	—	Satisfactory in all	—	Mean growth ratio to contralateral digit up to 85%	Results rated by Chen et al's[94] criteria: 44% excellent, 32% good, 8% moderate, 4% poor
Demiri et al,[51] 1995	Digits and major limb	12	18 mo–14 y	13	—	NA	—	—	—	—	Proximal bone: 94.5% of contralateral digit. Replanted part: 92.7% of contralateral digit	—

Tan & Teoh,[72] 1995	Digits	8	8 mo–13 y	6	4	100	100	—	—	—	—	75% with good to excellent functional use
Baker & Kleinert,[71] 1994	Digits	29	<34 mo	32	—	69	—	—	—	—	—	Favorable factors for survival include clean cut, weight >11 kg, vein repaired
Saies et al,[60] 1994	Digits and major limb	120	3 d–16 y	73	89	63	88	Avg TAM 155°	Avg 2PD 8 mm	—	—	72% survival of replant if after laceration and 53% if after crush or avulsion; 100% survival of revasc if laceration and 75% if crush or avulsion. Rate of survival was higher in patients <9. Rate of salvage was 10% for replants
Beris et al,[96] 1994	Major limb	18	2.5–16 y	13	5	77	80	—	—	—	—	Children underwent avg 2.8 additional procedures to improve function
Taras et al,[70] 1991	Digits and major limb	120	7 mo–16 y	162	—	77	—	—	—	—	—	—

(*continued on next page*)

Table 2
(*continued*)

Author, Year	Description	Patients	Ages	Replantations	Revasc (n)	Replant Survival (%)	Revasc Survival (%)	Active Motion	Sensation	Grip and Pinch	Bone Growth	Comments
Daigle & Kleinert,[68] 1991	Major limb	15	2–17 y, avg 9.8 y	15	—	87	—	All with elbow M3+ with good ROM	S2+ in lower extremity and S3 or more in upper extremity; 38% with 2PD <15 mm	Avg grip was 10 kg vs 45 kg (normal hand); 84% with useful key pinch (>1 kg)	—	Avg Carroll test score 59
Ikeda et al,[37] 1990	Digits	14	14 mo–9 y, avg 4 y	17	—	88	—	—	SW normal light touch 71%, diminished light touch 29%; 85% with 2PD 3 mm	—	Mean growth ratio to contralateral digit 86%	Avg Tamai[95] classification was 88%. Two patients with cold intolerance
Jaeger et al,[27] 1981	Digits and major limb	41	<16 y	60	0	85	—	TAM 0–90° in 15%, 90–180° in 61%, and 180–270° in 20%	All with protective sensibility. 15% with 2PD 5 mm	—	Growth assessed in 8 (20%) patients: 5 with equal growth, 2 with no growth, 1 with overgrowth	—
McC O'Brien et al,[67] 1980	Digits and major limb	31	13 mo–14 y, avg 6.8 y	22	15	65[a]	65[a]	—	Avg 2PD 4 mm	—	All show bony growth in digit	Guillotine injury 71% survival vs crush/avulsion injury with 47% survival

Abbreviations: Avg, average; DIP, distal interphalangeal; 2PD, 2-point discrimination; NA, not available; Replant replantation; Revasc, revascularization; ROM, range of movement; s2PD, static 2-point discrimination; SW, Semmes-Weinstein test; TAM, total range of motion.

[a] Total rate of survival for digital replantations and revascularizations, unable to differentiate between the two; all 4 major limb replants survived.

all patients had normal pulses and elbow function. Similar favorable early outcomes were confirmed by others,[78–80] but contradicted by Sabharwal and colleagues,[81] who reported on 6 patients with vascular repair, all of whom developed stenosis or reocclusion of the brachial artery at mean follow-up of 31 months. In a longer-term study with 14-year mean follow-up (7–21 years), Konstantiniuk and colleagues[26] noted patency of 12 out of 12 reconstructions, but 7 of the brachial arteries showed enlargement (6 concentric, 1 aneurysmal), with intramural calcification in 2 patients. In conclusion, vascular patency and functional outcomes are good but patients require long-term follow-up for early detection of vascular problems.

Access to care, and health disparities

Despite the evidence showing good results and the accepted indications for pediatric replantation, this procedure is performed in less than 50% of digital amputations in children in the United States. Berlin and colleagues[35] analyzed the Nationwide Inpatient Sample and found that the pediatric replantation rate was consistently between 16% and 27% of amputations over a 12-year period from 1999 to 2011. Assessing the Healthcare Cost and Utilization Project Kids' Inpatient Database, Squitieri and colleagues[82] found a replantation rate of 40% in the years 2000, 2003, and 2006. It is likely that the true rate lies somewhere in between these reported rates.[35] Nevertheless, given the broad indications for pediatric digital replantation, these rates seem to be lower than would be expected based on consensus recommendations. It is not clear how many of the amputations were truly replantable, especially given that most pediatric digital amputations occur at the fingertip. Nevertheless, both studies showed that the rate of pediatric replantation has been consistent over many years. This finding contrasts data in adults in whom a decline in attempted digit replantation has been observed recently.[35,83,84] The discrepancy likely indicates increasingly restrictive clinical indications for replantation in adults rather than lack of facilities or a shortage of competent surgeons.[82]

The Squitieri and colleagues[82] study uncovered 2 additional concerns in pediatric digital replantation. The first was that most (52%) pediatric replantation was being performed at hospitals with an annual volume of only 1 to 2 such cases per year. In addition, 86% of all the hospitals that performed these procedures were not children's hospitals. Given the technical expertise and resources needed for such cases (and follow-up procedures), it is difficult to imagine that the results obtained from low-volume centers will match those of higher-volume ones or others well-versed in pediatric microsurgery (eg, dedicated pediatric hospital). These findings argue for increasing regionalization to concentrate experience and resources, and for improving access to specialized centers, as has been proposed for adults. The second concerning finding was the disparity in race and insurance status. Black, Hispanic, and uninsured children were significantly less likely to undergo digital replantation than white children and patients with private insurance. Given the significant functional benefit that digital replantation can provide children, additional work is needed in this area to further understand and resolve these disparities in care.

Psychosocial considerations

Very little has been written about the psychosocial impact of traumatic amputations in children. Most of the literature on coping and adjustment to amputation comes from the oncological literature. Limited studies have shown remarkable resilience in the pediatric population after amputation for tumors.[85,86] The major difference in these two populations may be the additional time for preparation and coping before the amputation in the cancer population. Studies are needed to assess coping in children after traumatic amputations.

It has been the author's observation that young children's sense of loss after an amputation pales in comparison with what the parents experience. This aspect of care is uniformly neglected. Understanding the parental viewpoint and the psychology of loss is crucial in making sound decisions about the care of a child. Almost universally, parents want everything possible done, no matter how unrealistic, to avoid loss. This desire is part of the psychology of loss that has been so well characterized in behavioral economics.[87] It is not sensible to expect parents to make sound judgments about complex, unfamiliar issues under severe stress. Clinicians should remain level headed and carefully weigh the risks and benefits of salvage attempts.

Masses, Tumors, and Malformations

Masses, tumors, and malformations represent another, less common, group of conditions that necessitate microvascular revascularization in children. The most common scenario is extirpative surgery for a lesion that is intimately associated with an artery, and in which a distal functional limb will be spared. If the artery needs to be sacrificed, then reconstruction with a graft will be required to salvage the distal limb. There is no available literature about this scenario,

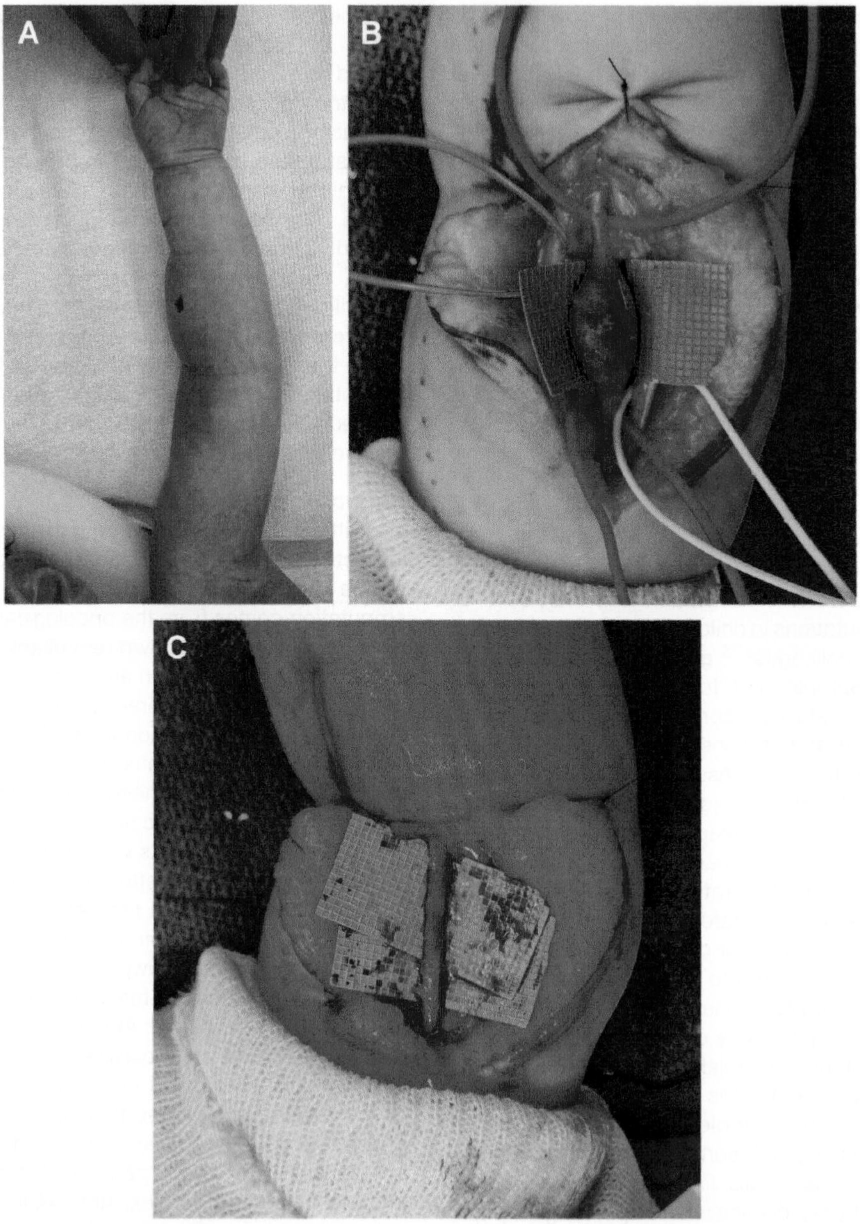

Fig. 10. (*A*) A 9-month-old girl was noted to have a pulsatile lump in the medial arm by her mother. There was no history of trauma or vascular access. Ultrasonography revealed a true aneurysm of the midbrachial artery. A work-up, which included a chest radiograph, abdominal ultrasonography, and a rheumatologic laboratory panel, was negative. (*B*) The aneurysm was resected and (*C*) reconstructed with a reverse vein graft. Pathologic examination revealed no underlying cause for the aneurysm. Two-years postoperatively, the patient maintained strong distal pulses and no evidence of dilatation or aneurysmal change on ultrasonography.

possibly aside from isolated procedures in larger microsurgical series. Nevertheless, microsurgical and revascularization principles and indications still apply. If a team approach is planned (eg, separate tumor and reconstructive teams), careful planning and communication is necessary to ensure efficiency and success. The most important determinant of success is performing revascularization in good-quality vessels that are uninjured from surgery and uninvolved with the lesion. In many cases, simultaneous soft tissue reconstruction and revascularization can be accomplished via a flow-through free tissue transfer.[88]

Vascular Disease

Even though there is a separate field of surgery for treating adults with vascular disease, none exists for children because the prevalence of pediatric vascular disease is very low. The literature focuses on a range of rare conditions including midaortic syndrome, fibromuscular dysplasia, Kawasaki disease, and aneurysms. Of these conditions, only aneurysms affect the extremities.

True aneurysms of the extremities in children are rare and are mostly attributable to congenital malformations or iatrogenic, inflammatory, or infectious processes.[89–93] On the extremities, aneurysms are usually discovered by parents or pediatricians, who may request an ultrasonography scan. Once discovered, a full work-up is necessary to rule out any systemic conditions and/or additional arterial disease elsewhere in the body. Although most patients are asymptomatic, early diagnosis and intervention are important to avoid complications. Arterial aneurysms pose significant morbidity, including thromboembolism with resultant ischemia, neurologic deficit from local nerve compression, and rupture with bleeding. The recommendation is to excise the diseased segment and reconstruct with vein grafts (**Fig. 10**). The entire diseased segment, including some arterial margin, should be taken to avoid recurrence. Arteries in children are very elastic and retract significantly once transected; thus, it is best to measure the length of the vein graft after resection of the lesion, not before. Long-term follow-up is necessary to ensure graft patency and proper limb growth.

SUMMARY

Replantation and revascularization in the pediatric extremity has unique clinical, technical, and psychosocial challenges that provide a fertile field of research and clinical experience. Because most children are free of significant premorbid conditions such as diabetes or atherosclerosis, they heal better and faster. Children regenerate peripheral nerves more rapidly, resulting in better sensory and motor function. The cortical plasticity of children allows them to adapt well to functional deficits and mismatch errors of reinnervation. However, the technical aspect of microsurgical care in children can be challenging because the structures are small. Because vessels are free of disease, the technical aspects of vascular reconstruction depend more heavily on survival of ischemic tissues. Additional technical challenges include preservation of growth centers, prevention of vasospasm, and protection of the reconstruction postoperatively. In addition, the psychosocial care of children (and their families) with extremity amputations can be challenging. Despite these challenges, pediatric replantation and revascularization procedures can be gratifying because children show excellent functional outcomes with minimal complications.

REFERENCES

1. Malt RA, McKhann C. Replantation of severed arms. JAMA 1964;189:716–22.
2. Malt RA, Remensnyder JP, Harris WH. Long-term utility of replanted arms. Ann Surg 1972;176(3): 334–42.
3. Upton J, Guo L. Pediatric free tissue transfer: a 29-year experience with 433 transfers. Plast Reconstr Surg 2008;121(5):1725–37.
4. Slutsky DJ. The management of digital nerve injuries. J Hand Surg 2014;39(6):1208–15.
5. Means KR, Rinker BD, Higgins JP, et al. A multicenter, prospective, randomized, pilot study of outcomes for digital nerve repair in the hand using hollow conduit compared with processed allograft nerve. Hand (N Y) 2016;11(2):144–51.
6. Rinker BD, Ingari JV, Greenberg JA, et al. Outcomes of short-gap sensory nerve injuries reconstructed with processed nerve allografts from a multicenter registry study. J Reconstr Microsurg 2015;31(5): 384–90.
7. Safa B, Buncke G. Autograft substitutes: conduits and processed nerve allografts. Hand Clin 2016; 32(2):127–40.
8. Hudson DA, Bolitho DG, Hodgetts K. Primary epineural repair of the median nerve in children. J Hand Surg Br 1997;22(1):54–6.
9. Bolitho DG, Boustred M, Hudson DA, et al. Primary epineural repair of the ulnar nerve in children. J Hand Surg 1999;24(1):16–20.
10. Lindsay WK, Walker FG, Farmer AW. Traumatic peripheral nerve injuries in children. Results of repair. Plast Reconstr Surg Transplant Bull 1962; 30:462–8.
11. Dautel G. Fingertip replantation in children. Hand Clin 2000;16(4):541–6.
12. Dautel G, Barbary S. Mini replants: fingertip replant distal to the IP or DIP joint. J Plast Reconstr Aesthet Surg 2007;60(7):811–5.
13. Zhu Z-W, Zou X-Y, Huang Y-J, et al. Evaluation of sensory function and recovery after replantation of fingertips at zone I in children. Neural Regen Res 2017;12(11):1911–7.
14. Faivre S, Lim A, Dautel G, et al. Adjacent and spontaneous neurotization after distal digital replantation in children. Plast Reconstr Surg 2003;111(1):159–65 [discussion: 166].

15. Wen G, Xu J, Chai Y-M. Fingertip replantation with palmar venous anastomoses in children. Ann Plast Surg 2017;78(6):692–6.
16. Hanna SA, Catapano J, Borschel GH. Painful pediatric traumatic neuroma: surgical management and clinical outcomes. Childs Nerv Syst 2016;32(7):1191–4.
17. Kim JYS, Brown RJ, Jones NF. Pediatric upper extremity replantation. Clin Plast Surg 2005;32(1):1–10, vii.
18. Duteille F, Lim A, Dautel G. Free flap coverage of upper and lower limb tissue defects in children: a series of 22 patients. Ann Plast Surg 2003;50(4):344–9.
19. Devaraj VS, Kay SP, Batchelor AG, et al. Microvascular surgery in children. Br J Plast Surg 1991;44(4):276–80.
20. Parry SW, Toth BA, Elliott LF. Microvascular free-tissue transfer in children. Plast Reconstr Surg 1988;81(6):838–40.
21. Fry WJ, Ernst CB, Stanley JC, et al. Renovascular hypertension in the pediatric patient. Arch Surg 1973;107(5):692–8.
22. Stanley JC, Ernst CB, Fry WJ. Fate of 100 aortorenal vein grafts: characteristics of late graft expansion, aneurysmal dilatation, and stenosis. Surgery 1973;74(6):931–44.
23. O'Neill JA. Long-term outcome with surgical treatment of renovascular hypertension. J Pediatr Surg 1998;33(1):106–11.
24. Berkowitz HD, O'Neill JA. Renovascular hypertension in children. Surgical repair with special reference to the use of reinforced vein grafts. J Vasc Surg 1989;9(1):46–55.
25. Cardneau JD, Henke PK, Upchurch GR, et al. Efficacy and durability of autogenous saphenous vein conduits for lower extremity arterial reconstructions in preadolescent children. J Vasc Surg 2001;34(1):34–40.
26. Konstantiniuk P, Fritz G, Ott T, et al. Long-term follow-up of vascular reconstructions after supracondylar humerus fracture with vascular lesion in childhood. Eur J Vasc Endovasc Surg 2011;42(5):684–8.
27. Jaeger SH, Tsai TM, Kleinert HE. Upper extremity replantation in children. Orthop Clin North Am 1981;12(4):897–907.
28. Borne A, Porter A, Recicar J, et al. Pediatric traumatic amputations in the United States: a 5-year review. J Pediatr Orthop 2017;37(2):e104–7.
29. Benson LS, Waters PM, Meier SW, et al. Pediatric hand injuries due to home exercycles. J Pediatr Orthop 2000;20(1):34–9.
30. Shah AS, Waters PM, Bae DS. Treatment of the "pink pulseless hand" in pediatric supracondylar humerus fractures. J Hand Surg 2013;38(7):1399–403 [quiz: 1404].
31. Badkoobehi H, Choi PD, Bae DS, et al. Management of the pulseless pediatric supracondylar humeral fracture. J Bone Joint Surg Am 2015;97(11):937–43.
32. Lim S, Javorski MJ, Halandras PM, et al. Epidemiology, treatment, and outcomes of acute limb ischemia in the pediatric population. J Vasc Surg 2018. https://doi.org/10.1016/j.jvs.2017.11.064.
33. Andraska EA, Jackson T, Chen H, et al. Natural history of iatrogenic pediatric femoral artery injury. Ann Vasc Surg 2017;42:205–13.
34. Soucacos PN. Indications and selection for digital amputation and replantation. J Hand Surg Br 2001;26(6):572–81.
35. Berlin NL, Tuggle CT, Thomson JG, et al. Digit replantation in children: a nationwide analysis of outcomes and trends of 455 pediatric patients. Hand (N Y) 2014;9(2):244–52.
36. Cheng GL, Pan DD, Zhang NP, et al. Digital replantation in children: a long-term follow-up study. J Hand Surg 1998;23(4):635–46.
37. Ikeda K, Yamauchi S, Hashimoto F, et al. Digital replantation in children: a long-term follow-up study. Microsurgery 1990;11(4):261–4.
38. Shi D, Qi J, Li D, et al. Fingertip replantation at or beyond the nail base in children. Microsurgery 2010;30(5):380–5.
39. Boulas HJ. Amputations of the fingers and hand: indications for replantation. J Am Acad Orthop Surg 1998;6(2):100–5.
40. Knobloch K, Lichtenberg A, Pichlmaier M, et al. Palmar microcirculation after harvesting of the radial artery in coronary revascularization. Ann Thorac Surg 2005;79(3):1026–30 [discussion: 1030].
41. Royse AG, Chang GS, Nicholas DM, et al. No late ulnar artery atheroma after radial artery harvest for coronary artery bypass surgery. Ann Thorac Surg 2008;85(3):891–4.
42. Shaw BA, Kasser JR, Emans JB, et al. Management of vascular injuries in displaced supracondylar humerus fractures without arteriography. J Orthop Trauma 1990;4(1):25–9.
43. Abzug JM, Herman MJ. Management of supracondylar humerus fractures in children: current concepts. J Am Acad Orthop Surg 2012;20(2):69–77.
44. Choi PD, Melikian R, Skaggs DL. Risk factors for vascular repair and compartment syndrome in the pulseless supracondylar humerus fracture in children. J Pediatr Orthop 2010;30(1):50–6.
45. Bloom JD, Mozersky DJ, Buckley CJ, et al. Defective limb growth as a complication of catheterization of the femoral artery. Surg Gynecol Obstet 1974;138(4):524–6.
46. Bassett FH, Lincoln CR, King TD, et al. Inequality in the size of the lower extremity following cardiac catheterization. South Med J 1968;61(10):1013–7.
47. Richardson JD, Fallat M, Nagaraj HS, et al. Arterial injuries in children. Arch Surg 1981;116(5):685–90.

48. Flanigan DP, Keifer TJ, Schuler JJ, et al. Experience with iatrogenic pediatric vascular injuries. Incidence, etiology, management, and results. Ann Surg 1983;198(4):430–42.
49. Buncke GM, Buntic RF, Romeo O. Pediatric mutilating hand injuries. Hand Clin 2003;19(1):121–31.
50. Hattori Y, Doi K, Ikeda K, et al. Significance of venous anastomosis in fingertip replantation. Plast Reconstr Surg 2003;111(3):1151–8.
51. Demiri E, Bakhach J, Tsakoniatis N, et al. Bone growth after replantation in children. J Reconstr Microsurg 1995;11(2):113–22 [discussion: 122–3].
52. May JW. Sterling Bunnell Traveling Fellowship report-1983. Amputation stump closure–a reconstructive procedure, not a failure. J Hand Surg 1984;9(6):828–9.
53. Eberlin KR, Busa K, Bae DS, et al. Composite grafting for pediatric fingertip injuries. Hand (N Y) 2015; 10(1):28–33.
54. Moiemen NS, Elliot D. Composite graft replacement of digital tips. 2. A study in children. J Hand Surg Br 1997;22(3):346–52.
55. Heistein JB, Cook PA. Factors affecting composite graft survival in digital tip amputations. Ann Plast Surg 2003;50(3):299–303.
56. Brent B. Replantation of amputated distal phalangeal parts of fingers without vascular anastomoses, using subcutaneous pockets. Plast Reconstr Surg 1979;63(1):1–8.
57. Arata J, Ishikawa K, Soeda H. Replantation of fingertip amputation by palmar pocket method in children. Plast Reconstr Surg 2011;127(3):78e–80e.
58. Lee PK, Ahn ST, Lim P. Replantation of fingertip amputation by using the pocket principle in adults. Plast Reconstr Surg 1999;103(5):1428–35.
59. Kim KS, Eo SR, Kim DY, et al. A new strategy of fingertip reattachment: sequential use of microsurgical technique and pocketing of composite graft. Plast Reconstr Surg 2001;107(1):73–9.
60. Saies AD, Urbaniak JR, Nunley JA, et al. Results after replantation and revascularization in the upper extremity in children. J Bone Joint Surg Am 1994; 76(12):1766–76.
61. Kotick JD, Taghinia A. Prolonged bleeding after a single leech application in pediatric hand surgery. J Hand Microsurg 2017;9(2):98–100.
62. Lu SY, Chiu HY, Lin TW, et al. Evaluation of survival in digital replantation with thermometric monitoring. J Hand Surg 1984;9(6):805–9.
63. Buckley T, Hammert WC. Anticoagulation following digital replantation. J Hand Surg 2011;36(8):1374–6.
64. Levin LS, Cooper EO. Clinical use of anticoagulants following replantation surgery. J Hand Surg 2008; 33(8):1437–9.
65. Arachchillage DRJ, Kamani F, Deplano S, et al. Should we abandon the APTT for monitoring unfractionated heparin? Thromb Res 2017;157:157–61.
66. Hanslik A, Kitzmüller E, Tran US, et al. Monitoring unfractionated heparin in children: a parallel-cohort randomized controlled trial comparing 2 dose protocols. Blood 2015;126(18):2091–7.
67. McC O'Brien B, Franklin JD, Morrison WA, et al. Replantation and revascularisation surgery in children. Hand 1980;12(1):12–24.
68. Daigle JP, Kleinert JM. Major limb replantation in children. Microsurgery 1991;12(3):221–31.
69. Yildiz M, Sener M, Baki C. Replantation in children. Microsurgery 1998;18(7):410–3.
70. Taras JS, Nunley JA, Urbaniak JR, et al. Replantation in children. Microsurgery 1991;12(3):216–20.
71. Baker GL, Kleinert JM. Digit replantation in infants and young children: determinants of survival. Plast Reconstr Surg 1994;94(1):139–45.
72. Tan AB, Teoh LC. Upper limb digital replantation and revascularisation in children. Ann Acad Med Singapore 1995;24(4 Suppl):32–6.
73. Lindfors N, Marttila I. Replantation or revascularisation injuries in children: incidence, epidemiology, and outcome. J Plast Surg Hand Surg 2012;46(5): 359–63.
74. Linnaus ME, Langlais CS, Kirkilas M, et al. Outcomes of digital artery revascularization in pediatric trauma. J Pediatr Surg 2016;51(9):1543–7.
75. Kirkilas M, Notrica DM, Langlais CS, et al. Outcomes of arterial vascular extremity trauma in pediatric patients. J Pediatr Surg 2016;51(11):1885–90.
76. Morão S, Ferreira RS, Camacho N, et al. Vascular trauma in children-review from a major paediatric center. Ann Vasc Surg 2018;49:229–33.
77. Schoenecker PL, Delgado E, Rotman M, et al. Pulseless arm in association with totally displaced supracondylar fracture. J Orthop Trauma 1996;10(6):410–5.
78. Reigstad O, Thorkildsen R, Grimsgaard C, et al. Supracondylar fractures with circulatory failure after reduction, pinning, and entrapment of the brachial artery: excellent results more than 1 year after open exploration and revascularization. J Orthop Trauma 2011;25(1):26–30.
79. Noaman HH. Microsurgical reconstruction of brachial artery injuries in displaced supracondylar fracture humerus in children. Microsurgery 2006; 26(7):498–505.
80. Alves K, Spencer H, Barnewolt CE, et al. Early outcomes of vein grafting for reconstruction of brachial arterial injuries in children. J Hand Surg 2018;43(3): 287.e1–7.
81. Sabharwal S, Tredwell SJ, Beauchamp RD, et al. Management of pulseless pink hand in pediatric supracondylar fractures of humerus. J Pediatr Orthop 1997;17(3):303–10.
82. Squitieri L, Reichert H, Kim HM, et al. Patterns of surgical care and health disparities of treating pediatric finger amputation injuries in the United States. J Am Coll Surg 2011;213(4):475–85.

83. Chen MW, Narayan D. Economics of upper extremity replantation: national and local trends. Plast Reconstr Surg 2009;124(6):2003–11.
84. Payatakes AH, Zagoreos NP, Fedorcik GG, et al. Current practice of microsurgery by members of the American Society for Surgery of the Hand. J Hand Surg 2007;32(4):541–7.
85. Teall T, Barrera M, Barr R, et al. Psychological resilience in adolescent and young adult survivors of lower extremity bone tumors. Pediatr Blood Cancer 2013;60(7):1223–30.
86. Yonemoto T, Kamibeppu K, Ishii T, et al. Psychosocial outcomes in long-term survivors of high-grade osteosarcoma: a Japanese single-center experience. Anticancer Res 2009;29(10): 4287–90.
87. Kahneman D. Thinking, fast and slow. 1st edition. New York: Farrar, Straus and Giroux; 2013.
88. Brandt K, Khouri RK, Upton J. Free flaps as flow-through vascular conduits for simultaneous coverage and revascularization of the hand or digit. Plast Reconstr Surg 1996;98(2):321–7.
89. Fann JI, Wyatt J, Frazier RL, et al. Symptomatic brachial artery aneurysm in a child. J Pediatr Surg 1994;29(12):1521–3.
90. Bahcivan M, Yuksel A. Idiopathic true brachial artery aneurysm in a nine-month infant. Interact Cardiovasc Thorac Surg 2009;8(1):162–3.
91. Sharp WV, Hansel JR. Aneurysm of the brachial artery. Case report of an unusual pathogenesis. Ohio State Med J 1967;63(9):1177–8.
92. Greenberg JI, Salamone L, Chang J, et al. Idiopathic true brachial artery aneurysm in an 18-month-old girl. J Vasc Surg 2012;56(5):1426.
93. Jones TR, Frusha JD, Stromeyer FW. Brachial artery aneurysm in an infant: case report and review of the literature. J Vasc Surg 1988;7(3):439–42.
94. Chen C, Qian Y, Yu Z. Extremity replantation. World J Surg 1978;2(4):513–24.
95. Tamai S. Twenty years' experience of limb replantation–review of 293 upper extremity replants. J Hand Surg Am 1982;7(6):549–56.
96. Beris AE, Soucacos PN, Malizos KN, et al. Major limb replantation in children. Microsurgery 1994; 15(7):474–8.

Recent Topics on Fingertip Replantations Under Digital Block

Isao Koshima, MD[a,*], Shuhei Yoshida, MD[a], Hirofumi Imai, MD[a], Ayano Sasaki, MD[b], Shogo Nagamatsu, MD[b], Kazunori Yokota, MD[b], Haruki Mizuta, MD[c], Mitsunobu Harima, MD[c], Jyunsuke Tashiro, MD[c], Shuji Yamashita, MD[c]

KEYWORDS

- Replantation • Fingertip replantation • Arteriovenous anastomosis • Delayed venous anastomosis
- Supermicrosurgery

KEY POINTS

- Reconstructive microsurgery has now evolved into a new stage of supermicrosurgery, whereby tiny (0.3 mm) vascular anastomoses are possible.
- The authors review successful fingertip replantations, which involve the use of arteriole (terminal branch of digital artery) anastomoses, arteriole graft obtained from the same fingertip defect, and reverse arteriole flow to subdermal venule.
- A new technique of delayed venular drainage for venous congestion with a high success rate is discussed.
- All replantations could be possible under digital block within 2 hours.

INTRODUCTION

There have been many prior studies investigating distal finger replantation.[1–7] However, as techniques continue to advance and the ability to perform more distal anastomoses improves, attention has turned to progressively smaller arterial anastomoses. In the past, fingertip amputation at the arteriole level distal to the digital arterial arch was difficult because of the challenges in reestablishing both the arteriole and subdermal venule systems. With the recent development of supermicrosurgery, these distal tiny branches (arterioles of 0.3 mm) of the digital artery and drainage system with subdermal venules can be anastomosed with or without vein grafts under a digital block.

This article describes successful fingertip replantations using terminal vessel anastomoses as

Disclosure Statement: The authors have no conflicts of interests to disclose.
This work was presented in part at the First World Reconstructive Microsurgery in Taipei on November 3, 2001, the 13th International Congress of the International Confederation for Plastic, Reconstructive and Aesthetic Surgery in Sydney on August 12, 2003, the 47th Annual Meeting of the Japanese Society of Plastic and Reconstructive Surgery in Tokyo on April 7, 2004, the 8th International Course on Perforator Flap in Sao Paulo on September 6, 2004, and the Korean Society of Plastic Reconstructive Surgery in May 2007.
[a] International Center for Lymphedema, Hiroshima University Hospital, 1-2-3, Kasumi, Minami-ku, Hiroshima City 734-8551, Japan; [b] Plastic and Reconstructive Surgery, Hiroshima University Hospital, 1-2-3, Kasumi, Minami-ku, Hiroshima City 734-8551, Japan; [c] Department of Plastic and Reconstructive Surgery, Graduate School of Medicine, The University of Tokyo, 1-3-7, Hongo, Bunkyo-ku, Tokyo 113-0011, Japan
* Corresponding author. International Center for Lymphedema, Hiroshima University Hospital, 1-2-3, Kasumi, Minami-ku, Hiroshima City 734-8551, Japan.
E-mail address: koushimaipla@gmail.com

Hand Clin 35 (2019) 179–184
https://doi.org/10.1016/j.hcl.2018.12.007

an example of supermicrosurgical arteriole replantation. The authors report their successful experience with the fingertip replantations under digital block with the use of reverse arterial inflow of the arteriole, arteriole-venular (AV) anastomosis using arteriole graft, and delayed establishment of subdermal venular drainage.

In the 1980s Yamano[1] in Japan reported fingertip replantations[2–7]; however, there was controversy over whether the fingers survived as free composite graft or were truly revascularized. Initially, success rates were lower presumably because of reestablishment of arterial inflow only without venous anastomosis. The success rate of later series increased with improved techniques of venous drainage. It is postulated that important factors that contribute to a higher survival rate are supermicrosurgical techniques, establishment of both arterial and venous systems, use of vein graft in cases with crush injuries, and rapid reexploration in cases of vascular obstruction.

DISTAL DIGITAL REPLANTATION

Materials and Methods

Since 1986, 50 patients underwent replantation of 65 fingers. There were 50 complete amputations and 15 incomplete amputations. The patients ranged from 1 to 72 years of age (average 36.4 years; 56 males and 9 females). Of the digits replanted, 31 were performed on the right hand and 34 on the left hand.

The injury mechanisms included sharp cuts in 9%, burn in 34%, crush in 44%, and avulsion in 11%. Replantation was carried out under digital block. Sixty percent of fingers underwent vein graft and 34% AV anastomoses.

Results

Overall survival was 68% in zone I and 75% in zone II for complete amputations. In the digits with arterial-only anastomosis, 78% of arterio-arteriole anastomosis and 72% of AV anastomosis survived. When considering the venous drainage, 78% of venular-venular anastomosis, 75% of AV anastomosis, and 58% of no anastomosis survived.

Case report of AV anastomosis

Case 1: AV anastomosis and arteriole graft for venous drainage A 47-year-old man sustained complete amputation of the left middle finger at the level of nail bed. Replantation was performed under digital block. After exploring the defect, the digital arterial arch was found to be preserved and four arterioles derived from the arch were transected. Two arterioles (terminal branch of digital artery, 0.3 mm each) in the proximal finger were anastomosed to the distal arteriole and the palmar subdermal venule in the volar aspect. Another distal subdermal venule (0.3 mm) was anastomosed to the proximal subdermal venule on its ulnar aspect with an arteriole graft, which was one of the proximal four arterioles in the proximal stump. All vascular anastomoses were performed with 11-0 nylon with a 50-μm needle.

Postoperatively, the fingertip survived completely without any venous congestion or arterial insufficiency (**Fig. 1**).

DELAYED VENOUS ANASTOMOSIS

Introduction

Success in distal finger replantation including crushed and avulsed types is still challenging because of problems with the venous drainage system that result in venous congestion.[1–3,8] Options for venous congestion include the use of fish-mouth incisions of the distal fingertip or removal of the nail bed,[8,9] medical leeches,[8,10,11] and the administration of heparinized saline.[8] However, these conservative treatments have limited effectiveness. Here the use of microsurgical techniques to establish distal venous outflow is described.[1,3,4]

Methods

Between April 1999 and April 2003, 16 distal phalanges of completely amputated fingers in 14 patients (11 males and 3 females) were replanted under digital block. Patients ranged in age from 15 to 72 years. All fingers reoperated on were successfully drained by additional single or double venous drainage with a vein graft (100% salvage rate). The 2 other congested fingers could not be reoperated on because of the level was too distal for reestablishment of venous outflow. The vein grafts (0.5 mm in diameter and <2 cm in length) used in primary and secondary operations were obtained from the volar side at the wrist joint under local anesthesia.

Results

Replantation was successful in 13 fingers (81.3% success rate). Among the 13 fingers, 7 showed postoperative venous congestion (43.8% of the total fingers) caused by venous insufficiency. Five of these 7 fingers were reoperated on and venous drainage was established under digital block.

AV anastomosis and delayed venous anastomosis

Reverse flow of arteriole to venule and delayed venous drainage A 28-year-old man sustained traumatic amputation of the left little finger at the

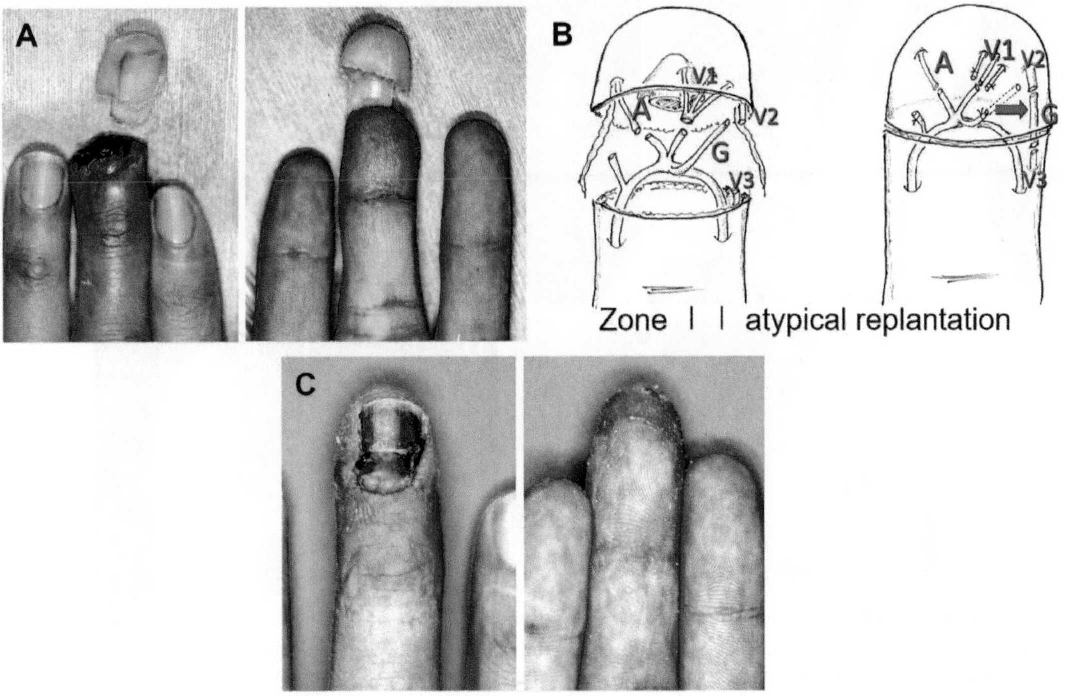

Fig. 1. (*A*) Case 1. A 47-year-old man with the fingertip amputation of the left middle finger. Dorsal view (*left*); volar view (*right*). (*B*) (*Left*) Preoperative schema (volar aspect). All the terminal arterioles and venules were completely transected at the distal of the digital arch. A, distal side of the anastomosed terminal arteriole; V1, distal terminal venule used for arteriovenous anastomosis; G, terminal arteriole used as a graft for venous drainage between both venules (V2, V3). (*Right*) After the completion of vascular anastomoses. The terminal arteriole (G) was grafted for venous drainage (V2, V3). (*C*) Two months after surgery (*left and right*). (*Adapted from* Koshima I. Atypical arteriole anastomoses for fingertip replantations under digital block. J Plast Reconstr Aesthet Surg 2008;61(1):85; with permission.)

level of distal interphalangeal joint caused by strong avulsion. The finger kept its connection with only the flexor tendon and the ulnar digital nerve, and had no blood flow.

Replantation was performed under a digital block. Because the ulnar digital artery was severely damaged as well as the ulnar digital nerve, it could not be used as a feeder for arterial inflow of the replanted finger. The radial digital artery was obstructed by thrombosis over a long span of the artery. Therefore, the tiny branch (arteriole, 0.3 mm in diameter) of the radial digital artery was transected and anastomosed to the distal subcutaneous venule as a source of reverse arterial inflow. However, as the arterial inflow was sluggish, little dermal bleeding of the replanted finger was detected after vascular anastomosis using 11-0 nylon with a 50-μm needle. Unfortunately, no other venule bleeding could be detected in the replanted finger. Therefore, no venous anastomosis could be achieved in the primary surgery. The replanted finger was pale and there was little bleeding with a pinprick test.

On the day after the primary replantation, the replanted finger was noted to be congested and reexploration was carried out under a digital block. A dilated subdermal venule was identified in the congested distal replanted finger. Venous drainage with a vein graft was achieved between the distal and proximal subdermal venules on the dorsal aspect of the finger. The vein graft (0.5 mm in diameter and 10 mm in length) was obtained from the dorsal foot under local anesthesia.

Postoperatively, venous congestion resolved and the finger survived (**Fig. 2**).

Case 2: delayed venous anastomosis A 66-year-old man sustained complete avulsion of the distal phalanx of the left little finger. Under digital block, one arterial anastomosis and one venous anastomosis with a vein graft from the volar side of the wrist were made. However, postoperative venous congestion of the replanted finger occurred. Five days after the primary replantation, additional venous drainage with a vein graft from the same donor site was performed under digital block. Postoperatively, congestion of the finger

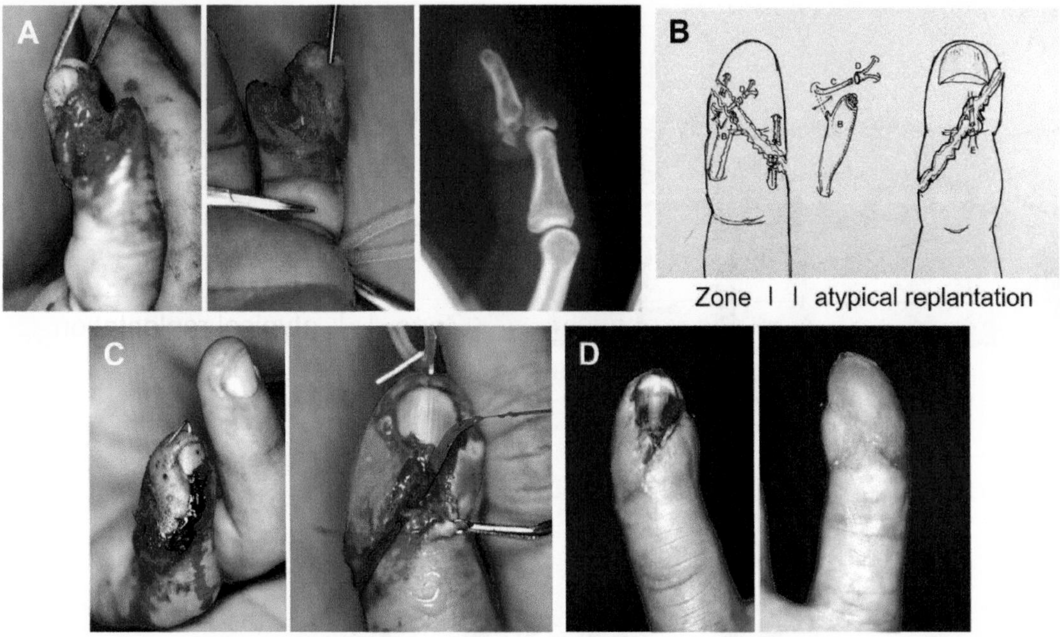

Fig. 2. (*A*) Case 2. A 28-year-old man with fingertip amputation of the left little finger. Doral view (*left*); volar view (*middle*); preoperative radiograph (*right*). (*B*) Schema of primary surgery under local anesthesia. Volar aspect (*left and center*). Reverse flow of transected tiny arteriole (C) of the thrombosed digital artery (B) was used to revascularize the replanted fingertip. D, subdermal venule. Dorsal aspect (*right*). Delayed venous drainage using a venular graft was effective the next day. E, cutaneous venule. (*C*) On the second day, venous congestion (*left*) was repaired with delayed venular drainage (*right*). (*D*) Two months after surgery (*left and right*). (*Adapted from* Koshima I. Atypical arteriole anastomoses for fingertip replantations under digital block. J Plast Reconstr Aesthet Surg 2008;61(1):86; with permission.)

decreased and it completely survived without any additional treatment (**Fig. 3**).

Technical aspects of fingertip replantation and lessons learned are as follows.

1. Never give up.
2. Venous congestion should be seen as another chance to successfully replant a digit.
3. Always prepare a revision operation quickly under digital block.
4. In cases with only arterial anastomosis, secondary (delayed) venous repair is a key method to salvage a fingertip replantation.

DISCUSSION

With the development of supermicrosurgery, it is now possible to perform anastomosis of 0.3-mm caliber vessels, and more distal fingertip replantations at the arteriole level, distal to the digital arterial arch. It was thought that replantation at this level was not feasible for fingertip replantation because many investigators have been concerned about weak arteriole inflow, technically difficult vascular anastomosis, and postoperative thrombosis of the digital arterioles and venules.

Case 1 demonstrates that fingertip replantation can be successfully carried out with arteriole and AV anastomoses as well as arteriole and venular grafts to reconnect subdermal venules of 0.3 mm for establishment of venous drainage. The arteriole graft was obtained from the same fingertip defect under digital block. This is a new ideal candidate for vascular graft because there is no need for additional local anesthesia.

Cases 2 and 3 demonstrate that anastomosis between tiny arteriole and venule (AV anastomosis) can be effective. An arteriovenous anastomosis between a tiny digital artery to the subdermal venules to establish an arterial and venous drainage system is important for fingertip replantations.[4] We previously reported that AV anastomosis is effective for distal phalangeal replantations.[4] We theorize that this is because there are no valves of the venules in the fingertip regions. In addition, reverse arteriole flow can be successful when a digital vessel is thrombosed.

Delayed Venous Anastomosis

Distal phalangeal replantations involving crushed and/or avulsed type injuries often result in venous

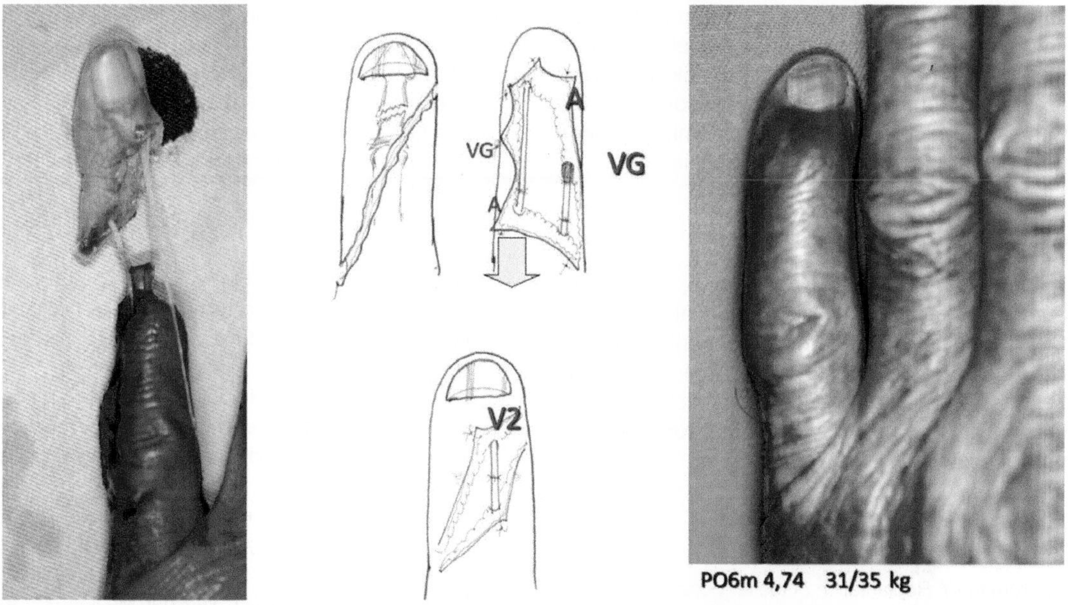

Fig. 3. Case 3. (*Left*) A 66-year-old man with avulsion of the left little finger. (*Middle*) Schema of replantation. Vascular anastomoses with an avulsed radial digital artery (A) and a palmar cutaneous vein with a vein graft (VG) were performed in the palmar side. However, because the vein was obstructed, new venous drainage (V2) was established in the dorsal aspect on the fifth day after the primary surgery. (*Adapted from* Koshima I, Yamashita S, Sugiyama N, et al. Successful delayed venous drainage in 16 consecutive distal phalangeal replantations. Plast Reconstr Surg 2005;115(1):149–54; with permission.)

congestion because establishment of smaller venous drainage is difficult during the primary surgery. Our results showed that nearly half (7 of 16 fingers, 43.8%) of the replanted distal phalanges had postoperative venous congestion. Without any treatment of this congestion, the distal replantation would have been unsuccessful. Other than the options of leeching and continued bleeding from the fingertip, there are few described options for venous outflow.

Regarding alternative forms of venous drainage, the use of the second digital artery as a venous outflow conduit has been described.[4,12–14] Another alternative is to allow bleeding from the amputated part with surgical[5,8,9] or medical leeches.[8,10,11] However, the results with this technique have been considered less than satisfying, and later there may be possible complications such as blood loss (within the 2–6 unit range[8]) and infections (in 7%–20% of cases of leech application for venous outflow problems[8]). Kim and colleagues[5] described a case series in which venous anastomosis was infeasible (49% of total cases), and the use of external bleeding with a topical heparinized saline solution with hyperbaric oxygen therapy led to a 64% survival rate.

Delayed venous drainage using subdermal venular anastomosis with a vein graft seems to be an effective strategy, given that all of the authors' reoperated fingers survived (5 of 5 fingers, 100%). With this delayed drainage, the total success rate was 81.3% (13 of 16 fingers). This high success rate is due to the fact that expanded venules in the congestive fingers became larger and had strong backflow (sometimes they had pulsatile bleeding during the secondary operation). Kamei and colleagues[15] reported the use of a venocutaneous fistula technique at the primary operation without drainage veins in the distal segment. This involved a temporary venous return bypass to prevent venous congestion with the use of a vein graft. Kamei mentioned that the vein graft continued to remain open until the fourth postoperative day. This method may be one solution for venous congestion during the primary operation.

Regarding the size of vein grafts used in this series, they were 0.5 mm in diameter and less than 2 cm in length. Such smaller veins could be obtained from the volar aspect of the wrist under local anesthesia. However, in young women and children, from the cosmetic point of view vein grafts may be obtained from a concealed area, such as the distal portion of the foot dorsum.

In conclusion, clinicians are now at a new stage of supermicrosurgery using vascular anastomoses for 0.3-mm caliber vessels. It is now technically possible for arterioles and venules to be recipient vessels for tissue transfers for finger defects. The authors also believe that fingertip replantations can be easily performed under digital block and that there is no need for axillary block or general anesthesia. In the future, new tissue transfers with supermicrosurgery (or nanomicrosurgery) will be possible under local anesthesia.

ACKNOWLEDGMENTS

The authors thank Dr Kouji Hirano, Orthopedic Surgery, Okayama Kyokuto Hospital, Okayama City, for his introduction of the patient in case 2, Dr Junichi Satoh, Kasaoka Dai Ichi Hospital in Kasaoka City, Okayama, and Dr Michihiro Oda, Onomichi City Hospital, Hiroshima, for their support of this work.

REFERENCES

1. Yamano Y. Replantation of the amputated distal part of the fingers. J Hand Surg 1985;10:211–8.
2. Suzuki K, Matsuda M. Digital replantations distal to the distal interphalangeal joint. J Reconstr Microsurg 1987;3:291–5.
3. Tsai T-M, McCave SJ, Maki Y. A technique for replantation of the finger tip. Microsurgery 1989;10:1–4.
4. Koshima I, Soeda S, Moriguchi T, et al. The use of arteriovenous anastomosis for replantation of the distal phalanx of the fingers. Plast Reconstr Surg 1992;89:710–4.
5. Kim W-K, Lim J-H, Han S-K. Fingertip replantations: clinical evaluation of 135 digits. Plast Reconstr Surg 1996;98:470–6.
6. Hattori Y, Doi K, Ikeda K, et al. Significance of venous anastomosis in fingertip replantation. Plast Reconstr Surg 2003;111:1150–8.
7. Koshima I, Yamashita S, Sugiyama N, et al. Successful delayed venous drainage in 16 consecutive distal phalangeal replantations. Plast Reconstr Surg 2005;115:149–54.
8. Pederson WC. Replantation. Plast Reconstr Surg 2001;107:823–41.
9. Gordon L, Leitner DW, Bunke HJ, et al. Partial nail plate removal after digital replantation as an alternative method of venous drainage. J Hand Surg 1985; 10A:360–70.
10. Nonomura H, Kato N, Ohno Y, et al. Indigenous bacterial flora of medicinal leeches and their susceptibilities to 15 antimicrobial agents. J Med Microbiol 1996;45:490–3.
11. Batchelor AGG, Davison P, Sully L. The salvage of congested skin flaps by the application of leeches. Br J Plast Surg 1984;37:358.
12. Smith AR, Sonneveld GJ, Van der Meulen JC. AV anastomosis as a solution for absent venous drainage in replantation surgery. Plast Reconstr Surg 1983;71:525–30.
13. Fukui A, Maeda M, Inada Y, et al. Arteriovenous shunt in digit replantation. J Hand Surg 1990;15A:160–5.
14. Suzuki Y, Ishikawa K, Isshiki N, et al. Fingertip replantation with an efferent A-V anastomosis for venous drainage: clinical reports. Br J Plast Surg 1993;46:187.
15. Kamei K, Sinokawa Y, Kishibe M. The venocutaneous fistula: a new technique for reducing venous congestion in replanted fingertips. Plast Reconstr Surg 1997;99:1771–4.

Flap Coverage of Dysvascular Digits Including Venous Flow-Through Flaps

Dong Chul Lee, MD*, Jin Soo Kim, MD, PhD,
Si Young Roh, MD, PhD, Kyung Jin Lee, MD,
Yong Woo Kim, MD

KEYWORDS

• Dysvascular digit • Replantation • Venous free flap • Immediate free flap • Thenar free flap
• Perforator flap

KEY POINTS

- It is essential to have careful and accurate planning based on an in-depth knowledge of the anatomy and physiology of the blood supply of the hand.
- The surgical indications of dysvascular digit with soft tissue loss are limited to cases that can expect a recovery of bone, joint, and tendon integrity.
- It is preferable to use the dominant digital artery in replantation, which is our priority, and the nondominant digital artery as the recipient vessel for the free flap.
- The venous free flap, thenar free flap, hypothenar free flap, second toe plantar free flap, and perforator-based flap can be used with replantation.
- The venous free flap is most commonly used and the best choice to reconstruct segmental defects in the digital artery and for simultaneous soft tissue coverage.

INTRODUCTION

The indications for replantation have historically been limited to clean guillotine-type injuries, but have expanded to include extensively injured fingers with soft tissue defects. This reconstruction is now possible owing to advancements in technique and experience.[1–6]

The goal of replantation and revascularization surgery is to restore viability to the digit and achieve the best aesthetic and functional result. Digital amputations are often caused by machine injuries, and such extensive trauma is commonly associated with vascular injuries, severely crushed soft tissue, and comminuted fractures.[6,7] Even though replantation is possible, immediate soft tissue coverage with a flap is sometimes needed.[5,8] It is advisable to cover the soft tissue defect, when present, with a flap, both to ensure survival of the finger and optimize function.[5,6]

Based on this principle, from a tactical point of view, the 2 arterial blood vessels on the digit have to be used wisely. Usually, the injured

Disclosure Statement: The authors have no financial interest in any of the products or devices mentioned in this article. This study did not have any funding sources. The Article Processing Charge was paid for by the authors.
Department of Plastic and Reconstructive Surgery, Gwangmyeong Sungae General Hospital, 36, Digital-road, Gwangmyeong, Gyeonggi-do 14241, South Korea
* Corresponding author.
E-mail address: ophand@gmail.com

Hand Clin 35 (2019) 185–197
https://doi.org/10.1016/j.hcl.2019.01.001

terminal aspect of the digit is given priority and provided with the dominant digital artery and vein, and the other vessel can be used for the flap. The blood supply has to be distributed to both the replanted digit and the flap used for the soft tissue coverage. A venous free flap can be used for digital artery reconstruction and soft tissue coverage simultaneously.[5] There are other free flap options and the best use for each is discussed thoroughly in this article.

INDICATION AND METHODS

A patient with an amputation is considered a desirable candidate for replantation when it is deemed possible to restore the structures (the bones, ligaments, and tendons) and function (range of motion [ROM] and sensation). It is often difficult to decide whether or not the dysvascular finger with soft tissue loss should be replanted, considering the need for free flap coverage. Replantation is relatively contraindicated in amputations caused by crush or avulsion mechanisms when there is substantial soft tissue loss.[9,10] However, owing to the pioneering efforts of many microsurgeons, techniques were developed that can save the finger with a flap and achieve a reasonable result.[1–3,5,7,11]

These injuries are usually severe. The goal of the surgery is meaningful function or aesthetical benefit, but not always achieved. This situation should be discussed with the patient before surgery. Planning of the surgery begins with preparation of the parts and hand, and carefully observing the arterial connections available in the amputated parts and available vessels for flap. In our practice, venous flaps are the main work horse flaps for defect coverage.[3,7,12]

Saving the dysvascular digit is the main goal of this surgery. If the flap fails but the digit survives, other options may be applied to address the soft tissue defect. The shortening of injured parts can be an option and has been used historically to gain relative length of the neurovascular structures, but in our experience, it is not particularly beneficial because it neither helps save time nor provides a structural benefit in terms of the final result.[13] Until now, there have been no definitive comparative studies on shortened replantation versus concomitant flap reconstruction. Covering the defect with a flap is more helpful in restoring the original geometry of the finger and functional outcomes.

In severe crush injuries, although it is a common belief that skin petechiae indicates the internal vascular injury of the amputation stump, our experience has found that it is difficult to predict the actual condition of the vessels based on skin petechiae.[10,14] Even severely injured fingers may have very good vascular conditions capable of nourishing the distal stump. However, severe crushing finger injuries may have more atrophic changes besides purely affecting ROM. The ROM is affected by the integrity of every structural component of the finger.[6]

The injured tissues must be cleaned then the structures must be assembled appropriately. We prefer fixation of bone using K-wires over other complex methods such as those involving plate and screw or wiring, because fracture complexity seems to dictate bone union more than fixation method.[15] Because the condition of the joint is key to the ultimate ROM, we try to minimize interventions that violate the interphalangeal joints.

For the flexor tendon repair, we prefer to repair both flexor digitorum superficialis and flexor digitorum profundus tendons in zone II. We believe that this optimizes secondary tendon surgery, such as tenolysis.[16]

After addressing the bony and tendon injuries, the crushed skin is redraped as closely as possible to its original position, and then the soft tissue defects and neurovascular status are carefully evaluated. In many cases, there may seem to be a skin defect that is larger than is truly present because of the retraction of the skin.

To restore perfusion to the injured digit, at least 1 artery and 1 vein should be repaired or reconstructed, and the same criterion is applied for the free flap, with careful planning of each vessel's direction whether it must go to the flap or to the stump.

Each finger has 2 digital arteries, one of which is dominant: thumb, index, and middle fingers usually have ulnar side dominance; the ring and little fingers have radial side dominance.

The diameter of the dominant side digital artery is approximately 1.4 to 1.8 mm and the nondominant side is 0.76 to 1.35 mm, with about a 30% difference between the dominant side and nondominant side.[17,18] Our interpretation of these data is that there is a larger amount of blood flow on the dominant side.[19] The dorsal veins of the finger are more dominant than the palmar side, but the palmar side vein has a width of 1.5 to 2.0 mm and is an appropriate recipient vessel.[17,20] The diameter of the palmar vein is 1. 5 to 2.0 mm and the dorsal side digital vein is usually bigger with both of these subcutaneous veins forming a pattern like a stepladder arrangement.[21,22]

After the bone and tendon repair, the skin defect, the artery, and the vein arrangement are assessed. The vascular defect size and skin flap dimensions are measured, and then the flap to be used is decided based on the available flap options.

The ideal flap is easy to harvest, malleable, the best match to the recipient skin color and texture, matches the defect size, has a pedicle size similar to the recipient vessel, and results in minimal donor site morbidity. In addition, the flap should be a reasonable size and not too large. In our experience, options for soft tissue reconstruction in these cases include venous free flaps, thenar free flaps, second toe plantar free flaps, and other conventional nominal skin flaps.

Principles of Flap Reconstruction of Dysvascular Digits

A. The dominant digital artery is preferentially chosen for digital revascularization.
B. The original tissue must be used as much as possible, and—if insufficient—a flap is used to cover the defect.
C. Repair the digital artery on both sides whenever possible.
D. A venous free flap is the primary choice for simultaneous vessel and skin replacement.
E. A venous free flap is not as reliable as a conventional free flap because of the risk of partial necrosis.
F. A thenar free flap is useful as a bridging-style free flap for finger revascularization.
G. A perforator-based small free flap is a favorable candidate for coverage, but it is limited by a relatively small pedicle size.

VENOUS FREE FLAP

Nakayama and colleagues[23] reported the viability of the venous free flap via animal experiments with various connections. The venous free flap is thin, pliable, and has low donor site morbidity. In addition, its vascular distributions are easy to identify with the naked eye, fast and easy to harvest, and versatile, and does not require sacrificing any major artery. Constructs include A-A style bridging or V-V stylė bridging.[23,24] Koch and colleagues[25] report clinical success using these techniques.

The arterialized venous flap may be supplied by arterial inflow and venous outflow (A-V-V) or arterial flow through (A-V-A). There are many design options based on the afferent and efferent vessel connections. **Fig. 1** shows variations of venous flaps. The venous pattern is not constant, so the surgeon can modify the connection as needed. It is obvious that more connection of the vessels can save more volume of this flap (see **Fig. 1**).

Small venous flaps will not include many vessels that can be repaired and careful identification of the network is essential to harvest. In the mid forearm, it depends on their suitable thickness; usually in the middle of the forearm we can find a suitable venous flap. At the wrist, there are more venous networks and connections, but the skin redundancy is often not great enough to close primarily. It can connect to a proximal artery, vein, or both, or have multiple vascular connections. It is obvious that multiple connections of vessels can provide more blood volume to this flap.[26]

The venous free flap has characteristics of both a skin flap and graft, which means that the vascular ingrowth from the wound edges is essential for its survival.[24,27–29] If the marginal skin is crushed or injured and not well-nourished, or a hematoma collects under the flap, the flap will be more prone to necrosis.[24,30] Therefore, it is better to save enough length and number of vessels from the flap during harvest to ensure flap survival.

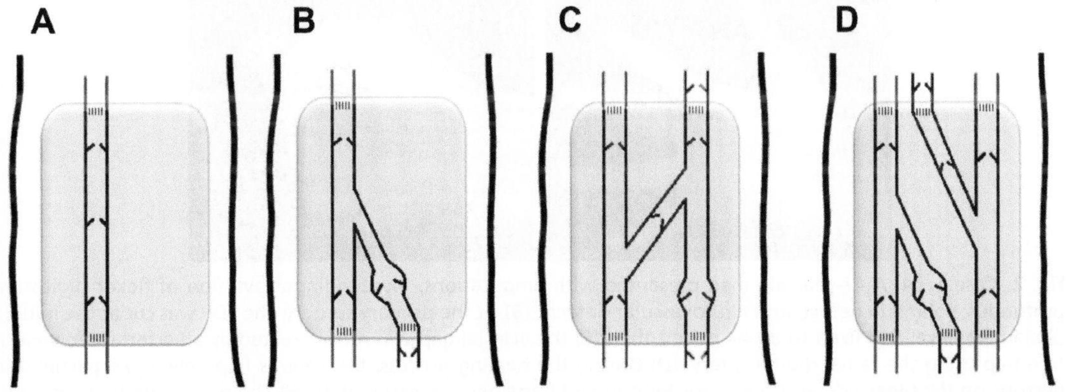

Fig. 1. (*A*) Commonly using pattern as A-A type connection of the venous flap. (*B*) With a straight arterial connection, the proximal vein connects to the proximal vein and it will expand owing to the internal pressure. (*C*) Connection of 2 parallel venous networks; the other side connects to a vein. (*D*) Complex connections of vein, which depend on the defect size and identified venous pattern.

Sometimes, single axial flow through a connection does not provide optimal perfusion to the flap. In these situations, using additional veins can be beneficial. Additional efferent vessels are better than afferent for an arterialized venous flap and veins drain better proximally than distally because an arterialized venous flap has higher pressure loads that might overload the venous outflow.[24]

To ensure a tension-free closure, the flap must be 10% to 20% bigger than the defect. A suprafascial harvest will provide a thinner flap.

The common donor sites for a venous free flap are the forearm and foot dorsum. We prefer the forearm because the venous network is abundant and easily identified. The foot dorsum has larger veins relative to digital vessels, which makes the anastomosis more difficult owing to this size discrepancy. If the size discrepancy is too great, it is better to harvest another flap that is a better match. The axial vessel of the flap that is going to be used to reconstruct the digital artery in replantation must be in the center of the flap.

In bilateral digital artery defects, we prefer to reconstruct the artery with a venous free flap on one side and vein graft on the other. Notably, we can reconstruct with a single venous free flap that has 2 parallel veins in it. However, if one draining vessel of the flap becomes obstructed for some reason, it could jeopardize both digital arteries, so we prefer to use the flap on one side using the venous flap. It is important to orient the vessel properly to make sure that the flow will not be impeded by valves in the vein.

After anastomosis, the venous flap will become congested and thereafter edematous with epidermolysis, and 20% to 40% of cases will have partial

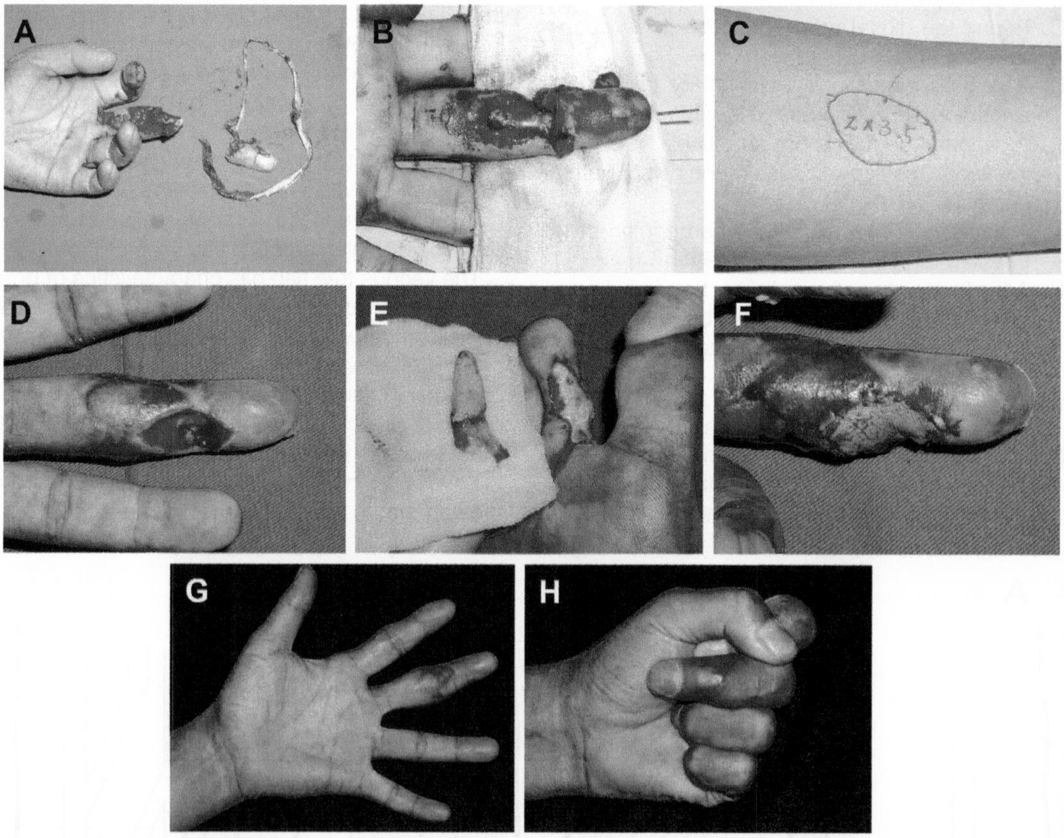

Fig. 2. Case 1. (*A*) A 47-year-old man presented with amputations, myotendinous avulsion of flexor digitorum profundus, volar skin defect, and neurovascular defects. (*B*) At the primary surgery, the FDP was cut at the middle phalangeal level and fixed to an A4 pulley, then (*C*) the arterial gap was reconstructed by an arterialized venous free flap using the radial digital artery. (*D*) During the healing process, the venous flap developed partial skin necrosis on the ulnar side and the flexor tendon and bone became exposed. (*E–H*) The patient underwent a second toe plantar neurovascular flap surgery to cover the ulnar side defect. After insetting the flap, the patient had excellent recovery of sensation at the ulnar finger pulp with 5 mm two-point discrimination at 18 months follow-up, but the contralateral side sustained a longer numbness period of the radial side of the finger pulp and end with 8 mm two-point discrimination.

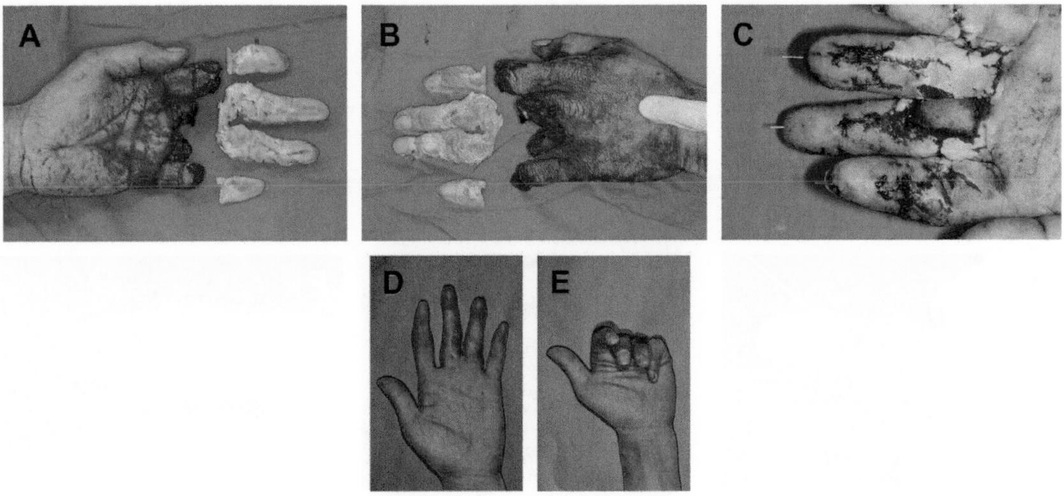

Fig. 3. Case 2. (*A–C*) A 32-year-old man had a severely crushed 4-finger amputation with a skin defect of the middle finger that was covered with a venous free flap using the ulnar digital artery and a vein graft for the radial side digital arterial gap. All the fingers sustained crushing injuries associated with comminuted fractures All fingers survived and the patient had minimal pain. (*D* and *E*) However, sensation was limited (two-point discrimination of 9–12 mm) there was TROM of 110-degrees.

or total skin necrosis even if the axial vessel remains patent. Once the blood flow and venous drainage normalize, the congestion will subside. The palmar side venous flap becomes darker in color, which is one of the disadvantages of this flap when it is used to reconstruct skin at the palmar aspect of the hand (**Figs. 2–5**).

One of the key factors that leads to successful salvage of the dysvascular digit is the experience of nursing staff in postoperative monitoring and their ability to detect any type of vascular insufficiency quickly and accurately.

SECOND TOE PLANTAR FREE FLAP

The second toe plantar free flap is an ideal skin flap for palmar skin defect coverage with neurovascular defects. This flap provides digital artery, nerve,

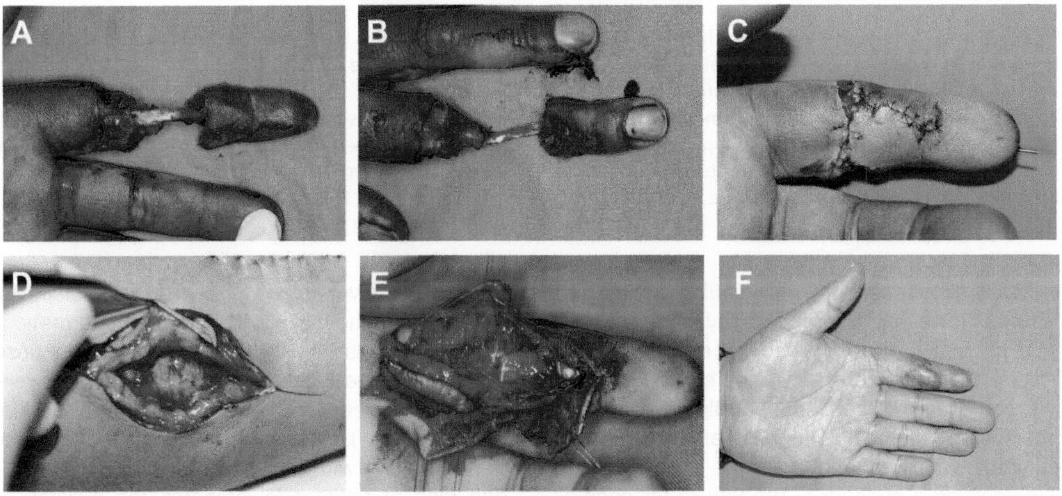

Fig. 4. Case 3. In a 39-year-old man, a venous free flap was used for volar tissue coverage and to address arterial insufficiency. (*A, B*) The patient underwent replantation and direct repair of the digital artery without a vein graft. (*C–E*) On the second day after the operation, the finger became cold and developed an abnormal discoloration, suggestive of arterial insufficiency, so the patient was brought emergently to the operating room and underwent decompression of the volar tissues and blood supply restoration by designing an arterialized venous free flap harvested from the forearm in a flow through fashion. (*F*) This procedure successfully rescued the threatened replantation.

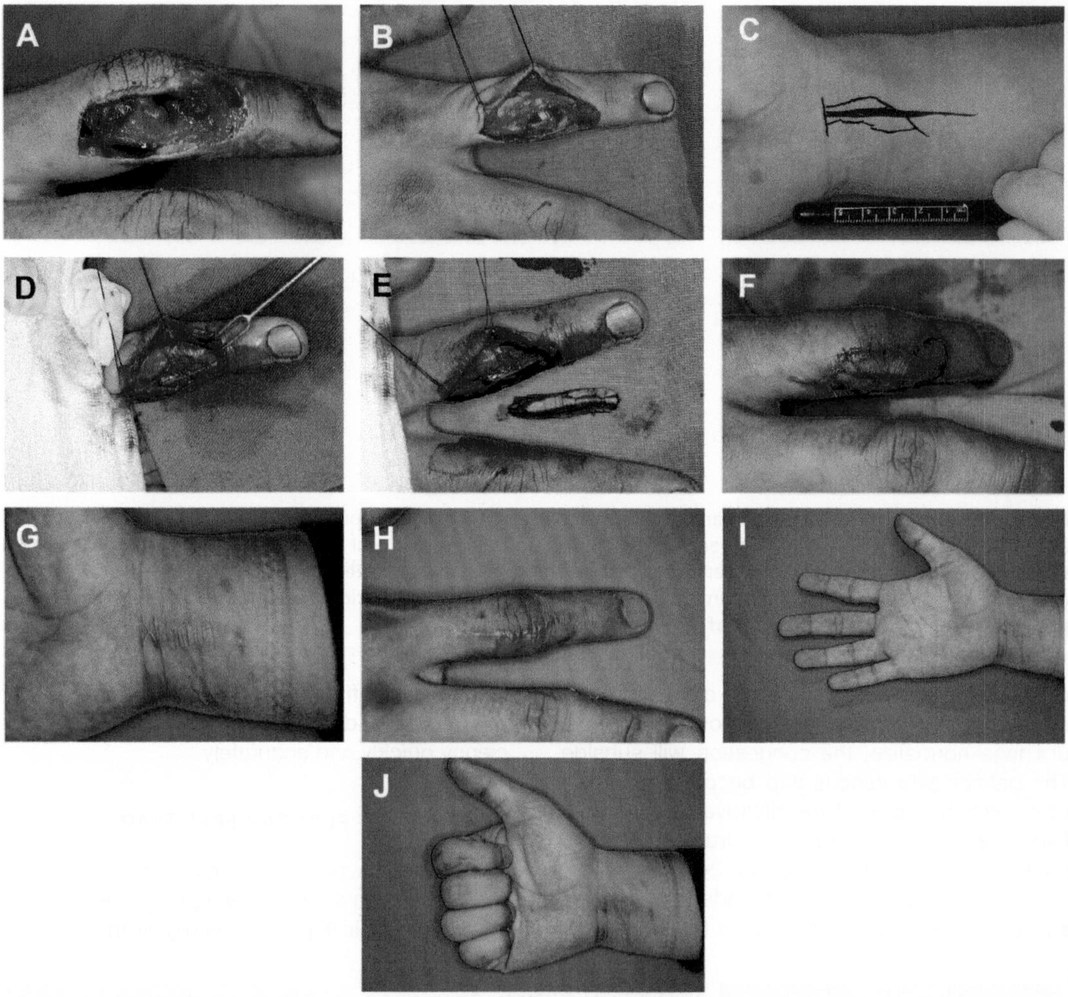

Fig. 5. Cases 4. A 19-year-old man with an injured index finger. (*A–C*) There is a defect of the dorsoulnar aspect of the digit, injury to the ulnar collateral ligament, and the partial loss of the extensor mechanism, which were reconstructed with a venous free flap and palmaris longus (PL) tendon graft. (*C, D*) After reconstructing the collateral ligament and the extensor tendon with the PL tendon, a narrow venous flap was used to cover the dorsal soft tissue defect in a V-V flow through type. (*E, F*) The dorsal venous flow is adequate to supply the venous skin flap. (*G–J*) Survival mechanisms of the venous flap depends on the vascular ingrowth from the wound edges and, for this to be optimum, the wound edge must be healthy as was observed in this case.

and skin simultaneously with similar quality and texture. However, it is limited by size and the need for a skin graft close to the donor site.[31,32] Despite these advantages, it has size limitations. It is considered a conventional skin flap in that proximal arterial and venous anastomosis is required to perfuse and drain the flap. This flap was used as a secondary procedure for case 1. It is important to note that harvesting too large of a large flap from the toe will lead to skin contracture of the plantar aspect of the toe, which will lead to difficulty with walking.[32]

There are several important technical points in harvesting that need to be considered. The deeper structures are very close to the skin, especially the plantar vein. The incision should be made meticulously and pass only through the dermis because the vein is immediately deep to this. When the vessels can be clearly seen with loupe magnification, the harvesting procedure is easier and safer. Also, during cutting with the scalpel the feeling of sudden loss of resistance indicates the incision of the dermis and the plantar vein that needs to be preserved as it becomes visible[32] (see **Fig. 2**).

Once the subcutaneous vein is identified, dissection progresses proximally, and then the dissection approaches the pretendinous layer. The digital artery on the medial side is preferred because it is the dominant vessel.[32] The digital artery is cut to the needed length and ligated. The plantar digital nerve is divided proximal to the metatarsophalangeal joint because there is abundant fatty tissue in this area to avoid the development of symptomatic neuromas. The donor site should be covered with a split thickness or full-thickness skin graft. We prefer a full-thickness skin graft to avoid contracture. Avoid applying the tie over the dressing too tightly, because this will jeopardize the donor area circulation and lead to graft failure.[32]

THENAR FREE FLAP (RADIAL ARTERY PERFORATOR FREE FLAP)

This flap is harvested from the thenar eminence, which is nourished by the radial artery palmar branch. The anatomic location is relatively constant, but the course and size are variable. According to Yang and associates,[33] there are at least 1 or 2 skin perforator branches in the wrist crease and then these branches penetrate the thenar muscle and connect to the superficial palmar arch.[33] Usually, the pedicle diameters of the thenar flap are similar those of the digital artery around the proximal phalanx level.

The radial artery perforator flap can be modified depending on the locations of the perforator to the skin. The volar wrist area is a complex anatomic structure with a palmaris longus tendon, cutaneous nerve, and arterial perforators, and it is the border of glabrous skin and hairy skin with a lot of small venous networks with thin pliable skin. These characteristics are advantageous, making it suitable to reconstruct the dorsum, palmar, side, and circumferential defect without donor site morbidity, while still following the principle of replacing like with like (**Figs. 6** and **7**).

FOURTH COMMON DIGITAL ARTERY PERFORATOR FLAP (HYPOTHENAR PERFORATOR FREE FLAP)

Hypothenar skin has many small skin perforators and it had been identified by the anatomic study and clinical reports. According to Han's description, the skin has quite constant skin perforators, which are located near ulnar eminences and their extensions. The author also had used this flap for a fingertip reconstruction in case of emergency base fingertip pulp reconstruction. Ulnar border skin is soft, and there is an abundant fatty pad on volar side and a thin skin paddle at the dorsal side. It is usually used as pulp skin coverage, so it will not need a longer pedicle. The author had isolated the skin perforator toward the origin and it had come from fourth common digital artery. According to Han's research, there is some anatomic variations of branch pattern and also constantly shows skin perforators. The naming of this flap does not have consensus, but the nutrient arterial originates from fourth common digital artery, hence the name. This flap was described by Kim and colleagues 2010,[34] but their description did not include a detailed course of the skin perforator.[35] In the authors' experience, we have found that the perforator arises from the fourth common digital artery, penetrates the fascia, and then supplies the dorsal ulnar skin (**Fig. 8**).

OTHER FREE FLAPS

Anconeus Free Flap

The anconeus is located at the lateral elbow area and helps to perform elbow extension and supination, but the muscle itself has limited functional importance.[36,37] It has a single dominant artery and a Mathes and Nahai classification type I.[37] The arterial pedicle has recurrent interosseous branches that penetrate the interosseous membrane. It runs deep to the muscle and provides vascular blood supply to the anconeus muscle by uniting with the lateral circumflex pedicle of the elbow.[37]

This flap is not commonly used because of drawbacks of a short pedicle and small vessel. However, there is minimal functional donor morbidity with flap harvest.[37] It may be used to treat defects arising from infection (**Fig. 9**).

Free-Style Muscle Perforator Flap

As mentioned elsewhere in this article, the authors prefer to use a conventional flap rather than a venous flap because, while designing a venous flap, one might accidentally come across a skin perforator coming through the forearm muscle (**Fig. 10**).

Wei and Mardini[38] describe a free-style free flap where the surgeon identifies the perforator and then transfers it to cover the defect. The most important aspect of the free-style flap is technical confidence to repair the vessel. This case was a 0.5-mm pedicle as an artery.

DISCUSSION

In 1912, Claude Guthrie wrote a book about his experiments of vascular repair and their consequences.[17] He declared rules for vessel repair: eversion, adequate tension, and equal intervals between stitches.[17,18] After the first digit replantation in 1965 by Tamai, many challenging trials of

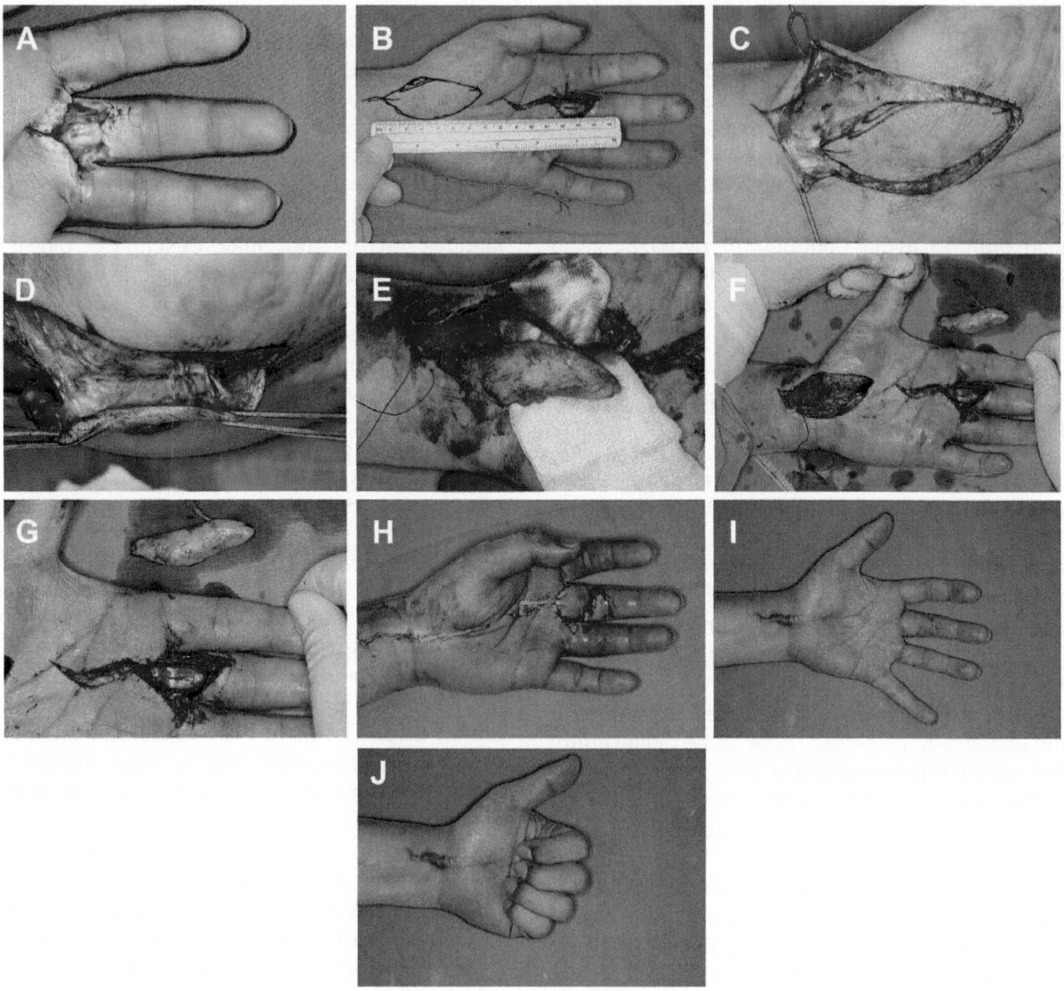

Fig. 6. Case 5. (*A*) In a 33-year-old man, a paint gun injection injury can be seen at the palmar metacarpophalangeal joint with injury to both digital arteries. In this case, there was much paint in the wound with compromise of the soft tissue bed. (*B*) Therefore, rather than using a venous free flap, we decided to cover with a thenar free flap. The flap was designed at thenar eminences and the incision line extended to the wrist. (*C*) After the incision was made along the designed line, the dissection was continued toward the radial artery near the styloid process area and then the superficial palmar branch was identified. (*D*) Flap elevation progressed toward the distal thenar crease then the skin perforator near scaphoid tubercle area was identified. In such cases, the arterial gap should be reconstructed with simultaneous skin coverage. (*E–H*) The digital artery was reconstructed using the pedicle of this flap in a flow through fashion. Venae comitans was repaired using the venae comitans of the second common digital artery. There were 2 venae comitans of the pedicle that we could use as the recipient vein (0.7 and 0.5 mm in width). (*I, J*) This patient demonstrated 220° of total range of motion.

replantation have been reported. Those reports describe technical improvement and limitations after replantation. The indications and contraindications for replantation continue to evolve, particularly with the development of supermicrosurgery techniques. The advancements include the physiology of ischemia, fine needles, sutures, microsurgical instruments, and microscopes that provide brighter and clearer vision. We continue to use the instruments developed by Dr Acland.[17,19,20]

The possibility of the recovery of digital function is the most important concern for finger replantation with free flap coverage. ROM is closely related to bone joint and tendon status along with sensation. The integrity of bone, joint, and tendon is directly related to functional outcome. The process of this surgery involves fixing the frame and repairing the artery and vein of the finger, then covering with a flap. Four successful vascular repairs can save the finger and flap. So, an accurate assessment of the vessel and

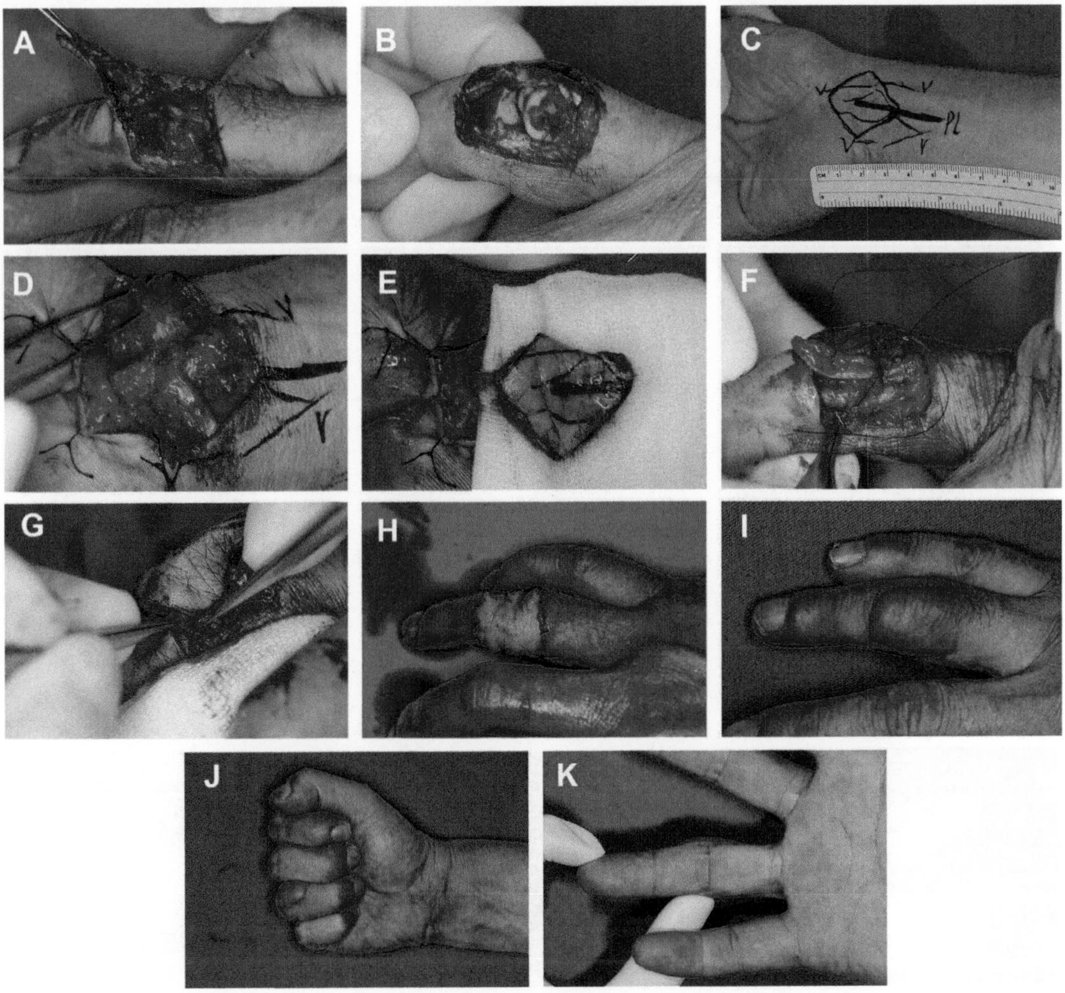

Fig. 7. Case 6. (*A, B*) In a 54-year-old man, an ulnar collateral ligament with partial extensor loss can be seen. (*C*) Initially, the plan was to cover the skin and simultaneously reconstruct the ulnar collateral ligament and extensor tendon by using a venous flap. The flap was designed at the wrist and the radial perforator region was intentionally dissected during the flap elevation, because it is preferable to retain the normal circulation than use a venous flap owing to its reliability. (*D*) At the radial side of the flap, there were direct skin perforators coming out from the radial artery perforator and it was 0.6 mm in diameter. This case reflects how precise anatomic understanding of the vascular structure and vessel repair techniques require intraoperative decisions between a venous flap and a perforator flap. There is a transverse branch from the digital artery near the distal interphalangeal joint that supplies the dorsal skin.[17] (*E–G*) The authors used it as a recipient artery because it was 0.5 mm in diameter. (*F*) The collateral ligament and extensor tendon were repaired by patch graft using a palmaris longus tendon and then the defect was covered with the perforator flap. (*H*) Venous repair was done at the proximal end of the flap. (*I–K*) He presented stable radial side stress of the proximal interphalangeal joint and 85° of range of motion.

following precise repair is the key to successful surgery.

In case 2 presented here, there was a crushed digit and soft tissue loss. In the amputated parts, skin was ruptured longitudinally, which appeared like a red line indicating vascular intimal injury. Based on our experiences, even severely crushed digits, with careful resection of the injured vessel segment, can be used for replantation.

Precise assessment of the injured vessel is necessary. Usually the artery is more vulnerable than the vein during injury, because the fixed point of side branches tear off from the main trunk and becomes a point of obstruction. So, arterial branching points near the amputation wound must be checked and repaired using a vein graft or venous flap if a defect is present.

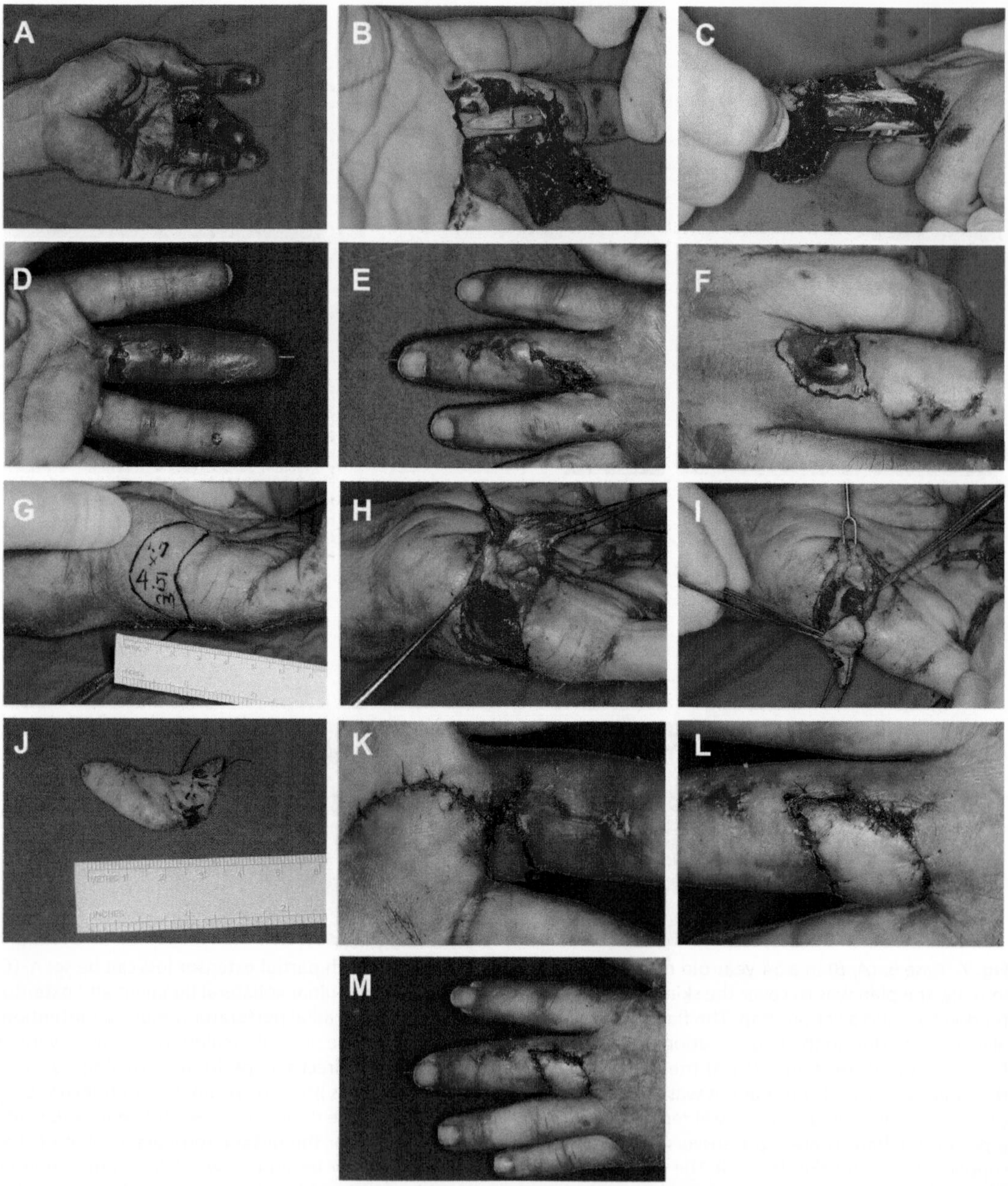

Fig. 8. Case 7. (*A–C*) A 59-year-old man had a severely crushed finger with soft tissue crushing resulting in a soft tissue defect with exposed tendon. (*D–F*) The skin could initially be redraped to cover the defect, but much of the marginal skin was lost. (*G*) The plan was to cover the soft tissue using a hypothenar perforator free flap.[34] (*H*) In this patient, the perforator come from the fourth common digital artery, traveled around the hypothenar mound, and terminated at the dorsal skin. (*I–J*) This patient had a volar and dorsal skin defect covered with this skin flap with the ulnar side digital artery reconstructed with a segmental artery coming from the fourth common digital artery. The donor vessel was repaired after placing a 5-mm segmental artery. This flap has a venous outflow at the dorsal–proximal area. (*K–M*) Therefore, this patient was a good candidate for ulnar side digital artery reconstruction and dorsal venous connection in the proximal direction.

Commonly, we find that the skin defect of a dysvascular finger can benefit from a small skin flap. For the replantation, flaps that are "flow through" and bring perfusion to the terminal segment are preferred; hence the venous free flap is commonly used for replantation. Second toe plantar flap, thenar, and hypothenar free flaps are useful for skin defect coverage and flow through relay of the blood flow. Often, we spend time deciding between the initial provision of greater inflow into the

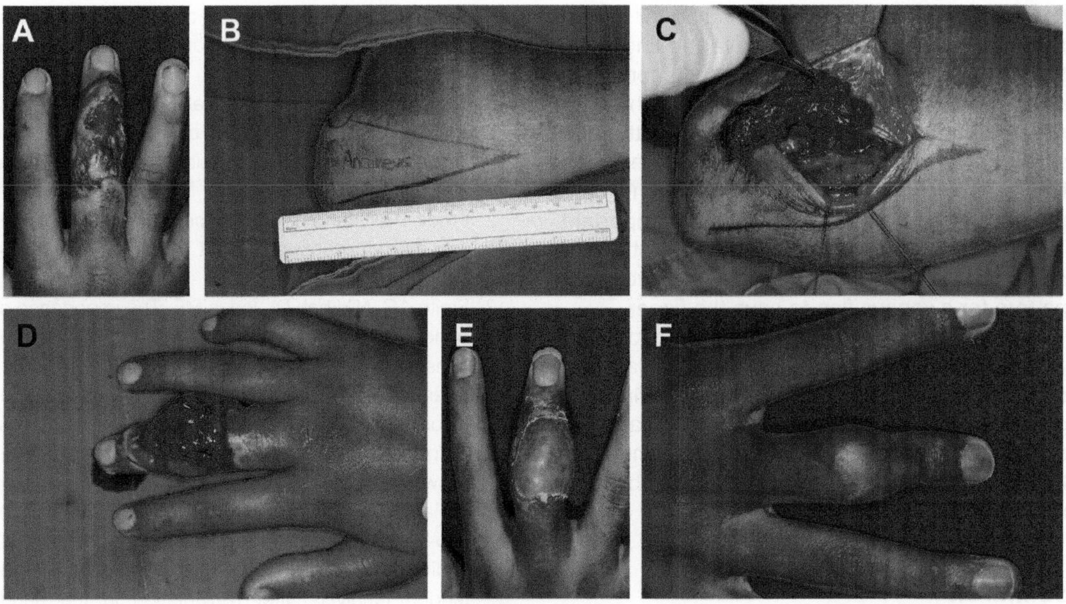

Fig. 9. Case 8. (*A*) A venomous snake bite on the middle finger led to dorsal skin necrosis, an exposed proximal interphalangeal joint, and bone necrosis. The patient was 11-years old and his father objected strongly to amputation. The infected tissues were removed except for the partially ischemic bone. (*B–D*) The wound was covered with an anconeus muscle flap, using the radial side digital artery and volar vein as a pedicle for the flap. The flap had covered the partially necrotic phalangeal bone and extensor tendon. The authors decided to postpone the skin graft over the muscle flap because of the possibility of infection. (*E*) The flap survived and, once the infection was controlled, the muscle flap was covered with split thickness skin graft. (*F*) After the skin graft was survived, the flap had shrunk. His finger survived, but the joint fused.

terminal digit and addressing the soft tissues secondarily. The most time-consuming step of replantation is the vessel repair stage; however, in our experience the hesitation to perform blood vessel repair takes more time than repair procedure itself.

As discussed elsewhere in this article, a venous free flap is an effective option for soft tissue

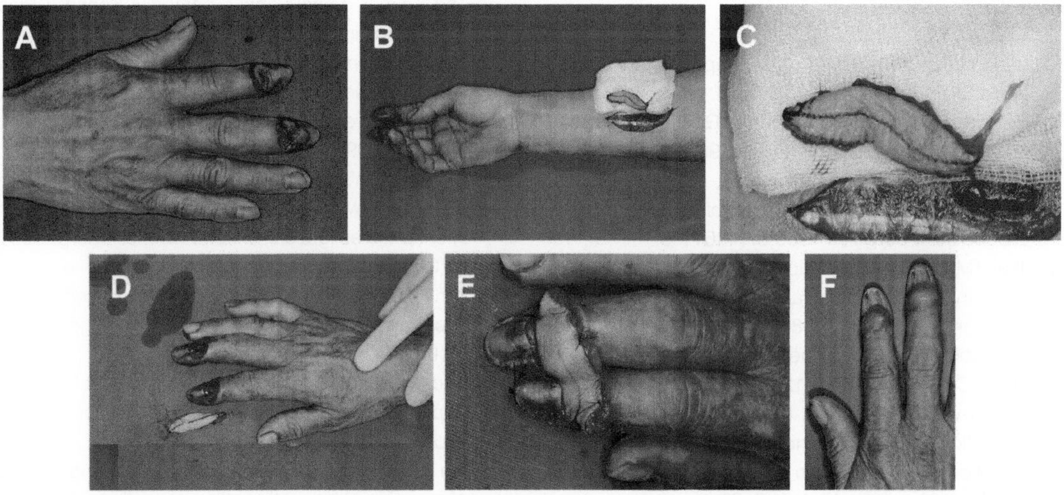

Fig. 10. Case 9. (*A*) In a 55-year-old woman, a plan to cover a dorsal burned wound with a venous flap from the forearm was made. (*B*) The authors serendipitously identified the volar skin perforator and, therefore, decided to use it. (*C, D*) The skin perforator was coming through the flexor digitorum superficialis muscle and the pedicle about 2 cm long was developed. The flap covered the index and middle finger dorsum in a bridged fashion and the arterial pedicle was used with the radial side branch of the index finger for arterial repair and the radial side subcutaneous vein as the draining vein. (*E, F*) The flap was divided 6 weeks after.

coverage with vascular reconstruction for replantation. It has the potential to save the finger and the skin defects can be subsequently concealed using a conventional skin flap among others. To save the venous free flap, a networking pattern inside of flap and more repair need to be made; however, for a successful replantation, rapid pass of the arterial blood flow is more important. Therefore, the axial vein must be directly connected instead of constructing the arborizing pattern for a venous flap to save the finger.

Repairing the vessel network may cloud the purpose of replantation. Therefore, the fact that this is a finger replantation, and not a flap surgery, must be kept in mind. In case of a dorsal side soft tissue defect, the venous connection loss can repair using a venous flap as a bridging material.

SUMMARY

Venous free flaps and other small perforator flaps like the thenar free flap have advanced the microsurgical care of dysvascular injuries to the digits. These procedures are technically complicated but have minimal donor site morbidity, and should be considered for dysvascular digits with soft tissue defects.

REFERENCES

1. Komatsu S, Tamai S. Successful replantation of a completely cut-off thumb. Plast Reconstr Surg 1968;42(4):374–7.
2. Kleinert HE, Jablon M, Tsai TM. An overview of replantation and results of 347 replants in 245 patients. J Trauma 1980;20(5):390–8.
3. Buncke HJ, Alpert BS, Johnson-Giebink R. Digital replantation. Surg Clin North Am 1981;61(2):383–94.
4. Urbaniak JR, Roth JH, Nunley JA, et al. The results of replantation after amputation of a single finger. J Bone Joint Surg Am 1985;67(4):611–9.
5. Tsai TM, Matiko JD, Breidenbach W, et al. Venous flaps in digital revascularization and replantation. J Reconstr Microsurg 1987;3(2):113–9.
6. Morrison WA, McCombe D. Digital replantation. Hand Clin 2007;23(1):1–12.
7. Zhong-Wei C, Meyer VE, Kleinert HE, et al. Present indications and contraindications for replantation as reflected by long-term functional results. Orthop Clin North Am 1981;12(4):849–70.
8. Saint-Cyr M, Wong C, Buchel EW, et al. Free tissue transfers and replantation. Plast Reconstr Surg 2012;130(6):858e–78e.
9. Pederson WC. Replantation. Plast Reconstr Surg 2001;107(3):823–41.
10. Sammer DM. Management of complications with flap procedures and replantation. Hand Clin 2015; 31(2):339–44.
11. Tamai S, Hori Y, Tatsumi Y, et al. Microvascular anastomosis and its application on the replantation of amputated digits and hands. Clin Orthop Relat Res 1978;(133):106–21.
12. Prucz RB, Friedrich JB. Upper extremity replantation: current concepts. Plast Reconstr Surg 2014; 133(2):333–42.
13. Smith AC, Nikkhah D, Jones ME. The importance of bone shortening in digital replantation. J Plast Reconstr Aesthet Surg 2016;69(10):1451–2.
14. Bueno RA Jr, Battiston B, Ciclamini D, et al. Replantation: current concepts and outcomes. Clin Plast Surg 2014;41(3):385–95.
15. Brown ML, Wood MB. Techniques of bone fixation in replantation surgery. Microsurgery 1990;11(3): 255–60.
16. Jupiter JB, Pess GM, Bour CJ. Results of flexor tendon tenolysis after replantation in the hand. J Hand Surg Am 1989;14(1):35–44.
17. Strauch B, de Moura W. Arterial system of the fingers. J Hand Surg Am 1990;15(1):148–54.
18. Leslie BM, Ruby LK, Madell SJ, et al. Digital artery diameters: an anatomic and clinical study. J Hand Surg 1987;12(5):740–3.
19. Hall JE. Guyton and Hall textbook of medical physiology e-Book. Elsevier Health Sciences; 2015.
20. Smith DO, Oura C, Kimura C, et al. The distal venous anatomy of the finger. J Hand Surg Am 1991;16(2): 303–7.
21. Nyström A, von Drasek-Ascher G, Fridén J, et al. The palmar digital venous anatomy. Scand J Plast Reconstr Surg Hand Surg 1990;24(2):113–9.
22. Endo T, Kojima T, Hirase Y. Vascular anatomy of the finger dorsum and a new idea for coverage of the finger pulp defect that restores sensation. J Hand Surg Am 1992;17(5):927–32.
23. Nakayama Y, Soeda S, Kasai Y. Flaps nourished by arterial inflow through the venous system: an experimental investigation. Plast Reconstr Surg 1981; 67(3):328–34.
24. Yan H, Brooks D, Ladner R, et al. Arterialized venous flaps: a review of the literature. Microsurgery 2010; 30(6):472–8.
25. Koch H, Scharnagl E, Schwarzl FX, et al. Clinical application of the retrograde arterialized venous flap. Microsurgery 2004;24(2):118–24.
26. Xiu Z-F, Chen Z-J. The microcirculation and survival of experimental flow-through venous flaps. Br J Plast Surg 1996;49(1):41–5.
27. De Lorenzi F, van der Hulst RR, den Dunnen WF, et al. Arterialized venous free flaps for soft-tissue reconstruction of digits: a 40-case series. J Reconstr Microsurg 2002;18(7):569–74.

28. Nichter LS, Haines PC. Arterialized venous perfusion of composite tissue. Am J Surg 1985;150(2):191–6.
29. Inoue G, Maeda N, Suzuki K. Resurfacing of skin defects of the hand using the arterialised venous flap. Br J Plast Surg 1990;43(2):135–9.
30. Yan H, Zhang F, Akdemir O, et al. Clinical applications of venous flaps in the reconstruction of hands and fingers. Arch Orthop Trauma Surg 2011;131(1):65–74.
31. Lee DC, Kim JS, Ki SH, et al. Partial second toe pulp free flap for fingertip reconstruction. Plast Reconstr Surg 2008;121(3):899–907.
32. Cho YJ, Roh SY, Kim JS, et al. Second toe plantar free flap for volar tissue defects of the fingers. Arch Plast Surg 2013;40(3):226–31.
33. Yang JW, Kim JS, Lee DC, et al. The radial artery superficial palmar branch flap: a modified free thenar flap with constant innervation. J Reconstr Microsurg 2010;26(8):529–38.
34. Kim KS, Kim ES, Hwang JH, et al. Fingertip reconstruction using the hypothenar perforator free flap. J Plast Reconstr Aesthet Surg 2013;66(9):1263–70.
35. Han HH, Choi YS, Kim IB, et al. A perforator from the ulnar artery and cutaneous nerve of the hypothenar area: an anatomical study for clinical application. Microsurgery 2017;37(1):49–56.
36. Schmidt CC, Kohut GN, Greenberg JA, et al. The anconeus muscle flap: its anatomy and clinical application. J Hand Surg Am 1999;24(2):359–69.
37. Jeon BJ, Jwa SJ, Lee DC, et al. The anconeus muscle free flap: clinical application to lesions on the hand. Arch Plast Surg 2017;44(5):420–7.
38. Wei F-C, Mardini S. Free-style free flaps. Plast Reconstr Surg 2004;114(4):910–6.

Revascularization and Replantation in the Hand
Ectopic Banking and Replantation

Brian H. Cho, MD[a], James P. Higgins, MD[b,*]

KEYWORDS

• Ectopic banking • Replantation • Amputation • Trauma • Upper extremity salvage

KEY POINTS

- Ectopic banking is a useful technique that allows delayed replantation in settings when conventional immediate replantation is not feasible.
- The period of ectopic banking permits staged wound preparation for the subsequent delayed replantation.
- The anatomic location of ectopic banking should be selected based on considerations such as ease of access to donor vessels, ability to protect or splint the banked part, additional disability to the injured patient, and ease of 2-team approach for second-stage surgery. The contralateral upper extremity provides many of these ideal characteristics.
- Duration of temporary banking is selected based on considerations such as degree of wound contamination, systemic health of the patient, technique used for wound bed preparation, and overall period of patient disability. Delayed replantation should be performed as soon as feasible to maximize functional recovery and minimize duration of disability.

INTRODUCTION

Since first described by Godina and colleagues[1] in 1986, temporary ectopic banking of amputated parts for subsequent replantation is a technique that has evolved in its use for extremity salvage and reconstruction. First described for the use of banking amputated fingers and hands in nonanatomical positions, several case reports have expanded its use for a variety of other amputated parts.[2,3] Ectopic banking and replantation remains an innovative and valuable surgical technique in select cases of trauma and amputation. The purpose of this article was to review the literature and provide an update on the clinical indications, banking location and duration, treatment considerations in ectopic banking, and replantation for upper extremity amputations.

CLINICAL INDICATIONS FOR ECTOPIC BANKING

The reports of ectopic banking by Godina and colleagues[1] describe its use in cases of devastating segmental injuries or amputation of the extremities, where the distal part requires replantation, but the amputation bed requires radical debridement. To achieve adequate wound debridement to permit immediate replantation, critical structures would require significant shortening, such that the functional result would be compromised. Godina and colleagues[1] advocated that ectopic

Disclosure: All authors have approved the article and its submission. The authors have no relevant disclosures or conflicts of interest.
[a] Curtis National Hand Center, 3333 North Calvert Street, Johnston Professional Building, 2nd Floor, Baltimore, MD 21218, USA; [b] The Curtis National Hand Center, MedStar Union Memorial Hospital, 3333 North Calvert Street, Johnston Professional Building, 2nd Floor, Baltimore, MD 21218, USA
* Corresponding author.
E-mail address: anne.mattson@medstar.net

Hand Clin 35 (2019) 199–206
https://doi.org/10.1016/j.hcl.2019.01.002

banking allows conservative debridement and open wound management of the proximal stump, which could aid in the preservation of limb length and vital structures.

Since its initial description, the indication for ectopic banking has been expanded to scenarios in which patients are severely injured and may not tolerate immediate replantation of the amputated part, such as in cases of multisystem trauma and hemodynamic instability.[4] In comparison with immediate replantation, ectopic banking requires significantly less operative time given that it typically requires only vascular anastomosis and is performed at a nontraumatized region of the body. In addition, initial ectopic banking may be performed concurrently with life-preserving surgeries in the acute trauma setting.[5] Definitive replantation and reconstruction can then be planned electively at a later date when the patient's overall condition is stabilized.

Beyond ectopic banking of the entire amputated part, several investigators have described a variation in this technique in which spare parts, or portions, of the amputated part are banked for future reconstruction. This is especially useful in cases of severe limb amputations in which the amputated part is so critically injured that an attempt at traditional replantation is unlikely to succeed. In these cases, spare parts or free fillet flap techniques may be used to harvest any salvageable tissue for ectopic banking and potential reconstruction. Jennings and Murphy[6] described the use of this technique in a case report in which a free radial forearm flap was harvested from a patient who sustained severe upper extremity amputation. The flap was harvested from the amputated forearm and the vessels were anastomosed to the subscapular vessels with the flap banked in the axilla. The proximal stump was then serially debrided until the proximal stump was clean and ready for reconstruction or soft tissue coverage. At this time, the banked radial forearm free flap was transferred over the open stump in a pedicled manner to provide delayed soft tissue coverage. The close proximity of the ectopic banking site (ipsilateral axilla) allowed transfer of the flap without the need for an additional microvascular anastomosis.

Beyond its indications for upper extremity salvage and reconstruction, ectopic banking techniques have been expanded to amputations of other areas of the body. Although beyond the scope of this article, several investigators have described cases in which amputated lower extremities, scalp, and genitals are ectopically banked for delayed replantation or soft tissue reconstruction.[2–4,7–12]

Although the indications for this technique have expanded since its original description, the global experience of published cases demonstrated that most cases are performed when the following scenarios are encountered:

- The amputated part is of adequate quality and value to warrant replantation.
- Conventional immediate replantation is not feasible due to the degree of contamination or tissue loss of the amputation stump.
- Serial debridement or soft tissue reconstruction of the amputation stump would enable delayed replantation.
- Most commonly, the amputated parts involved are digits or an amputated hand.[2]

PREOPERATIVE COUNSELING

As with the treatment of any devastating injury, it is important to discuss the process and expectations regarding upper extremity salvage and replantation with the patient and/or family. With advances in microsurgical techniques and aggressive wound management, the rates of replant survival after banking and replantation remain reasonably high.[2,13–15] Regardless, ectopic banking and replantation is an arduous process. Patients should be counseled ahead of time that they will likely require multiple surgeries, an extended hospital stay, and lengthy rehabilitation. These considerations are similar to conventional replantation. Additional counseling should be provided to candidates for ectopic banking regarding the proposed site of banking. The planned site of banking (ipsilateral limb, contralateral limb, upper or lower extremity, or torso) and duration of banking will have implications for period of recovery, dependence on family or other caregivers, difficulty with ambulation, feeding, and self-care (eg, bathing, personal hygiene).

Even with successful replantation, patients with forearm-level amputations often have limited functional use of the replanted part.[16] Regardless, studies have shown that patients who sustained upper extremity amputation reported more favorable patient-reported outcomes after successful replantation compared with revision amputation and prosthetic rehabilitation.[17]

ECTOPIC BANKING LOCATION

In their first reported case, Godina and colleagues[1] described banking several amputated fingers in the groin of the patient. The initial banking was successful, and the parts remained viable for several days; however, the banked fingers were ultimately lost due to disruption of the microsurgical anastomosis because of patient flexion at the hip. This experience led to their recommendation of using banking sites that allow for stable immobilization and protection of the vascular anastomosis. They suggest the axilla as a convenient banking site for postoperative care and early rehabilitation therapy of the banked part.

Several reports have since described successful temporary banking in the groin, lower extremity, and upper extremity.[4,5,16,18] Common donor vessels used at these locations include the deep inferior epigastric artery, superficial circumflex iliac artery, descending branch of the lateral circumflex femoral artery, dorsalis pedis artery, and the radial or ulnar arteries (**Fig. 1**). Regardless of the site, the authors believe that the banking site must encompass several key characteristics that are summarized in **Box 1**.

Yang and colleagues[19] described a unique technique of ectopically banking an amputated thumb on the ipsilateral distal forearm with subsequent pedicled transfer to its native position. They report that the amputated thumb can be anastomosed to the radial artery proximal to the radial styloid. This allows sufficient pedicle length to rotate the ectopically banked thumb to the proximal stump at the time of delayed replantation. This technique obviates the need for microsurgical anastomoses at the second surgery. The major disadvantage to this technique is the mandatory sacrifice of the radial artery.

In our experience, with upper extremity salvage and reconstruction, the contralateral distal upper extremity has been an ideal site for ectopic banking. The contralateral forearm has easily accessible donor vessels that are suitable for either an end-to-side or end-to-end anastomosis. The contralateral upper extremity is often spared from trauma and provides a banking location that is far from the zone of injury and facilitates the use of a 2-team approach. In addition, splints can be easily constructed to include the banked part and upper extremity to provide protection and support. Last, the use of the upper extremity banking optimizes a patient's mobility and allows early participation with physical and occupational therapy with less concern for compromising the banked part. It is worth considering, however, that the use of the contralateral upper extremity exposes an uninjured limb to surgical risks including infection, stiffness, and scarring.

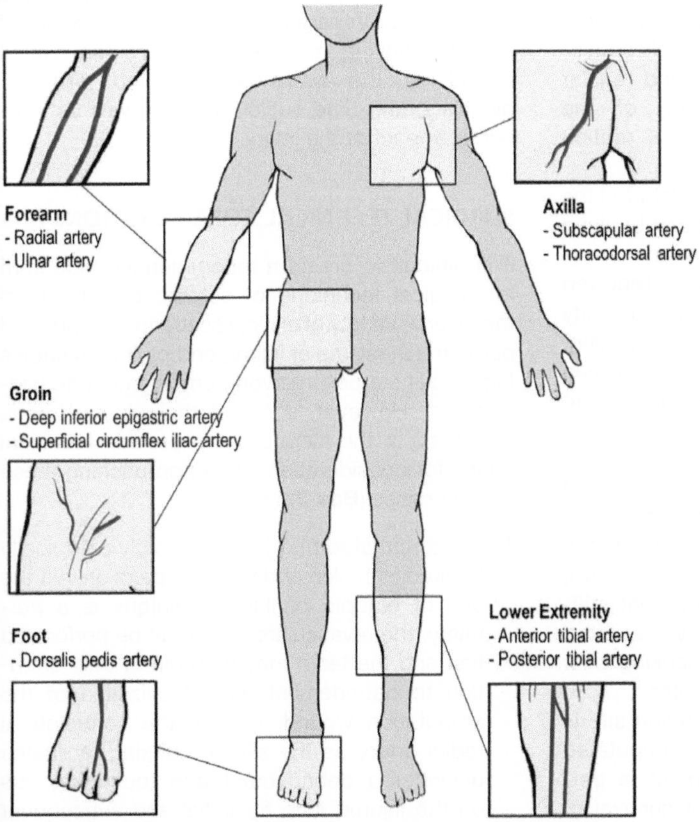

Fig. 1. Ectopic banking locations and recipient donor vessels. (*Courtesy of* M. Seu, BA, Chicago, IL.)

Box 1
Summary of the characteristics to the ideal ectopic banking location

- Reliable donor vessels of sufficient vessel caliber
- Amenable to splinting or immobilization of the banked part
- Outside the zone of injury
- Allows for the use of a 2-team approach
- Permissible to patient rehabilitation and mobility during the banking period

DURATION OF ECTOPIC BANKING AND PROXIMAL WOUND MANAGEMENT

There has been significant debate regarding the ideal duration of banking before replantation of the amputated part. In their report, Godina and colleagues[1] emphasized the importance of a prolonged delay before replantation. In their described case, the amputated forearm was banked in the axilla for 66 days before replantation back onto the proximal stump. They commented that a prolonged period of banking ensures complete healing of the proximal stump and that perhaps, in their case, an even longer delay might have resulted in decreased hypertrophic scarring. Equally important, Godina and colleagues[1] emphasized the importance of early and regular passive physiotherapy and splinting of the banked part to maintain joint range of motion and suppleness.

Since this report, investigators have debated the necessity, and the presumed benefits, of banking amputated parts for long durations. A recent systematic review by Tu and colleagues[2] reported that in 31 cases there was considerable variability in the literature regarding the duration of banking. They found that 23% were banked for less than 1 month, 32% for 1 to 3 months, 32% 3 to 6 months, and 13% for longer than 6 months. Suggestions for earlier replantation have been advocated in the literature due to reports of decreased functional results after prolonged banking.[20] Suboptimal results include tendon shortening, proximal nerve retraction and fibrosis, decreased joint range of motion, and joint stiffness. Accordingly, several cases have reported successful outcomes after shorter banking over the span of several weeks versus months.[2,21]

Heavy contamination of the amputation site is an indication for ectopic banking of the amputated part. In this setting, serial debridement is performed to maximize the chances of survival of the part after delayed replantation.[1,22] In the original report of Godina and colleagues,[1] the goal of wound management was to achieve healing by secondary intention and skin grafting before delayed replantation. Subsequent investigators have used other techniques to prepare the wound bed for replantation. Free flap reconstruction has been used simultaneously with the delayed replantation. This technique delivers uninjured tissue to provide coverage of vital structures such that the replantation need not be performed as a subsequent staged procedure. Negative pressure wound therapy (NPWT) also provides a useful adjunct in the treatment extremity salvage. NPWT maintains wound homeostasis and reduces wound exudate and soft tissue edema.[23] Studies also have shown that NPWT with instillation further enhances wound healing and expedites the debridement of acute and chronic wounds.[24] Use of NPWT on the amputation stump may shorten the delay from initial ectopic banking to subsequent delayed replantation.

Minimizing the delay between ectopic banking and subsequent delayed replantation has many potential benefits. Early definitive replantation allows healing to begin earlier, which expedites nerve regeneration and tendon rehabilitation. The banking period should last only the duration needed to achieve adequate debridement and wound bed preparation. Limiting the period of ectopic banking may help minimize the overall period of the patient's perceived "illness," disability, and time out of work, as well as economic impact of the injury.

SURGICAL TECHNICAL CONSIDERATIONS

It is difficult to create a recommended algorithm for surgical technique of ectopic banking from the diverse variety of clinical scenarios, amputated parts, mechanisms of injury, and patient variables (eg, social support network, employment considerations). However, some of the general trends described in the literature can provide technical pearls for consideration when approaching these difficult cases (**Box 2**):

1. The amputated part may be rapidly ectopically banked with skin and vessel repairs only. If the use of ectopic banking technique is a certainty, the revascularization may be performed first and the team may then direct their attention to debridement and stabilization of the amputation wound. Use of the contralateral radial artery as the site of banking facilitates unhindered debridement and tourniquet use on the injured limb for initial and subsequent

Box 2
Technical tips when harvesting and replanting banked parts

- Preserve previously performed arterial and venous anastomosis
- Harvest the entire length of the ectopic recipient artery and vein
- Reconstruct arterial defect at the banking location with autologous vein graft
- End-to-side anastomoses should be used when possible

staged debridements without risk to the banked part. This can be performed as end-to-side or end-to-end into the radial artery (**Figs. 2–5**). Alternatively, branch vessels of the ulnar or radial artery can be used as inflow and source if caliber-matched end-to-end anastomoses are preferred (ie, palmar branch of radial artery).

2. Debridement of the amputated stump can be pursued with the goal of preservation of length and critical structures in a manner that would be impossible if immediate replantation was pursued. For example, exposed and viable bone or nerve may be preserved throughout debridements with planned delayed coverage at the time of reconstruction. This wound can then be managed with open wound dressing technique or negative pressure dressing technique while serial debridements may be performed.
3. When the amputation stump is deemed ready for closure, consideration should be given to simultaneous soft tissue reconstruction and replantation of the ectopic part to minimize the total duration of disability for the patient. This rapid return of the part to its native position also may be beneficial for nerve regeneration[25] and the ability to perform primary tendon repairs.
4. When harvesting the ectopically banked part, the previously performed arterial venous anastomosis should be preserved if possible, using the entire length of the ectopic recipient artery and vein as harvested conduits for transfer to the amputation stump. This provides the ease of harvest of the banked part without dissection in the potentially vulnerable region of prior microanastomoses. These anastomoses may be left undisturbed in their healing process and vessel dissection can occur at a remote "upstream" site. This would alleviate the need for additional microvascular anastomoses, and permit the revascularization of the orthotopic replanted part to be performed proximal to the amputation stump, potentially out of the zone of injury. It also permits greater ease of microvascular reconstruction due to the larger-caliber anastomoses of the upstream vessels.[22]
5. Reconstruction of the arterial defect in the banked extremity (ie, contralateral radial artery)

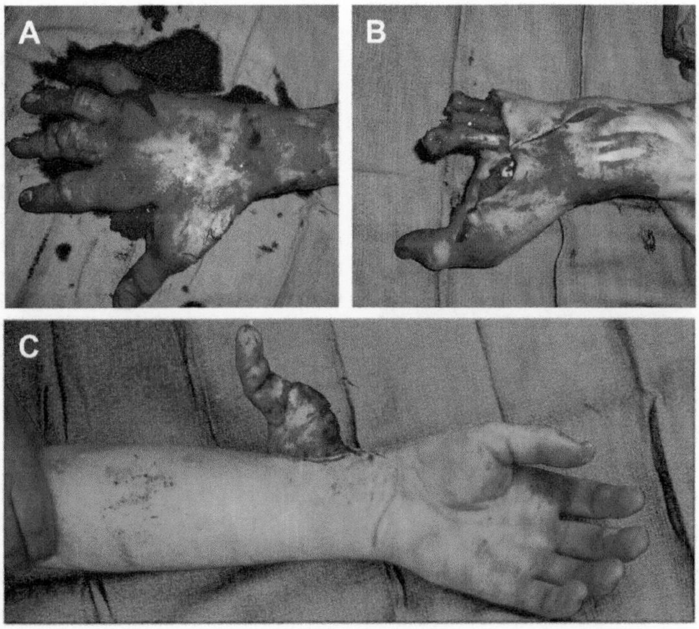

Fig. 2. A 17-year-old boy sustained an avulsion injury to the right hand secondary to a corn-picking machine accident. (*A*) Severe crush and avulsion injury to the right hand. (*B*) Right hand after serial debridement and an index ray amputation. (*C*) The amputated right small finger was salvaged at initial surgery and banked in the contralateral forearm. The digital vessels were anastomosed in an end-to-side fashion to the left radial artery.

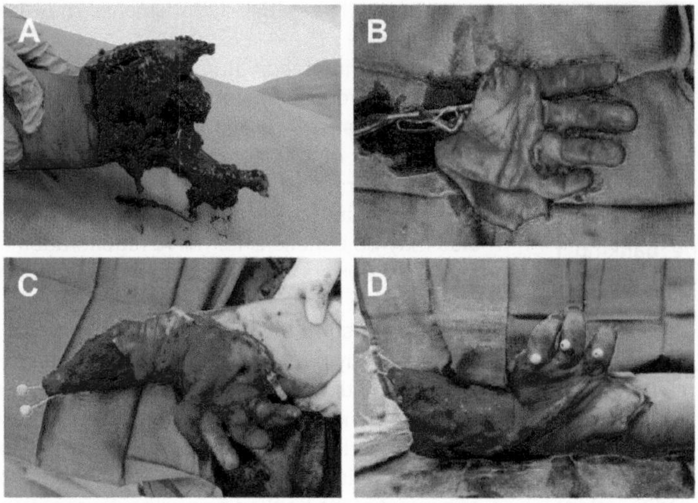

Fig. 3. An adult man sustained a trans-metacarpal avulsion amputation of the left hand when he caught his hand in agriculture machine. (*A*) Proximal stump of the left hand. (*B*) Amputated part. (*C, D*) The amputated hand was ectopically banked into the left forearm. The common digital arteries were anastomosed in an end-to-side fashion to the radial artery. (*Courtesy of* I. K. Fox, MD, St Louis, MO.)

may occur at the time of delayed orthotopic replantation. This may minimize morbidity to the extremity that serves as the site of banking.[26] This decision can also be made based on the preoperative assessment of perfusion to the extremity (ie, Doppler Allen test).

6. If definitive soft tissue coverage will be provided by free flap reconstruction, anastomoses should be performed in an end-to-side fashion to allow for preservation of the distal blood flow to the radial and ulnar arteries to the extremity, as well as to serve as a source for sequential anastomosis for the delayed replantation of the ectopic part. This is most easily achieved using the ipsilateral radial artery because of its superficial location throughout the forearm. The delayed replanted part, harvested with a long segment of arterial and venous pedicles (ie, the radial artery and cephalic vein from the contralateral arm) can then be easily anastomosed into the radial artery in the atraumatic proximal forearm end-to-side, and the cephalic vein end-to-end. The free flap used for simultaneous soft tissue reconstruction can readily be anastomosed into the radial artery downstream end-to-side in a location that permits maximal insetting.

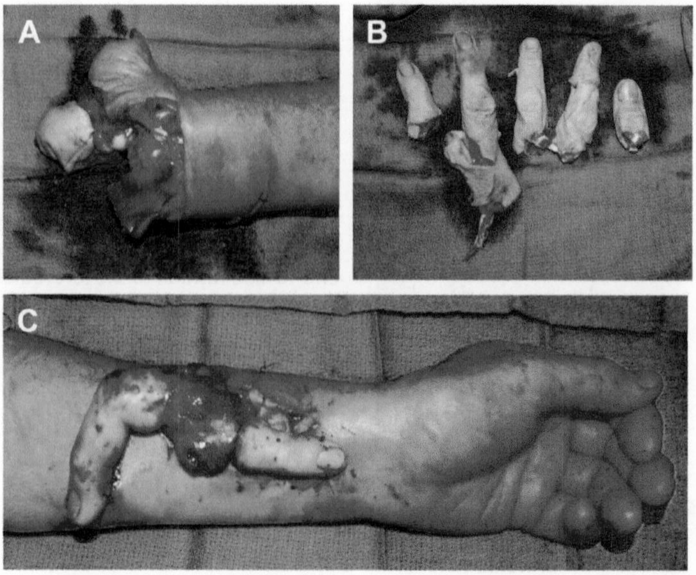

Fig. 4. An adult man sustained a crush amputation at the radiocarpal level when his hand was caught in a bowling ball return. (*A*) The proximal stump of the right upper extremity. (*B*) Retrieved digits. (*C*) The long and index fingers were deemed salvageable and were ectopically banked on the contralateral forearm. Both digital vessels were anastomosed in an end-to-side fashion to the radial artery. (*Courtesy of* R. D. Katz, MD, Baltimore, MD.)

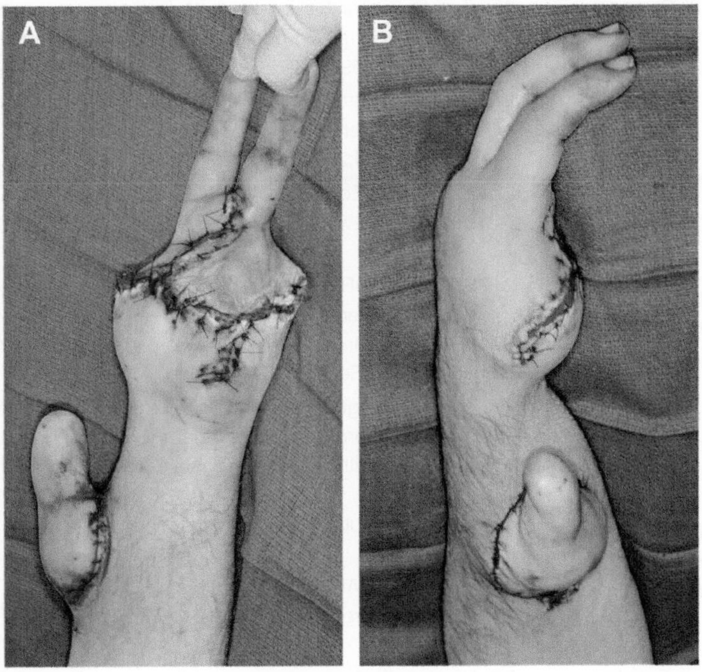

Fig. 5. A 27-year-old right-handed man sustained a traumatic amputation of the right small finger, ring finger crush injury, midshaft metacarpal-level thumb amputation, and a near-complete amputation through the proximal left lower leg secondary to a ballistic projectile. (*A*, *B*) After a left below-knee amputation, the left great toe was ectopically banked on the left forearm. The dorsal intermetatarsal artery was anastomosed in an end-to-side fashion to the radial artery.

SUMMARY

Although the treatment of major upper extremity amputation remains a difficult challenge, advances in techniques of ectopic banking and microvascular replantation has allowed patients the prospect of replantation when not previously possible. Furthermore, there has been greater emphasis on not only replantation survival, but optimization of the long-term patient-reported outcomes after replantation. This is especially pertinent given the advancements and the associated functional improvements in the fields of limb prosthetics and upper extremity allotransplantation. As we look forward, our efforts should be directed not only toward replantation viability but whether the resulting replanted limb can provide outcomes that are superior to other viable alternatives.

REFERENCES

1. Godina M, Bajec J, Baraga A. Salvage of the mutilated upper extremity with temporary ectopic implantation of the undamaged part. Plast Reconstr Surg 1986;78(3):295–9.
2. Tu Y, Lineaweaver WC, Culnan DM, et al. Temporary ectopic implantation for salvaging amputated parts: a systematic review. J Trauma Acute Care Surg 2018;84(6):985–93.
3. Jin Y, Hua C, Hu X, et al. Microsurgical replantation of total avulsed scalp: extending the limits. J Craniofac Surg 2017;28(3):670–4.
4. Wang JN, Wang SY, Wang ZJ, et al. Temporary ectopic implantation for salvage of amputated lower extremities: case reports. Microsurgery 2005;25(5):385–9.
5. Chernofsky MA, Sauer PF. Temporary ectopic implantation. J Hand Surg Am 1990;15(6):910–4.
6. Jennings JF, Murphy RX Jr, Chernofsky MA, et al. Amputation stump salvage using a "banked" free-tissue transfer. Ann Plast Surg 1991;27(4):361–3.
7. Xu H, Zhang Y, He J, et al. Ectopic implantation of an avulsed scalp with a tissue expander on a forearm for combined total scalp avulsion and spine injuries: a case report. Microsurgery 2017;37(7):819–23.
8. Matloub HS, Yousif NJ, Sanger JR. Temporary ectopic implantation of an amputated penis. Plast Reconstr Surg 1994;93(2):408–12.
9. Kayikcioglu A, Agaoglu G, Nasir S, et al. Crossover replantation and fillet flap coverage of the stump after ectopic implantation: a case of bilateral leg amputation. Plast Reconstr Surg 2000;106(4):868–73.
10. Valerio IL, Hui-Chou HG, Zelken J, et al. Ectopic banking of amputated great toe for delayed thumb reconstruction: case report. J Hand Surg Am 2014;39(7):1323–6.
11. Sanger JR, Logiudice JA, Rowe D, et al. Ectopic scalp replantation: a case report. J Plast Reconstr Aesthet Surg 2010;63(1):e23–7.
12. Ramdas S, Thomas A, Arun Kumar S. Temporary ectopic testicular replantation, refabrication and orthotopic transfer. J Plast Reconstr Aesthet Surg 2007;60(7):700–3.

13. Nazerani S, Vaseghi H, Hesami S, et al. Ectopic major transplantation for salvage of upper and lower extremity amputations. Chin J Traumatol 2013;16(6):330–3.
14. Ng WK, Kaur MN, Thoma A. Long-term outcomes of major upper extremity replantations. Plast Surg (Oakv) 2014;22(1):9–13.
15. Brown M, Lu Y, Chung KC, et al. Annual hospital volume and success of digital replantation. Plast Reconstr Surg 2017;139(3):672–80.
16. Bakhach J, Katrana F, Panconi B, et al. Temporary ectopic digital implantation: a clinical series of eight digits. J Hand Surg Eur Vol 2008;33(6):717–22.
17. Pet MA, Morrison SD, Mack JS, et al. Comparison of patient-reported outcomes after traumatic upper extremity amputation: replantation versus prosthetic rehabilitation. Injury 2016;47(12):2783–8.
18. Nazerani S, Motamedi MH. Ectopic single-finger transplantation, a novel technique for nonreplantable digits: assessment of 24 cases–presenting the "piggyback" method. Tech Hand Up Extrem Surg 2009;13(2):65–74.
19. Yang J, Yang W, Cao S, et al. Local ectopic implantation for salvaging an amputated thumb: an anatomical study and a case report. Ann Plast Surg 2013;70(2):187–91.
20. Graf P, Groner R, Horl W, et al. Temporary ectopic implantation for salvage of amputated digits. Br J Plast Surg 1996;49(3):174–7.
21. Li J, Ni GH, Guo Z, et al. Salvage of amputated thumbs by temporary ectopic implantation. Microsurgery 2008;28(7):559–64.
22. Higgins JP. Ectopic banking of amputated parts: a clinical review. J Hand Surg Am 2011;36(11):1868–76.
23. Schlatterer DR, Hirschfeld AG, Webb LX. Negative pressure wound therapy in grade IIIB tibial fractures: fewer infections and fewer flap procedures? Clin Orthop Relat Res 2015;473(5):1802–11.
24. Kim PJ, Attinger CE, Steinberg JS, et al. The impact of negative-pressure wound therapy with instillation compared with standard negative-pressure wound therapy: a retrospective, historical, cohort, controlled study. Plast Reconstr Surg 2014;133(3):709–16.
25. Birch R, Raji AR. Repair of median and ulnar nerves. Primary suture is best. J Bone Joint Surg Br 1991;73(1):154–7.
26. Higgins JP. A reassessment of the role of the radial forearm flap in upper extremity reconstruction. J Hand Surg Am 2011;36(7):1237–40.

Outcomes Following Replantation/ Revascularization in the Hand

Hoyune E. Cho, MD*, Sandra V. Kotsis, MPH,
Kevin C. Chung, MD, MS

KEYWORDS

- Digit replantation • Outcomes after replantation in the hand • Functional outcomes
- Patient-reported outcomes • Outcome measures

KEY POINTS

- There is a great deal of heterogeneity in the literature for measurement tools and reported outcomes for replantation in the hand.
- Both functional outcomes and patient-reported outcomes together facilitate a comprehensive assessment of the benefits of replantation for amputation injuries in the hand.
- Recommended parameters to measure are digit survival, arc of motion, sensation, grip strength, return to work, complications, and patients' perspectives on overall hand function, activities of daily living, pain, work performance, aesthetics, and satisfaction.
- Factors influencing outcomes include patient age, comorbidities, specific digits injured, level of injury, mechanism of injury, surgeon skill and experience, and hospital volume.
- Establishing a recommended set of outcomes, outcome measures, and ways to report them will improve the quality of evidence that permits patients to make informed decisions.

INTRODUCTION

Traumatic digit amputation impacts 45,000 people's lives every year.[1] Although usually not life threatening, it decreases the patient's ability to do the same preinjury tasks and causes psychological stress. Moreover, most patients with traumatic digit amputation are young and of working age. Treatment options include revascularization or replantation of the amputated segment and revision amputation of the stump.

The most commonly accepted indications for replantation are thumb injuries, multiple digits involved, and injuries in children.[2,3] For injuries of other digits, there is a perception that replantation is not worthwhile because the functional gain is too small for the cost and efforts required in comparison to revision amputation.[4,5] However, an increasing number of studies have reported noninferiority of functional and patient-reported outcomes after replantation of single digits.[1,5–7]

Funding: Funding for this work was supported by a Midcareer Investigator Award (2 K24-AR053120-06) to Dr K.C. Chung from the National Institute of Arthritis and Musculoskeletal and Skin Diseases, USA of the National Institutes of Health and a Surgical Scientist Training Grant in Health Services and Translational Research (2 T32-GM008616-16A1) for Dr H.E. Cho from the National Institutes of Health, USA Ruth L. Kirschstein National Research Service Award Institutional Research Training Grant at the University of Michigan Medical School, USA.
Disclosure Statement: The authors did not have any relationship with a commercial company with a financial interest in the subject discussed in this article.
Section of Plastic Surgery, Department of Surgery, University of Michigan Medical School, 1500 East Medical Center Drive, 2130 Taubman Center, SPC 5340, Ann Arbor, MI 48109-5340, USA
* Corresponding author.
E-mail address: hoyunech@med.umich.edu

Hand Clin 35 (2019) 207–219
https://doi.org/10.1016/j.hcl.2018.12.008

hand.theclinics.com

In addition to clinical indications, the decision to replant or not should require a thorough deliberation of the possible surgical outcomes. In other words, patients need a reasonable understanding of the expected level of functional and aesthetic recovery, commitment for rehabilitation, and time required for recovery after replantation before an informed decision is made between replantation and revision amputation.[8] Those who need to return to work quickly or have limited financial resources may be better served with a revision amputation procedure.[9]

Rigorous evaluation of outcomes after replantation or revascularization is difficult because there are many confounding variables. Moreover, the variability in the types of outcomes reported and the methods used to obtain those outcomes deter a meaningful comparison across studies. Lack of detail for injury characteristics, such as complete versus subtotal amputation, level of injury and mechanism of injury, and subjective criteria of evaluation, further complicate assessment.[10] These challenges in understanding outcomes after replantation need to be considered to establish a standard way to measure and report outcomes to improve the ability to make an evidence-based decision.

In this article, the authors review the concepts and the recommended ways to measure

- Initial vascular success
- Functional outcomes
- Patient-reported outcomes
- Factors that influence outcomes

INITIAL VASCULAR SUCCESS OF DIGIT REPLANTATION

In the immediate postoperative period, close monitoring of vascular patency is a key to the survival of the replanted digit.[8] Perfusion should be monitored by examining the color, pulp turgor, capillary refill, and temperature of the replanted digit.[11] A soft, pale fingertip with delayed capillary refill of more than 2 seconds indicates arterial occlusion, and an edematous, blue fingertip with rapid capillary refill indicates venous occlusion. Lower temperature in the replanted digit greater than 2°C is a discouraging sign for digit viability. To improve perfusion, constrictive sutures and dressings should be taken down first (**Fig. 1**). Leeches and heparin-soaked pledgets can be attempted to allow for egress of blood from the digit. Last, the patient can be taken back to the operating room for exploration of the vascular anastomoses. The expected survival rate for digital replantation and revascularization is 50% to 85%.[11]

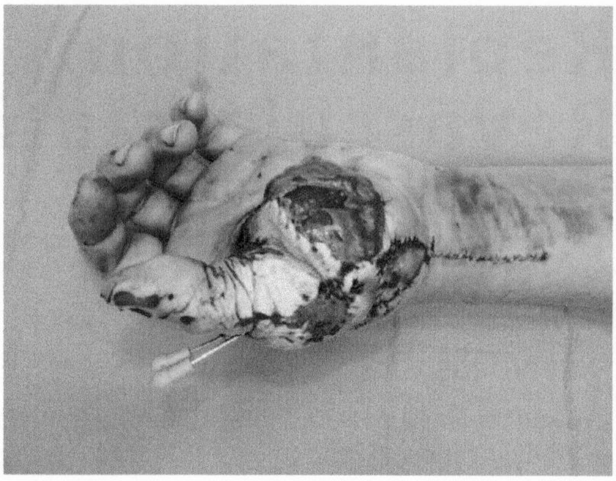

Fig. 1. Release of constrictive sutures to improve perfusion.

In the literature, the reported rates of initial vascular success vary widely, depending on the follow-up period, types of digits evaluated, and the characteristics of the injury. In fact, the definition of successful replantation differs between different study designs. Owing to the limits of coding scheme and data structure, the rates of successful replantation reported by many database studies are actually rates of initial vascular survival of the replanted digit. For instance, a national-level investigation using the largest inpatient database from 1998 to 2012 found a 79% rate of success for thumb and 67% for other digits, but was unable to perform subgroup analyses by individual digit type or mechanism of injury because of the lack of information in the database.[12] In addition, it is unclear whether these data capture late revision amputations. Similarly, another retrospective database study found a 70% rate of survival from 2008 to 2012 but did not provide rates for subcategories of digit types or injury types.[13]

On the other hand, studies based on clinical data can report detailed results. For example, in a study of 121 digit replantations over a 14-year period between 1997 and 2010 at large academic level I trauma centers, Fufa and colleagues[14] defined survival as digit viability for a minimum of 21 days and found a 57% rate of survival. They found higher survival rates for the thumb (68%), index (63%), and long (65%) fingers compared with the ring (35%) or small (36%) fingers. Regarding the mechanism of injury, sharp injuries (55%) had a similar rate of survival as avulsion injuries (56%), which were unexpectedly lower than the survival rate for crush injuries (68%). When classified by level of amputation, Tamai level V (most proximal) showed the highest rate of survival at 80%, followed by level II (67%), level IV (55%), and level III (53%).[14,15] Replantation in nonsmoking patients showed a higher rate of survival (65%) than those who smoked (45%). Replantation procedures that included multiple venous repairs showed higher rates (64%) than those with 0 or 1 venous repair (46%). As surgeon years in practice increased, the rates of survival increased as well. Replantation cases performed by surgeons with less than 5 years of experience had a 49% rate of survival, whereas 68% of the cases survived when performed by those with more than 10 years of experience.[14]

Clinical studies can provide detailed information that may help with surgical decision making, but there are many factors that influence the surgical outcome, such as patients' comorbidities, smoking status, and injury severity.[2] The results of one clinical study may not be generalizable, that is, the findings are not relevant to patients at another hospital for various reasons. For instance, patients' characteristics, the level of expertise of surgeons, the operative staff, and inpatient care resources may differ from one institution to another.

A systematic review compiles and tabulates data from multiple studies to diminish selection bias and thus may be more appropriate for evidence-based clinical decision making. A meta-analysis of 8 clinical studies compiled data from 1803 digit replantations in 1299 patients, to examine how different factors affect survival rates (**Table 1**).[16] Rates of survival were similar for injury levels from distal interphalangeal (DIP) joint to proximal phalanx (88%–89%) but were lower for distal phalanx (78%) and metacarpophalangeal (MCP) joint (79%). Middle (83%), ring (83%), and little fingers (89%) had higher survival rates than thumb (68%) or index finger (75%). Clean injuries survived at a higher rate (91%) than crush (68%) or avulsion injuries (66%). A systematic review solely assessing digit replantation after avulsion injuries found a 68% rate of survival for thumb avulsion injuries and a 78% rate of survival for finger avulsion injuries.[17] Another systematic review of 2273 distal digit replantations found the overall survival rate to be 86%, with no difference between Tamai level I and II amputations.[6] Clean cut injuries survived at a much higher rate (92%) than crush (80%) or avulsion-type injuries (75%) (**Fig. 2**), and those with vein repair showed higher survival rates for both Tamai level I (92% vs 83%) and level II (88% vs 78%) amputations.[6]

Table 1
Rates of survival by injury characteristics

Injury Characteristics	Subcategory	Rate of Survival (%)
Mechanism of injury	Clean	91.4
	Crush	68.4
	Avulsion	66.3
Zone of injury	Distal phalanx	77.7
	DIP joint	88.9
	Middle phalanx	87.7
	PIP joint	88.7
	Proximal phalanx	88.9
	MCP joint	78.9
Digit injured	Thumb	68.1
	Index	75.0
	Middle	82.8
	Ring	82.8
	Little	88.9

Data from Dec W. A meta-analysis of success rates for digit replantation. Tech Hand Up Extrem Surg 2006;10(3):124–9.

The rates of digit survival found in the literature vary greatly, but a meaningful comparison is difficult because database studies lack details on injury characteristics, and results from single institutions are not generalizable. The authors recommend that the survival of the replanted digit be assessed at least 21 days after the operation to ensure definitive viability, and specific injury characteristics be reported to generate high-quality evidence.

FUNCTIONAL OUTCOMES AFTER REPLANTATION

Although many studies discuss successful replantation, the term should be reserved for cases that demonstrate satisfactory functional outcomes and not merely digit survival.[2] Success should convey a meaningful contribution of the replanted

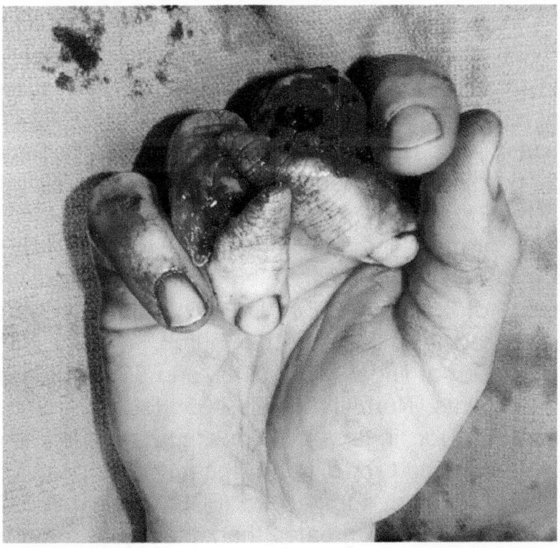

Fig. 2. Crush injury by industrial pressing machine.

digit to the patient's level of functional capacity, measured at least 1 year after the surgery to account for any secondary procedures and further improvement in function.[10] In other words, replantation cannot be deemed successful until adequate function is restored.[11] The traditional measures of functional outcome measurement after digit replantation include range of motion, sensation, and grip/pinch strength.

The scoring system constructed by Tamai is designed to evaluate functional outcomes as well as patient-reported outcomes after digit replantation, by including categories such as activities of daily living, patient satisfaction, and subjective symptoms (**Table 2**).[15] Each outcome category is evaluated for a numerical score, and the total score ranges between −10 and 140. Although this scoring system provides an objective measurement, the scoring process is highly subjective, with criteria such as mild, moderate, and severe, without any specific definitions. Another scoring system, Chen's criteria, quantitatively evaluates 4 outcome parameters (return to work, range of motion, sensory, and motor recovery) for a grade I through IV, but still calls for a subjective assessment without a specified standard method of measuring outcomes (**Table 3**).[10] One study compared the 2 scoring tools by applying them to evaluate functional outcomes after transmetacarpal replantation and concluded that Tamai's scores represent realistic function of the hand despite being more complicated to use.[18]

In this section, the authors review the recommended parameters for an objective, quantifiable outcomes evaluation.

Arc of Motion

The authors recommend that the range of motion be reported by measuring total active motion (TAM) in degrees, because it takes into consideration any joints that were fused, range of motion of remaining joints, and flexor and extensor functions. TAM, as described by the American Society for Surgery of the Hand, is the sum of active range of motion measured with a goniometer in the MCP joint, proximal interphalangeal (PIP) joint, and DIP joint for each individual digit (**Fig. 3**). Normal active range of motion is 80° at DIP joints of finger and interphalangeal joint of the thumb, 100° at PIP joints, 90° at finger MCP joints, and 55° at thumb MCP joints. Normal TAM is 135° for the thumb and 270° for fingers.[19,20] For amputation injuries in flexor zone I, or distal to the insertion point of flexor digitorum superficialis (FDS), the expected arc of motion is greater than the injuries more proximal because the FDS tendon is intact and uninjured.[2,21,22] Similarly, ring avulsion injuries with damage to skin and the vasculature only show good motor recovery if the FDS is intact.[2] In the literature, the reported values of TAM depend on the level of injury and the digit injured (**Tables 4** and **5**).[5,17,18,23–28] The mean TAM appears to decrease as the injuries are more proximal (**Fig. 4**).

Sensation

The authors recommend assessment of sensory recovery of the replanted digit using a 2-point discrimination (2PD) test or by Semmes-Weinstein Monofilament (SWF) testing. 2PD test is the most commonly used tool to measure sensory outcome after nerve repair.[29] It examines tactile gnosia, the replanted segment's sensory function to discern that 2 nearby objects in contact with the skin are 2 distinct points of touch. The standard way of assessment is for the examiner to find the shortest distance between 2 points of touch using calipers, by starting wider than the expected value and moving the 2 points closer and closer.[30] The normal values in the hand are thumb (2.5–5 mm), index (3–5 mm), other digits (4–6 mm), palm (11 mm), and dorsal metacarpal (7–12 mm).[29] SWF is a commonly used tool to detect peripheral neuropathy for the loss of protective sensation.[31] The monofilaments are applied to skin perpendicularly until the fiber bends slightly, for approximately 1.5 seconds. The patients report whether they can feel the monofilament or not.[32] There are various monofilament sizes (1.65–6.65) with different amounts of target force calibrated. The clinician records the smallest monofilament size that the patient is able to detect.

Among studies that reported sensory recovery outcome measured by 2PD test, some reported the actual distance measured and others the percentage of cases that fell into distance groups. Boeckx and colleagues[23] reported that 59% of 34 single-digit replantations were categorized to have 2PD of greater than 15 mm, and 34% show a fair to bad recovery of sensory function (6–15 mm). Only 3% showed normal sensibility of less than 6 mm. In another study of single-digit replantation cases, Chen and colleagues[26] also categorized their results in groups: 17% of cases were in less than 6-mm category, 47% were in the 6- to 10-mm category, 17% were in the 11- to 15-mm category, and 20% were in the greater than 15-mm category. The actual distances reported by other studies are presented in **Tables 6** and **7**.[6,17,18,23–26,28,33–35]

There were 2 studies that reported sensibility testing using SWF. Paavilainen and colleagues[18]

Table 2
Tamai scoring system

Range of motion (0–40)		
Thumb	Opposition: possible (10), difficult (5), impossible (0) Total range of motion: >50% of normal (10), <50% of normal (5), stiff (0)	
Fingers	Total range of motion: >151° (20), 111°–150° (15), 71°–110°(10), <70°(5), stiff (0)	
Activities of daily living (0–20)		
Pushing, tapping, hanging, or drawing, grasping soft material, grasping hard material, power grasp, picking up a coin, picking up a needle, wringing a towel, dipping up water, washing face, knotting, buttoning, writing, scissoring, hammering, using screwdriver, using clothespin, fumbling in pocket, showing rock, paper, scissors		For each category, easy (1), difficult (0.5), impossible (0)
Sensation (grading by British Medical Research Council) (0–20)		
No recovery of sensibility (S0) (0)	Recovery of superficial pain sensibility (S1) (4)	Recovery of superficial pain and some touch sensibility (S2) (8)
Recovery of pain and touch sensibility with disappearance of overresponse (S3) (12)	S3 level of recovery but localization of stimulus is good with imperfect recovery of 2PD (S3+) (16)	Complete recovery (S4) (20)
Subjective symptoms (0–20)		
Pain, cold intolerance, numbness, paresthesia, tightness, and so forth		Severe (−3), moderate (−2), mild (−1)
Cosmesis (0–20)		
Atrophy, scar, color change, deformities (angulation, rotation, mallet, swan neck, buttonhole, and so forth)		Severe (−3), moderate (−2), mild (−1)
Patient satisfaction (0–20)		
Highly satisfied (20), fairly satisfied (15), satisfied (10), poorly satisfied (5), not satisfied (0)		
Job status (− 10–0)		
Same job (0), changed (−5), cannot work (−10)		

Adapted from Sebastin SJ, Chung KC. Challenges in measuring outcomes following digital replantation. Semin Plast Surg 2013;27(4):176; with permission.

Table 3
Chen's criteria

Grade	Return to Work	Range of Motion	Sensory Recovery	Motor Recovery
I (Excellent)	Resume original job	>60% of normal	Normal	4–5 out of 5
II (Good)	Resume suitable work	>40% of normal	Near normal	3–4 out of 5
III (Fair)	Independent activities of daily life	>30% of normal	Partial recovery	3 out of 5
IV (Poor)	No recovery of useful function			

Adapted from Sebastin SJ, Chung KC. Challenges in measuring outcomes following digital replantation. Semin Plast Surg 2013;27(4):176; with permission.

found 55% of transmetacarpal replantation cases to fall within the normal range (2.83–3.61), with diminished protective sensation (4.31) in 22%, loss of protective sensation (4.56) in 14%, and loss of sensation in 9%. Instead of reporting the monofilament size, Chen and colleagues[26] reported the target force applied by the different-sized monofilaments. They reported a normal sensation of touch (0.07 g) for 27% of digit replantation cases, 0.4 g in 33%, 2 g in 30%, 4 g in 3%, and loss of sensation (300 g) in 7%.

Grip Strength

The authors recommend that grip strength be measured with a Jamar hydraulic hand dynamometer (ASP Global, Atlanta, GA), because it is a reliable and validated instrument.[10,36] The Jamar dynamometer has adjustable handles with 5 different positions, with different distances between the instrument body and the handle. Different handle positions influence the measured grip strength. The authors recommend handle position 2 (4.8 cm distance), because it was shown to produce maximal grip strength in the participants.[36,37] Patients should sit in a straight-backed chair, feet flat on the ground, shoulder adducted, elbow flexed at 90°, and forearm and wrist in a neutral position (**Fig. 5**).[37,38] Dynamometers measure strength in weight (kilograms or pounds). The authors recommend reporting the ratio of measurements, between the affected side and normal side.[10] Reporting ratios take into

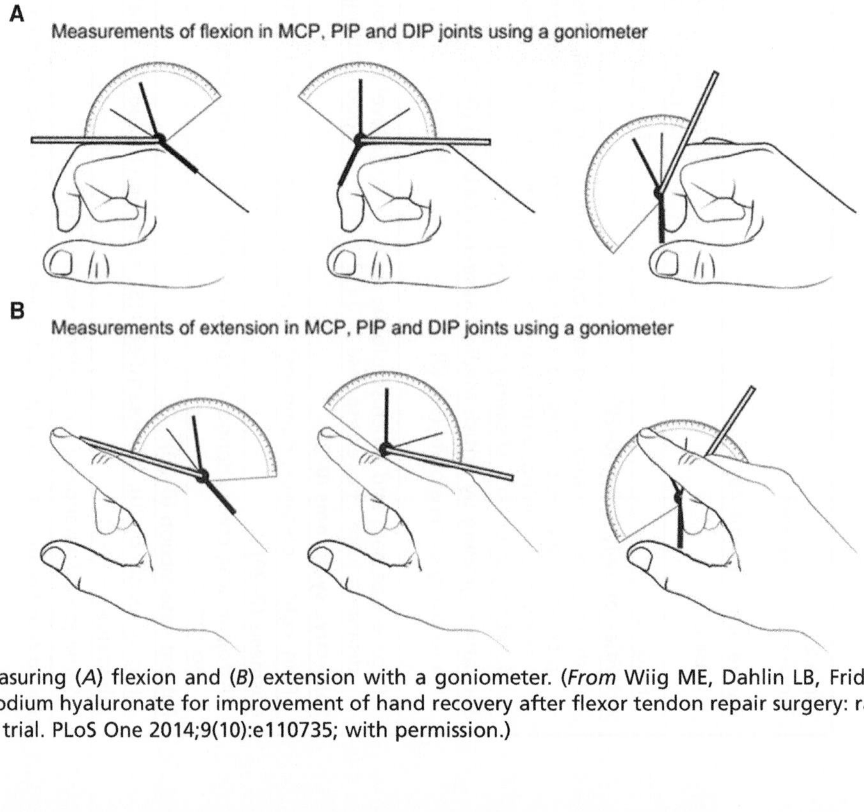

Fig. 3. Measuring (*A*) flexion and (*B*) extension with a goniometer. (*From* Wiig ME, Dahlin LB, Fridén J, et al. PXL01 in sodium hyaluronate for improvement of hand recovery after flexor tendon repair surgery: randomized controlled trial. PLoS One 2014;9(10):e110735; with permission.)

Table 4
Total arc of motion (°), by level of injury

Authors	Flexor I	Middle Phalanx	PIP Joint	Proximal Phalanx	Flexor II	Metacarpus	Metacarpus to Distal Forearm
Boeckx et al,[23] 1992	—	151	106	95	—	109	—
Buntic et al,[5] 2008	170	—	—	—	133	—	—
Adani et al,[24] 2013	180	—	—	—	—	—	—
Paavilainen et al,[18] 2007	—	—	—	—	—	154	—
Assouline et al,[25] 2017	—	—	—	—	—	—	203

consideration the individual variability of strengths among patients, because what is normal for one patient may be considered decreased power for another patient.

For an overall assessment among digit replantation cases (nonspecific of digit injured or level of injury), the mean grip strengths reported were 20 kg[35] and 39.6 kg (91% of normal side).[26] Rosberg[39] analyzed 326 digit replantations and reported grip strength as a ratio to the normal side, by digit type and level of injury: thumb 84%, fingers 64%, mid hand 56%, wrist 28%, and proximal to wrist 26%. For fingertip replantation, Hattori and colleagues[7] found 83% grip strength in their review of 23 cases. For transmetacarpal replantation, the mean grip strength measured was 56% among 33 cases.[18] For more proximal injuries, the mean grip strength was 39% of normal.[25]

Return to Work

Patients may have an easier time returning to jobs that require less manual and digit function. To control for this variability, the authors recommend assessing this parameter by categorizing whether the patient was able to return to the same job, had to get a different job, or was not able to work at all.[10]

There were several studies that used scoring systems by Tamai and Chen to evaluate the functional outcomes after replantation, but none of them reported specific results for each variable within the scoring systems.[18,25,35] A systematic review of distal digit replantation by Sebastin and Chung[6] evaluated 30 studies for working status, but did not mention whether the patients had returned to their original work or not. The authors found 3 studies specifically mentioned the job status of the patients.[23,25,33] The study by Assouline and colleagues[25] reported Chen's grade for each patient but mentioned the job status for only 5 of their 11 cases; 3 patients returned to their original job and 2 patients were classified as disabled. Boeckx and colleagues[23] reported that 8 out of 13 patients returned to same job, 2 changed jobs, and 2 did not return to work. Wu and

Table 5
Total arc of motion (°), by digit type

Authors	Overall	Thumb	Fingers	Index	Middle	Ring	Small
Chen et al,[26] 2018	—	75	145	—	—	—	—
Zhu et al,[27] 2018	—	136	192	—	—	—	—
Boeckx et al,[23] 1992	112	—	—	104	105	131	145
Adani et al,[24] 2013[a]	—	—	—	—	—	185	—
Sears and Chung,[17] 2011[a]	—	—	—	—	—	174	—
Bamba et al,[28] 2018[ab]	—	—	—	—	—	179	—

[a] These studies only studied ring avulsion injuries.
[b] Subgroup analysis showed mean TAM of 201° for Urbaniak class I (circulation adequate) injuries, 187° for class II (circulation inadequate), and 168° for class III (complete degloving or complete amputation).

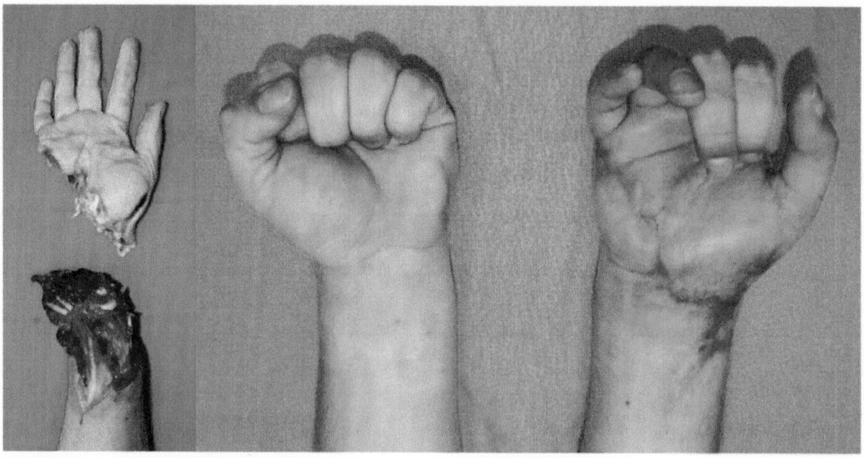

Fig. 4. Decreased range of motion after replantation at proximal level of injury.

colleagues[33] found that all of the 33 patients who worked before their injuries returned to their original workplace.

Complications

There are numerous potential complications after replantation with a variety of different ways to measure them. Thus, it is difficult to compare results between studies. Categories such as severe, moderate, and mild rely on subjective assessment of the evaluator, and this introduces a great deal of bias. Therefore, the authors recommend reporting complications as present or absent. Among the possible complications, such as pain, tightness, color change, and scarring, the authors recommend reporting on cold intolerance, pulp atrophy, and nail deformity as a minimum set.[10]

In the literature, the authors found that studies varied greatly in their report of both the type of complications assessed and the method used to evaluate them. Hahn and Jung[34] reported that out of 468 successful digit replantations, 117 fingers had nail deformity (25%), 46 developed a nonunion (10%), 47 had pulp atrophy (10%), 41 had paresthesia (8%), and 14 patients had intractable pain (3%). Chen and colleagues[26] applied the Cold Intolerance Severity Scoring Scale (0–100) to measure the severity of cold intolerance and found a mean score of 31 among 30 cases of single-digit replantations.[26] Wu and colleagues[33] used their own scoring system and found that, among 35 patients, 25 patients reported no cold intolerance, 5 with mild intolerance, 3 with moderate, and 1 with severe symptoms. In a systematic review of distal digit replantation (flexor zone 1) studies, Sebastin and Chung[6] found 87 cases reporting pulp atrophy and 156 cases of nail deformity among 683 cases with long-term follow-up. Hattori and colleagues[7] assessed for presence of pain (2), paresthesia (7), and cold intolerance (8) for 23 successful replantation cases of injury at Tamai zones I or II. For transmetacarpal replantation, 100% of patients with some recovery of sensibility reported experiencing

Table 6
Two-point discrimination test results (mm), by level of injury

Authors	Tamai I	Distal Phalanx	Middle Phalanx	PIP Joint	Proximal Phalanx	Metacarpus	Metacarpus to Distal Forearm
Boeckx et al,[23] 1992	—	—	15.9	24.9	17.5	18.5	—
Wu et al,[33] 2018	7.7	—	—	—	—	—	—
Hahn and Jung,[34] 2006	7	—	—	—	—	—	—
Sebastin et al,[6] 2011	—	7	—	—	—	—	—
Paavilainen et al,[18] 2007	—	—	—	—	—	14.7	—
Assouline et al,[25] 2017	—	—	—	—	—	—	14.1

Table 7
Two-point discrimination test results (mm), by digit type

Authors	Overall	Ring Finger
Woo et al,[35] 2015	11.7	—
Chen et al,[26] 2018	10.4	—
Adani et al,[24] 2013[a]	—	185
Sears and Chung,[17] 2011[a]	—	174
Bamba et al,[28] 2018[ab]	—	179

[a] These studies only studied ring avulsion injuries.
[b] Subgroup analysis showed mean 2PD of 5.6 mm for Urbaniak class I (circulation adequate) injuries, 8.3 mm for class II (circulation inadequate), and 10.5 mm for class III (complete degloving or complete amputation).

cold intolerance, but 50% reported diminishing symptoms within 5 years.[18]

PATIENT-REPORTED OUTCOMES AFTER REPLANTATION

Patient-reported outcome measures provide an insight to patients' experience and their subjective evaluation of the care received. It is especially important for interventions such as digit replantation that takes the wish of patient into consideration for surgical decision making.[40] By evaluating a patient's experience, providers can assess the benefits of treatment from the perspective of the very recipients of the treatment.[41] Important data, such as the ability to perform activities of daily living, quality of life, and satisfaction, can only be obtained from the patient.[42] Assessment of patient-reported outcomes is essential for a complete evaluation of the efficacy of digit replantation.

There are numerous questionnaires to measure patient-reported outcomes in health care, with varying levels of appropriateness for different diseases and interventions. For instance, there are more than 15 different types of health-related quality-of-life scales that can be used in hand surgery.[10] Among many, the Michigan Hand Outcomes Questionnaire (MHQ)[43] and the Disabilities of the Arm and Shoulder (DASH) Questionnaire[44] have been found to be valid and reliable in the assessment of patient-reported outcomes related to care received for hand trauma.[45] For a robust collection and comprehensive analysis of data, these questionnaires should be administered at multiple time points during the treatment process.

The Michigan Hand Outcomes Questionnaire

The MHQ is a 37-item questionnaire with individual scales for overall hand function, activities of daily living, work performance, pain, aesthetics, and satisfaction with hand function. In each scale, higher scores denote better hand performance, with the exception of the pain scale that equates high scores with greater pain. The raw scale score for each of the 6 scales is the sum of responses normalized by numerical normalizing algorithms. The raw score can be converted to a score ranging between 0 and 100. Each hand is assessed separately. If both hands are affected, the right hand scores and left hand scores can be averaged.[43]

Zhu and colleagues[27] assessed patient-reported outcomes via the MHQ for single-digit replantation by digit type and level of injury (**Table 8**). They found higher scores for more distal level of injury for each digit. They also compared the MHQ scores of each subgroup to the amputation cases that underwent revision amputation and found superior results for thumb and index finger at all levels of injury, and at more proximal levels for middle (level II–V) and ring (level IV and V) finger replantation. Similar results were seen in the study by Kamarul and colleagues,[46] with mean MHQ scores for digit level injuries (thumb 67.6 and

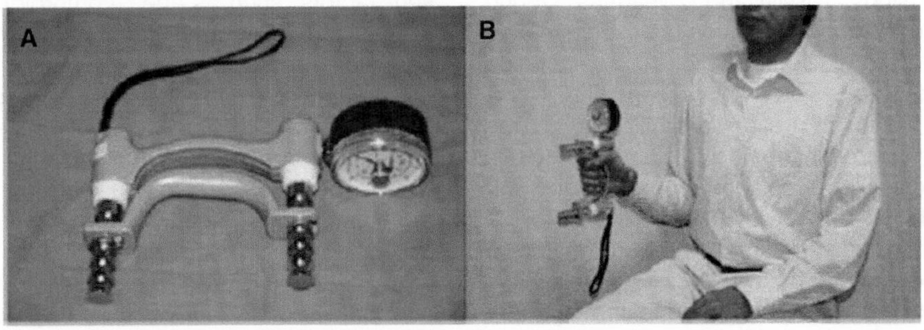

Fig. 5. Measuring grip strength with a Jamar dynamometer. (*A*) Instrument at position 2. (*B*) Standard patient position. (*From* Han SH, Nam KS, Cho YS, et al. Normative data on hand grip strength. J Nov Physiother 2011;1:102; and *Courtesy of* ASP Global, Atlanta, GA.)

Table 8
Patient-reported outcomes by injured digit and level of injury

	Thumb		Index		Middle		Ring		Small	
Tamai Level[a]	Cases (N)	MHQ Score	Cases (N)	MHQ Score	Cases (N)	MHQ Score	Cases (N)	MHQ Score	Cases (N)	MHQ Score
I	11	91.3 ± 5.6	5	95.4 ± 4.1	6	94.5 ± 4.7	5	96.5 ± 6.1	4	95.6 ± 4.9
II	27	92.1 ± 6.8	8	96.1 ± 3.7	7	95.1 ± 4.8	12	95.7 ± 6.2	10	95.2 ± 7.9
III	41	88.9 ± 8.2	11	88.2 ± 9.6	9	88.5 ± 11.2	10	87.2 ± 6.8	11	91.3 ± 6.8
IV	0	—	15	85.4 ± 12.9	14	84.3 ± 9.9	11	84.1 ± 13.5	12	91.3 ± 7.8
V	33	83.0 ± 10.5	11	83.5 ± 12.1	8	84.1 ± 7.6	6	82.9 ± 4.7	23	88.6 ± 11.5

[a] Higher MHQ scores indicate better hand function.

From Zhu H, Bao B, Zheng X. A comparison of functional outcomes and therapeutic costs: single-digit replantation versus revision amputation. Plast Reconstr Surg 2018;141(2):244e–9e; with permission.

fingers 72.0) being higher than proximal injuries at the palm (50.0) or at the wrist (52.8).

The Disabilities of the Arm and Shoulder

The DASH questionnaire consists of 30 questions that assess the symptoms and functional status of patients with upper extremity diseases or injuries, on a 5-point Likert scale. The components included for symptoms are pain, weakness, stiffness, and paresthesia. A physical performance evaluation is based on the patient's ability to perform daily activities, house/yard chores, shopping/errands, recreational activities, self-care, dressing, eating, sleep, and sports/performing arts. For social functional status evaluation, the questions address family care, occupation, and socializing with friends and relatives. Psychological well-being is assessed by self-image. There are assigned values for each of the possible responses, and they can be summed and converted to a score between 0 and 100, with higher scores indicating more severe disability.[47]

A review of 30 single-digit replantation cases by Chen and colleagues[26] found the mean DASH score to be 6.6, indicating good hand functionality. In another study, Tessler and colleagues[48] found superior scores for replantation (24.0) versus revision amputation (21.9). Within the replantation group, dominant side replantation (29.7) was found to result in greater disability compared with the non-dominant-side replantation (18.0). For more distal level replantation, Hattori and colleagues[7] found a mean DASH score of 2 for 23 successful fingertip replantation cases. This result echoes the findings by the studies that used the MHQ, that distal digit replantations show greater functional recovery than those more proximal. In comparison with the scores from the revision amputation group (mean DASH score 7), the successful replantation was correlated with better functional status.

Some studies used the Quick DASH questionnaire, an abbreviated version of the DASH with adequate validity and reliability. The Quick DASH also generates a score between 0 and 100, with 100 indicating greater disability.[47] Rosberg[39] used this tool to evaluate 326 replantation cases and found a mean score of 11.4. In subgroup analyses, higher Quick DASH scores were found for more proximal levels (wrist 43.2, proximal to wrist 29.5) compared with middle hand level (13.6). There was no difference in Quick DASH scores for thumb (9.1) and finger (9.1) replantations. Kamarul and colleagues[46] showed lower Quick DASH scores for finger (26.3) than thumb (30.1), but the digit level replantations were associated with better functional status than more proximal level replantations (palm 60.2, wrist 56.3).

FACTORS INFLUENCING OUTCOMES AFTER REPLANTATION

There are multiple factors that influence the outcome of replantation surgery in the hand. Patient factors, such as age,[4] comorbidities, especially those that compromise peripheral perfusion, such as diabetes, autoimmune diseases, and collagen vascular diseases,[2,49] have been reported to influence outcomes. Hustedt and colleagues[50] found that patients with more than 3 comorbidities had a significantly higher rate of failed replantation, and greater relative risk of failure among patients with peripheral vascular diseases. Multiple studies found significant difference in rate of replant survival for patients who smoked and those who did not,[49,51] with 3 times higher odds of successful replantation for non-smokers.[14]

Level of injury and the mechanism of injury have also been mentioned by multiple expert hand surgeons to influence outcomes after replantation.[2,4,8,15] In fact, the characteristics of the amputation heavily influence the level of clinical indication for replantation.[4,8] Soucacos[2] stated that functional outcomes after replantation for injury in flexor zone 1 and 3 tend to be better than those in zone 2, because of intact FDS in zone 1 and better vascular supply by superficial or deep palmar arch in zone 3 compared with common digital arteries in zone 2 (**Fig. 6**). Multiple studies have found superior outcomes for arc of motion, grip strength, and subjective functional recovery for distal digit replantation compared with more proximal injuries.[5,7,17,23,24,27,39] Clean-cut, or guillotine, amputations have been noted to produce better outcomes.[2–4,15,51]

Many experts have stated that ischemia time heavily influences the survival of replant and the long-term functional outcomes.[2,3,46,51] In digit replantation consideration, Soucacos suggested a maximum of 8 hours for warm ischemia and 30 hours for cold ischemia. However, with advances in microsurgery, more recent studies have published noninferior outcomes for cases with prolonged ischemia times.[22] Rather than conducting the replantation procedure during the night when the surgeon is tired or the team assembled is not familiar with the instrumentation, delayed elective replantation in working hours provides the most optimal condition for performing this tedious and intricate procedure. Woo and colleagues[35] have found that total survival rate in delayed replantation (88%) was not statistically different from the survival rate in immediate replantation (84%). Furthermore, they evaluated the delayed replantation cases by Chen's criteria and found good (grade II) and excellent (grade I) functional recovery. Cavadas and colleagues[52] analyzed 597 digit replantation cases and found similar survival rates between the immediate replantation group (91%) and delayed replantation group (93%).

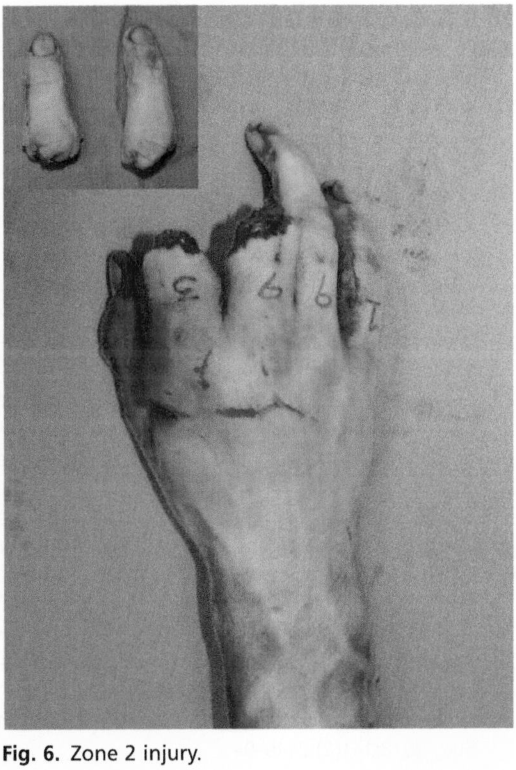

Fig. 6. Zone 2 injury.

Factors on the provider side, such as surgeon skill and experience and facility's level of excellence, have been noted to influence outcomes after replantation.[2,4,7,8] Surgeons with more than 10 years of experience had higher rate of survival (68%) in digit replantation compared with surgeons with 5 to 9 years of experience (57%) and less than 5 years of experience (49%).[14] Related to surgical expertise, Hahn and Jung[34] found that higher number of vascular anastomoses completed during replantation correlated with higher rates of survival. They reported a 68% rate of survival for 1 arterial anastomosis group, 82% for 1 arterial and 1 venous anastomoses group, 95% for 1 arterial and 2 venous anastomoses group, and 99% for 2 or more arterial and 2 venous anastomoses group.

Hospitals with high case volume have demonstrated higher rates of replant survival, along with higher odds of success.[12,13,53,54] For thumb replantation, hospitals with 20 cases or more showed 2 times higher odds of success.[53] Moreover, digit replantation performed by high-volume surgeons (>5 cases per year) at high-volume hospitals (>20 cases per year) had 2.5 times greater likelihood of survival.[12] Brown and colleagues[13] showed that a minimum of 3 cases per year was required for a hospital to achieve a 70% rate of success with digit replantation. Efforts toward regionalization for replantation in the hand will likely improve outcomes.

A patient's level of commitment and adherence to rehabilitation protocols can directly influence the outcomes of replantation. In addition, it appears that validated outcomes are strongly influenced by depression and anxiety.[55,56] Depression is correlated with the severity of trauma perception after replantation.[57] A recent study by Efanov and colleagues[58] showed that use of patient-advisors in the rehabilitation period helped improve functional recovery and quality of life, because the group of patients with patient-advisors showed superior DASH scores (29.6 vs 34.8).

SUMMARY

Functional outcomes and patient-reported outcomes together assess the benefits of replantation for amputation injuries in the hand. However, the current literature does not provide high-quality evidence, owing to the variability in the outcomes reported, instruments used to measure, and means of reporting data. In addition, many studies do not include details of the confounding factors that influence outcomes. Establishing a standard for outcomes evaluation and reporting will help patients and surgeons make informed treatment decisions based on evidence.

REFERENCES

1. Giladi AM, McGlinn EP, Shauver MJ, et al. Measuring outcomes and determining long-term disability after revision amputation for treatment of traumatic finger and thumb amputation injuries. Plast Reconstr Surg 2014;134(5):746e–55e.
2. Soucacos PN. Indications and selection for digital amputation and replantation. J Hand Surg Br 2001; 26(6):572–81.
3. Mulders MA, Neuhaus V, Becker SJ, et al. Replantation and revascularization vs. amputation in injured digits. Hand (N Y) 2013;8(3):267–73.
4. Weiland AJ, Villarreal-Rios A, Kleinert HE, et al. Replantation of digits and hands: analysis of surgical techniques and functional results in 71 patients with 86 replantations. Clin Orthop Relat Res 1978;(133):195–204.
5. Buntic RF, Brooks D, Buncke GM. Index finger salvage with replantation and revascularization: revisiting conventional wisdom. Microsurgery 2008; 28(8):612–6.
6. Sebastin SJ, Chung KC. A systematic review of the outcomes of replantation of distal digital amputation. Plast Reconstr Surg 2011;128(3):723–37.
7. Hattori Y, Doi K, Ikeda K, et al. A retrospective study of functional outcomes after successful replantation versus amputation closure for single fingertip amputations. J Hand Surg Am 2006;31(5):811–8.
8. Bueno RA Jr, Battiston B, Ciclamini D, et al. Replantation: current concepts and outcomes. Clin Plast Surg 2014;41(3):385–95.
9. Ozer K, Kramer W, Gillani S, et al. Replantation versus revision of amputated fingers in patients air-transported to a level 1 trauma center. J Hand Surg Am 2010;35(6):936–40.
10. Sebastin SJ, Chung KC. Challenges in measuring outcomes following digital replantation. Semin Plast Surg 2013;27(4):174–81.
11. Charles HM, Thorne GCG, Chung KC, et al. Grabb and Smith's plastic surgery. 7th edition. Philadelphia: Wolters Kluwer; 2013.
12. Hustedt JW, Bohl DD, Champagne L. The detrimental effect of decentralization in digital replantation in the united states: 15 years of evidence from the national inpatient sample. J Hand Surg Am 2016;41(5):593–601.
13. Brown M, Lu Y, Chung KC, et al. Annual hospital volume and success of digital replantation. Plast Reconstr Surg 2017;139(3):672–80.
14. Fufa D, Calfee R, Wall L, et al. Digit replantation: experience of two U.S. academic level-I trauma centers. J Bone Joint Surg Am 2013;95(23):2127–34.
15. Tamai S. Twenty years' experience of limb replantation–review of 293 upper extremity replants. J Hand Surg Am 1982;7(6):549–56.
16. Dec W. A meta-analysis of success rates for digit replantation. Tech Hand Up Extrem Surg 2006; 10(3):124–9.
17. Sears ED, Chung KC. Replantation of finger avulsion injuries: a systematic review of survival and functional outcomes. J Hand Surg Am 2011;36(4):686–94.
18. Paavilainen P, Nietosvaara Y, Tikkinen KA, et al. Long-term results of transmetacarpal replantation. J Plast Reconstr Aesthet Surg 2007;60(7):704–9.
19. Pratt AL, Ball C. What are we measuring? A critique of range of motion methods currently in use for Dupuytren's disease and recommendations for practice. BMC Musculoskelet Disord 2016;17:20.
20. Adams LS, Topoozian E, Green LW. Range of motion. In: Casanova JS, editor. Clinical assessment recommendations. 2nd edition. Chicago (IL): American Society of Hand Therapists; 1992.
21. Urbaniak JR, Roth JH, Nunley JA, et al. The results of replantation after amputation of a single finger. J Bone Joint Surg Am 1985;67(4):611–9.
22. Jazayeri L, Klausner JQ, Chang J. Distal digital replantation. Plast Reconstr Surg 2013;132(5): 1207–17.
23. Boeckx W, Jacobs W, Guelinckx P, et al. Late results in replanted digits. Is replantation of a single digit worthwhile? Acta Chir Belg 1992;92(4): 204–8.
24. Adani R, Pataia E, Tarallo L, et al. Results of replantation of 33 ring avulsion amputations. J Hand Surg Am 2013;38(5):947–56.
25. Assouline U, Feuvrier D, Lepage D, et al. Functional assessment and quality of life in patients following replantation of the distal half of the forearm (except fingers): a review of 11 cases. Hand Surg Rehabil 2017;36(4):261–7.
26. Chen J, Zhang AX, Chen QZ, et al. Long-term functional, subjective and psychological results after single digit replantation. Acta Orthop Traumatol Turc 2018;52(2):120–6.
27. Zhu H, Bao B, Zheng X. A comparison of functional outcomes and therapeutic costs: single-digit replantation versus revision amputation. Plast Reconstr Surg 2018;141(2):244e–9e.

28. Bamba R, Malhotra G, Bueno RA Jr, et al. Ring avulsion injuries: a systematic review. Hand (N Y) 2018; 13(1):15–22.
29. Lundborg G, Rosen B. The two-point discrimination test–time for a re-appraisal? J Hand Surg Br 2004; 29(5):418–22.
30. Rea P. Spinal tracts – ascending/sensory pathways [Chapter 8]. In: Rea P, editor. Essential clinical anatomy of the nervous system. San Diego (CA): Academic Press; 2015. p. 133–60.
31. Shaffer S, Harrison A, Brown K, et al. Reliability and validity of Semmes-Weinstein Monofilament testing in older community-dwelling adults. J Geriatr Phys Ther 2005;28(3):112–3.
32. Feng Y, Schlösser FJ, Sumpio BE. The Semmes Weinstein monofilament examination as a screening tool for diabetic peripheral neuropathy. J Vasc Surg 2009;50(3):675–82, 682.e1.
33. Wu F, Shen X, Eberlin KR, et al. The use of arteriovenous anastomosis for venous drainage during Tamai zone I fingertip replantation. Injury 2018;49(6):1113–8.
34. Hahn HO, Jung SG. Results of replantation of amputated fingertips in 450 patients. J Reconstr Microsurg 2006;22(6):407–13.
35. Woo SH, Cheon HJ, Kim YW, et al. Delayed and suspended replantation for complete amputation of digits and hands. J Hand Surg Am 2015;40(5):883–9.
36. Trampisch US, Franke J, Jedamzik N, et al. Optimal jamar dynamometer handle position to assess maximal isometric hand grip strength in epidemiological studies. J Hand Surg Am 2012;37(11):2368–73.
37. Roberts HC, Denison HJ, Martin HJ, et al. A review of the measurement of grip strength in clinical and epidemiological studies: towards a standardised approach. Age Ageing 2011;40(4):423–9.
38. Han SH, Nam KS, Cho YS, et al. Normative data on hand grip strength. J Nov Physiother 2011;1:102.
39. Rosberg H-E. Disability and health after replantation or revascularisation in the upper extremity in a population in southern Sweden – a retrospective long time follow up. BMC Musculoskelet Disord 2014;15:73.
40. Anker SD, Agewall S, Borggrefe M, et al. The importance of patient-reported outcomes: a call for their comprehensive integration in cardiovascular clinical trials. Eur Heart J 2014;35(30):2001–9.
41. Weldring T, Smith SMS. Patient-reported outcomes (PROs) and patient-reported outcome measures (PROMs). Health Serv Insights 2013;6:61–8.
42. Deshpande PR, Rajan S, Sudeepthi BL, et al. Patient-reported outcomes: a new era in clinical research. Perspect Clin Res 2011;2(4):137–44.
43. Chung KC, Pillsbury MS, Walters MR, et al. Reliability and validity testing of the Michigan Hand Outcomes Questionnaire. J Hand Surg Am 1998;23(4):575–87.
44. Hudak PL, Amadio PC, Bombardier C. Development of an upper extremity outcome measure: the DASH (disabilities of the arm, shoulder and hand) [corrected]. The Upper Extremity Collaborative Group (UECG). Am J Ind Med 1996;29(6):602–8.
45. Alderman AK, Chung KC. Measuring outcomes in hand surgery. Clin Plast Surg 2008;35(2):239–50.
46. Kamarul T, Mansor A, Robson N, et al. Replantation and revascularization of amputated upper limb appendages outcome and predicting the factors influencing the success rates of these procedures in a tertiary hospital: an 8-year retrospective, cross-sectional study. J Orthop Surg (Hong Kong) 2018; 26(1). 2309499017749983.
47. The DASH outcome measure. Institute for Work & Health. Available at: http://www.dash.iwh.on.ca/. Accessed July 15, 2018.
48. Tessler O, Bartow MJ, Tremblay-Champagne MP, et al. Long-term health-related quality of life outcomes in digital replantation versus revision amputation. J Reconstr Microsurg 2017;33(6):446–51.
49. Shale CM, Tidwell JE 3rd, Mulligan RP, et al. A nationwide review of the treatment patterns of traumatic thumb amputations. Ann Plast Surg 2013;70(6):647–51.
50. Hustedt JW, Chung A, Bohl DD, et al. Evaluating the effect of comorbidities on the success, risk, and cost of digital replantation. J Hand Surg Am 2016;41(12): 1145–52.e1.
51. Waikakul S, Vanadurongwan V, Unnanuntana A. Prognostic factors for major limb re-implantation at both immediate and long-term follow-up. J Bone Joint Surg Br 1998;80(6):1024–30.
52. Cavadas PC, Rubi C, Thione A, et al. Immediate versus overnight-delayed digital replantation: comparative retrospective cohort study of survival outcomes. J Hand Surg Am 2018;43(7):625–30.
53. Mahmoudi E, Chung KC. Effect of hospital volume on success of thumb replantation. J Hand Surg Am 2017;42(2):96–103.e5.
54. Mahmoudi E, Huetteman HE, Chung KC. A population-based study of replantation after traumatic thumb amputation, 2007-2012. J Hand Surg Am 2017;42(1):25–33.e6.
55. Niekel MC, Lindenhovius AL, Watson JB, et al. Correlation of Dash and QuickDASH with measures of psychological distress. J Hand Surg Am 2009; 34(8):1499–505.
56. Ring D, Kadzielski J, Fabian L, et al. Self-reported upper extremity health status correlates with depression. J Bone Joint Surg Am 2006;88(9):1983–8.
57. Gokce A, Bekler H, Karacaoglu E, et al. Anxiety and trauma perception and quality of life in patients who have undergone replantation. J Reconstr Microsurg 2011;27(8):475–80.
58. Efanov JI, Papanastasiou C, Arsenault J, et al. Contribution of patient-advisors during rehabilitation for replantation of digits improves patient-reported functional outcomes: a presentation of concept. Hand Surg Rehabil 2018. https://doi.org/10.1016/j.hansur.2018.04.002.

Postoperative Management and Rehabilitation of the Replanted or Revascularized Digit

Adnan Prsic, MD[a,*], Jeffrey B. Friedrich, MD, MC[b]

KEYWORDS

• Replantation • Revascularization • Rehabilitation • Postoperative care

KEY POINTS

- Survival of a replanted digit without function does not equal success. Successful replantation includes a digit with adequate stability, range of motion, and sensibility.
- Completion amputation or ray amputation should be considered seriously if replantation will lead to an unstable, stiff, and insensate digit.
- Postoperative monitoring is performed with clinical examination with a focus on temperature, skin color, turgor, edema, and vascular patency, using a hand-held arterial and venous Doppler.
- Vigilance in the postoperative period is critical for the survival of the replanted digit. Arterial occlusion should be expediently explored in the operating room with revision of the vascular anastomosis.
- Digital motion rehabilitation should start after 5 to 7 days of digital viability and splinting of the affected digit. Early protective motion protocol is implemented to maintain digital motion with emphasis on tendon glide and joint motion while preventing micromotion of the osteosynthesis site.

INTRODUCTION

Major advances have been made in digital replantation since the early days when Susumi Tamai[1] of Nara, Japan, performed the first successful digital replantation by vascular anastomosis on July 7, 1965. Current literature cites survival rates of replanted digits anywhere from 57% to 90%, with most replantations being performed at urban academic centers.[2–4]

The purpose of digital replantation and revascularization should be to provide functional outcomes that allow purposeful utilization of the digit with adequate stability, range of motion, and sensibility. On the 1 hand, survival of a replanted digit by itself may be a triumph of surgical technique or careful case selection. On the other hand, one could argue that survival without adequate function does not equal a success but rather a failure in reconstruction. It is, therefore, prudent that postoperative care, including potential complications, rehabilitation, expected function, and limitations, are discussed with the patient preoperatively. The alternative treatment that some may elect is a completion amputation or even ray amputation of the affected digit, and possibly a prosthetic replacement.

The postoperative management begins with preoperative evaluation and informed consent. A

Disclosure Statement: No disclosures.

[a] Plastic and Reconstructive Surgery, Yale School of Medicine, PO Box 208041, New Haven, CT 06520-8041, USA; [b] Orthopaedics, Division of Plastic Surgery, University of Washington, Harborview Medical Center, Seattle Children's Hospital, 325 9th Avenue, Box 359796, Seattle, WA 98104, USA

* Corresponding author. Boardman Building, 3rd Floor, 330 Cedar Street, New Haven, CT 06510.

E-mail address: adnan.prsic@yale.edu

Hand Clin 35 (2019) 221–229

https://doi.org/10.1016/j.hcl.2019.01.003

0749-0712/19/

standard informed consent should include a discussion about postoperative outcomes ranging from successful replantation to arterial and/or venous thrombosis, which could result in necrosis of the digit. The patient should also be informed about more severe complications, such as stroke, myocardial infarction, and even death. Emphasis should be placed on creating an appropriate plan based on the condition or extent of damage of the amputated segment, intraoperative findings, and the technique used for revascularization (eg. primary anastomosis vs vein graft). The postoperative approach for sharp amputations with minimal crush or avulsion components consists of close monitoring and aggressive intervention. One should be equally vigilant about postoperative monitoring and aggressive with operative exploration for pediatric patients, thumb replantations, and multiple digit replantations (**Figs. 1** and **2**).

For injuries of multiple digits and/or thumbs with extensive endothelial damage and large zones of injury that have high probability of failure even after exploration or vascular anastomosis revision, the hand surgeon might be less aggressive in the postoperative period and not consider reexploration as an option in the event of thrombosis. The hand surgeon must ensure that the patient is aware of the prognosis and agrees with the postoperative plan before proceeding with the replantation.

IMMEDIATE POSTOPERATIVE MONITORING PROTOCOL

Patients are typically admitted to a general inpatient floor unless there are concerns for systemic medical issues, in which event the patients are admitted to a higher care level unit, such as an intermediate unit or a surgical intensive care unit. Clinical examination for evaluation of temperature, skin color, turgor, edema, and vascular patency with a handheld arterial and venous Doppler are performed hourly during the first 48 hours, then every 2 hours during postoperative day 3, according to the authors' protocol. Examinations are performed by trained nursing staff, house-staff (residents and fellows), and surgeons.

IMMEDIATE POSTOPERATIVE PHARMACOLOGIC AND ENVIRONMENTAL SUPPORT

Postoperative environmental conditions during the first 72 hours and beyond consist of a comfortable room temperature setting for the patient. The use of heated rooms and other warming adjuncts, such as heating lamps, pads, or forced air warming blankets, is discouraged. There is no evidence to support improved success rates in microsurgical procedures with environmental heating. On the contrary, the risk of burns have been reported with use of thermal lamps in hand surgery.[5]

Similarly, there is only anecdotal evidence of caffeine intake leading to peripheral vasoconstriction, decreased tissue perfusion, and subsequent loss of replanted digits. No evidence against caffeine has borne out of studies (although existing studies are not adequately powered to demonstrate clinical equivalence). The authors do not enforce a strict caffeine-free diet postreplantation.[6–8]

Clinical observations have suggested that antithrombotic therapy reduces the morbidity after microsurgical free tissue transfers.[9] It was proposed as early as 1978 by Ketchum[10] that the outcome of microvascular free tissue transfer could be improved by the addition of agents that decrease platelet function, increase blood flow, decrease blood viscosity, and counteract the effects of thrombin on platelets and fibrinogen. Literature shows that microvascular venous thrombi contained more fibrin than platelets and the opposite in arterial thrombi, theoretically making aspirin

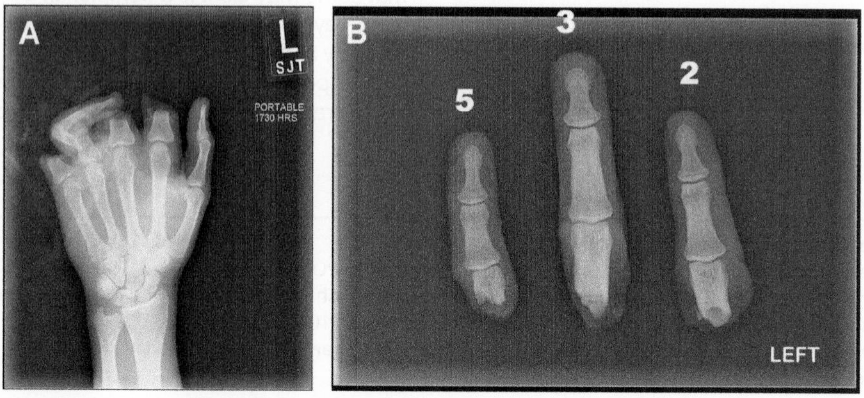

Fig. 1. Multiple digit amputation. (*A*) AP radiograph of left hand. (*B*) Radiograph of amputated digits.

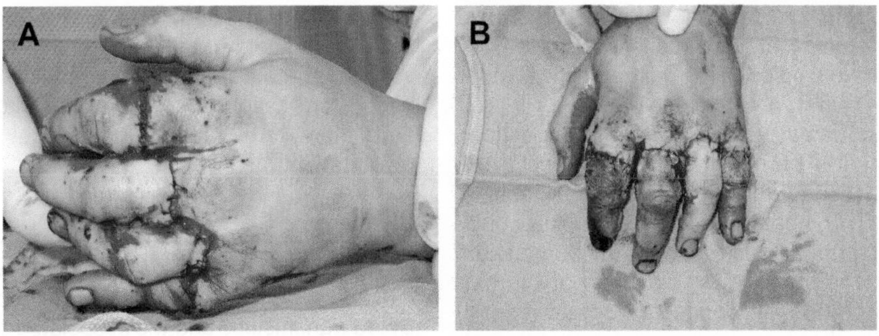

Fig. 2. Intraoperative photographs of replanted digits (*A*) with adequate perfusion, (*B*) with congestion and failure of index finger.

the preferred agent for arterial thrombosis and heparin the better anticoagulant for venous thrombosis.[11,12] The authors follow Buckley and Hammert's[13] recommended daily administration of 325 mg of aspirin and, if not contraindicated due to systemic illness, subcutaneous heparin or low molecular weight heparin for deep venous thrombosis prophylaxis.

COMPLICATIONS

Complications of replantation leading to replant failure or functional impairment can be grouped into 2 categories: early (<72 h) and late (>72 h). Acute problems may include failure to reestablish venous outflow, no reflow or ischemia reperfusion injury, venous occlusion, and arterial occlusion. Late or chronic complications are infections, such as cellulitis, localized abscess, and osteomyelitis. Nonunion and tendon adhesions requiring tenolysis are also long-term complications arising after replantation. However, the most common complications are arterial and venous thrombosis. Arterial thromboses are found in some series to be 3 times as common as venous but have favorable outcomes in the setting of complications.[14] The salvage rate of digital replantations complicated by arterial thrombosis is noted to be 30%, whereas it is only 7% for venous occlusion.[14]

Venous Occlusion or Congestion

Venous occlusion and congestion is caused by intrinsic occlusion or extrinsic compression of the vascular anastomosis and areas distal or proximal to it. In cases of intrinsic occlusion, venous thrombi form at the anastomosis or at other areas within the zone of injury (**Fig. 3**). When there is intraoperative venous insufficiency, one should explore and revise the venous anastomosis. Meticulous technique is necessary because trauma to the blood vessel and exposure of subendothelial structures to blood flow within the microvasculature leads to increase in thrombus formation.[15] In some instances after intraoperative revision of venous anastomosis, the hand surgeon may add subcutaneous or intravenous heparin as a postoperative agent. A retrospective study in free flaps by Khouri and colleagues[16] has shown decrease incidence of flap failure with subcutaneous heparin injection. This has, however, not been confirmed in digital replantation.[17,18] Despite common use of intravenous heparin by many centers, the data on the benefit of heparin administration in digital replantation are lacking.

Algorithms for pharmacologic thromboprophylaxis for free flaps and microsurgical anastomoses are published based on reviews of level 3, level 4, and level 5 evidence.[19] The lack of data and well-executed studies on the efficacy of such agents on replantation, free tissue transfers, and microvascular anastomoses does not justify routine administration.[20] Additionally, the increased risk of complications, such as bleeding with heparin, and cerebral or pulmonary edema and anaphylaxis with dextran, make them unattractive candidates for routine thromboprophylaxis.[18,21] Based on

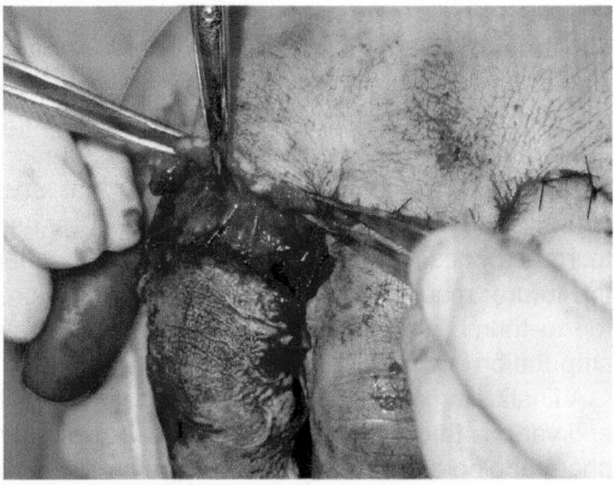

Fig. 3. Thrombosis of distal dorsal vein of index finger at anastomotic site.

published data on dextran complications, and because of complications experienced by the authors, we have ceased using dextran as a postreplantation adjunct.

With postoperative signs of venous congestion, the first step is the removal of the dressing or splint and, subsequently, skin sutures to release any extrinsic compression of the veins that could be causing outflow obstruction. Mild congestion can also be improved with elevation of the extremity. For moderate congestion that does not resolve with these measures, one may attempt leech therapy to reduce venous pressure, assist with the outflow, and exploit the mechanism of hirudin in the inhibition of thrombin and formation of microvascular thrombi. If congestion worsens or does not resolve with leech therapy, the patient may be returned to the operating room for exploration. In general, we reexplore venous-congested thumb and hand or arm replantations but, typically, do not reexplore venous congested digits that are not thumbs. We also reexplore any replantation with signs of arterial compromise.

Arterial Occlusion

Arterial occlusion can be extrinsic or intrinsic. As with venous congestion, one's first step should be the removal of dressing or splint and, subsequently, skin sutures to release any extrinsic compression of the vessels. Optimization of blood pressure, blood volume, and hydration status should also be considered. Capillary refill, skin temperature, and vascular Doppler monitoring is used in such cases to confirm the lack or presence of blood flow. If no increase in blood flow is achieved by optimizing these measures, the patient is returned to the operating room for exploration. Arterial ischemia due to thrombosis is an emergency and requires exploration and likely revision of the anastomosis to salvage the digit. This is typically accomplished with resection of the thrombosed area with subsequent primary anastomosis or vein graft. In the case of thrombus requiring a large area of resection not suitable for vein grafting, we perform a completion amputation with a loose closure. Careful debridement and preservation of surrounding soft tissue, periosteum or bones, tendons, and nerves is essential for future reconstruction, whether pollicization, toe-to-thumb transfer, or simply a digital ray amputation is considered.

A final treatment option in the salvage of arterial and venous thrombosis is the use of intravascular pharmacologic thrombolysis with agents such as streptokinase, urokinase, recombinant tissue plasminogen activator, and acylated plasminogen-streptokinase-activator complex. The authors currently do not recommend treatment with intravascular thrombolysis because most evidence is based on case reports for free flap salvage and there are none for salvage of digital replantation.[22–28]

Bleeding

Digital replantation can be associated with significant intraoperative and postoperative blood loss. Blood transfusions and the associated adverse effects (eg, viral transmission, allergic or febrile reactions, acute hemolysis) can result from large blood volume replacement. Buntic and Brooks[29] showed that, with artery-only replantations of the distal fingertip in which iatrogenic bleeding was maintained for venous outflow, 58% of subjects received blood transfusions. The average transfusion was 1.8 units ranging from 0 to 9 units. In such cases, close monitoring of hemoglobin or hematocrit and vital signs is recommended. Multiple daily examinations of the replanted digit should also be made part of the treatment plan because blood can be concealed in bulky dressings. Continued administration of anticoagulants for baseline comorbidities or, specifically, for the replantation of a digit or digits can contribute to increased bleeding. In a study by Furnas and colleagues,[30] multiple-agent anticoagulation therapy in addition to administration of aspirin was shown to produce a greater drop in the hematocrit than single-agent therapy (15% vs 6%). Only 2% of the subjects receiving a single agent had a blood transfusion compared with 53% of the subjects receiving multiple agents. Similar findings were also published by Nikolis and colleagues,[18] in which routine use of intravenous heparin following digital replantation and revascularization was found to have increased rate of side effects but was found to have similar outcomes in subjects not receiving intravenous heparin.

Replant Failure

In cases of distal replantation in which replant failure is obvious by ischemia and development of necrosis, the digit is often allowed to fully demarcate before performing a completion amputation or plan for further reconstruction (**Fig. 4**). In cases of single distal replantation failure that is not for a thumb, a delayed ray resection after revision amputation is recommended. That is, we do not routinely perform immediate ray amputation and prefer to perform a completion amputation and then consider a ray resection secondarily. For more proximal replant failures, an immediate revision amputation is considered. For replantation

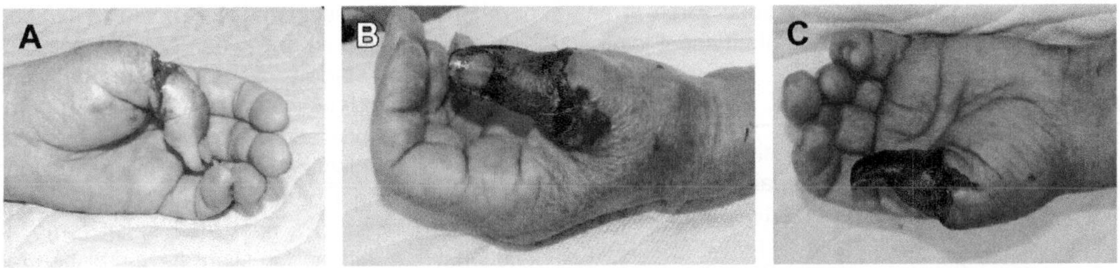

Fig. 4. Revascularization failure of thumb. (*A*) Preoperative photograph. (*B, C*) Necrosis or mummification of the thumb.

failures of the thumb, treatment options to be considered are toe-to-thumb transfer or a prosthetic for low-demand patients (**Fig. 5**).

Infection

The exact incidence of infectious complications in digital replantations has not been established. Given the contaminated nature of the injuries that result in amputation, the hand surgeon should be on high alert for infection, which typically is most common at postoperative days 5 to 7. Generally, replantation patients are administered antibiotic prophylaxis for 48 hours unless there is heavy contamination, in which case 7 days of antibiotics are administered. Venous thrombosis can occur in the setting of infection if not quickly discovered and treated. Specifically, infections secondary to leech therapy in the early course can lead to loss of the replanted digit and even septicemia.[31] Recent publications have reported increasing antibiotic resistance of *Aeromonas hydrophila.*[32,33] Therefore, high suspicion should be kept even in the setting of prophylactic treatment with ciprofloxacin.

Pin track infections remain common with the use of Kirschner wires (K-wires) because they are a common mode of fixation for digital replantations. The rate of infections noted in the literature ranges from 7% for buried versus 17.6% for exposed K-wires. Long-term complications, such as osteomyelitis, are not common but should be considered in chronic wounds with a history of pin track infections.[34,35]

Skeletal Complications

Skeletal stability is an essential component for a successful replantation. Therefore, nonunion can hinder rehabilitation and lead to significant functional impairment. Nonunion is cited to occur anywhere from 3% to 31% of the time based on the location of the injury.[36–40] Replanted bone is somewhat slow to heal, as seen on radiographs. For this reason, the authors typically wait at least 3 months before considering revision osteosynthesis if the bone is not healing appropriately. Revision surgery with bone grafting or shortening should be performed for optimal functional results. A suggested method of fixation is with crossing K-

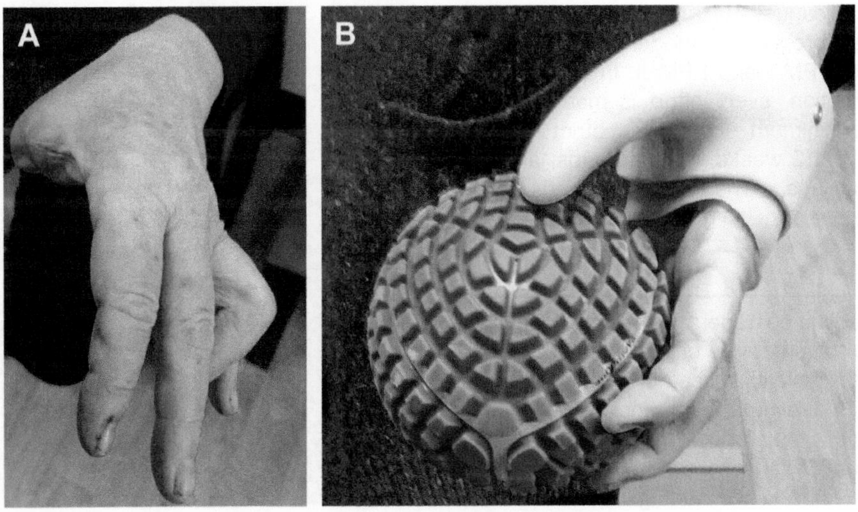

Fig. 5. (*A*) Patient after thumb completion amputation. (*B*) Patient with prosthesis.

wires (extraarticular) or interosseous wires in an attempt to avoid immobilization of adjacent joints.

Tendon Complications

Extensor and flexor tendon adhesions postreplantation can cause significant impairment in digital motion and render the replantation a functional failure. Eggli and colleagues[41] performed both extensor and flexor tenolysis. Complications of flexor tendon ruptures were reported but extensor tenolysis was found to be safe without any complications. Jupiter and colleagues[42] found tenolysis provided significant functional improvement only in replanted fingers. Replanted thumbs had poor functional outcomes even after tenolysis.

POSTOPERATIVE IMMOBILIZATION AND REHABILITATION

The goal of any digital replantation is function for daily use with adequate stability, range of motion, and sensibility. Stability and sensibility are achieved with good surgical technique and healing; however, range of motion can only be achieved with aggressive rehabilitation. Close communication between the therapist and the surgeon is also essential and requires a detailed report about the osteosynthesis, vascular repair, and tendon repair. Knowing the boundaries of rehabilitation during early stages of healing allows maximum utilization of the therapy modalities.

In the early days of digital replantation, varying philosophies on the timing of digital range of motion rehabilitation were published. Some have proposed as late as 3 to 4 weeks postoperatively to as early as 1 day.[38,43,44] An evidence-based model of early protected motion (EPM) in digital revascularization and replantation was developed by Silverman and colleagues.[45,46] The protocol is based on a graded progressive model of hand therapy in 2 stages: EPM I and EPM II. In addition to a focus on motion, every effort is made to keep edema to a minimum, starting with strict elevation during the first 2 weeks, edema wraps, and soft tissue massage when the wounds have adequately healed.

Splinting

In the immediate postoperative period, the guiding principle is to immobilize only the affected joints. The patient is typically placed in a temporary volar resting plaster splint in the intrinsic plus position, allowing sufficient room for edema to avoid compression of venous outflow and creation of dried blood cast in the setting of postoperative bleeding wounds or leech administration. Gauze or other bulky dressing material should be avoided between digits so as not to compress anastomoses. When the viability of the replanted digit has been established, typically 5 to 7 days postoperatively, the postoperative splint is converted to a custom thermoplastic splint (**Fig. 6**). In situations that require longer periods of immobilization, the patient is placed in a cast after splint removal. The wrist is positioned in slight flexion or neutral, the metacarpophalangeal (MCP) joints placed in maximum tolerated flexion (typically 30°–40°), and the interphalangeal (IP) joints placed in extension. This position facilitates easy adjustment over the course of rehabilitation as further range of motion gains are made. Soft Velcro bands are used to support the wrist, MCP, proximal interphalangeal (PIP), and distal interphalangeal (DIP) joints with the splint. Alternatively, if dorsal splints are not comfortable and create compression, a volar splint or further modifications can be made together with the therapist.

Early Protective Motion Program

Hand therapy varies among centers and depends on injury elements. Patients with a tenuous flexor tendon repair in zone 2 will have a different

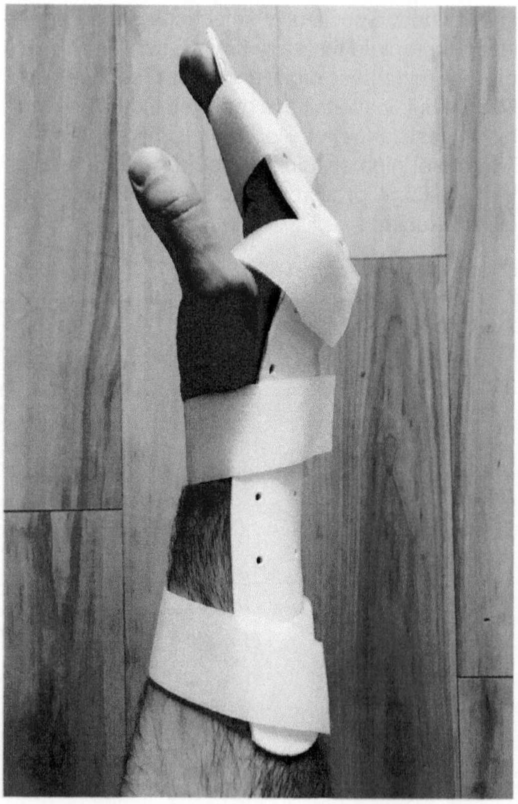

Fig. 6. Rehabilitation splint.

rehabilitation than patients with a zone 1 injury with a robust flexor digitorum profundus repair. Despite these subtleties, we generally use a 2-part EPM program, EPM I and EPM II, described by Silverman and colleagues[45,46] (see later discussion).

EPM I is based on the following treatment goals: to protect all repaired structures, maintain and improve MCP collateral ligament length, prevent joint stiffness, control edema, monitor wound care, educate the patient, and aid in psychological adjustment to disease. Typical exercises are started with controlled tenodesis consisting of assisted wrist flexion with simultaneous extension of MCP and IP joints alternating with assisted wrist extension allowing limited MCP and IP joint flexion. This is continued for 7 to 14 days, depending on the type of injury, level of edema, wound healing, and ability of the patient to adhere to the frequency and duration of the exercises.

EPM II is based on the following treatment goals: to protect all repaired structures, maintain intrinsic muscle function, prevent PIP joint stiffness, minimize tendon adhesions, provide differential gliding of tissues, and improve tendon tensile strength. EPM II consists of 2 phases: passive and active. After conclusion of EPM I, the EPM II passive phase is initiated with wrist motion passively assisted to neutral and passive extension of MCP joints with simultaneous passive flexion of IP joints, depending on the injury. PIP joints are limited to 60° of flexion and DIP joints to approximately 10° to 30°. Up to this point, no active contraction of extrinsic extensor or flexors is used. Starting with EPM II, the active phase combines active contraction of both extrinsic extensors and flexors. Active and assisted MCP joint extension is performed while IP joint flexion is performed simultaneously. Additionally, active and assisted MCP flexion is performed in conjunction with IP joint extension. Exercises are performed under the close supervision of the therapist and, when comfortable, the patients are placed on a home regimen. A typical home regimen consists of 5 to 10 repetitions of each exercise every 2 hours while awake.

No composite finger flexion (simultaneous MCP, PIP, DIP joint flexion) is allowed for at least 4 to 6 weeks postoperative. Thereafter, full flexion and extension exercises are added, allowing simultaneous MCP, PIP, and DIP joint flexion. Dynamic flexion splints or PIP extension-assist splints can also be fashioned to aid in mobilization but are not necessary if the patient is doing well (**Fig. 7**).

Strengthening

Strengthening exercises for pinch and grip strength are begun at 8 weeks postoperatively, depending on the progress of the patient. At this point, all temporary osteosynthesis methods, such as K-wires, are expected to be (or have been) removed. Functional use of the hand is liberated according to progress, pain level, and healing as assessed by tissue quality, tendon excursion, and radiographic evaluation of the osteosynthesis site.

Desensitization and Pharmacologic Augmentation for Hypersensitivity

Scar massage and desensitization are started after wounds have adequately healed, as early as 3 to 4 weeks. Although no trials have yet proven the efficacy of gabapentin in reducing chronic postoperative pain and hypersensitivity in digital replantation, the authors use it as an adjunct, based on published postsurgical treatment data and its potential use for chronic postoperative pain in upper extremity transplantation.[47,48]

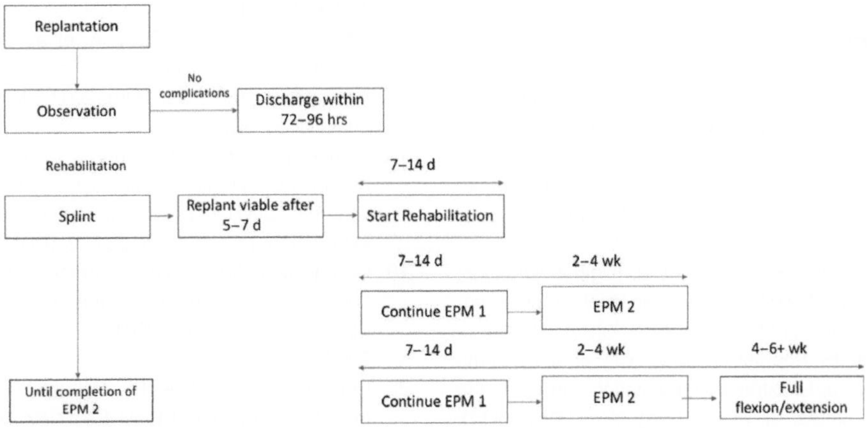

Fig. 7. Rehabilitation timeline.

SUMMARY

Digital replantation still remains among the more complex reconstructive operations in hand surgery. Given the traumatic mechanism of these injuries, the functional recovery can vary according to the severity. With a wide range of complexity of cases requiring replantation and/or revascularization, it is not surprising that a single postoperative protocol has not been created or adapted by reconstructive hand surgeons.

Maintaining the patency of arteries and veins by pharmacologic means has been a widely researched topic. Unfortunately, the data on postoperative anticoagulation and prevention of arterial and venous thrombosis in digital replantation have not proven any drug to favorable and, therefore, the selection of the agent rests with the surgeon. Despite advances in microsurgery and digital replantation, the surgeon must rely heavily on the physical examination and the appearance of the digit. Vigilance is required to note early replant failure and intervene accordingly.

Similarly, the same vigilance is required of the hand therapist in the immediate and long-term follow-up. Ensuring that the patient maintains tendon glide with appropriate rehabilitation exercises and observing the digit for imminent problems, such as infection or failure of osteosynthesis, is required for success. Although the creation of postoperative protocols has been adapted by many specialties, unsurprisingly, the postoperative management and rehabilitation of the replanted or revascularized digit remains guided by individual surgeon's preferences as higher quality data are gathered.

Digital replantation and revascularization can have excellent outcomes. Although the intraoperative technique is important, the postoperative period is equally critical to the survival and functional success of the replanted digit.

REFERENCES

1. Komatsu S. Successful replantation of a completely cut-off thumb: case report. Plast Reconstr Surg 1968;42:374–7.
2. Boulas HJ. Amputations of the fingers and hand: indications for replantation. J Am Acad Orthop Surg 1998;6(2):100–5.
3. Fufa D, Calfee R, Wall L, et al. Digit replantation: experience of two U.S. academic level-I trauma centers. J Bone Joint Surg Am 2013;95(23):2127–34.
4. Friedrich JB, Poppler LH, Mack CD, et al. Epidemiology of upper extremity replantation surgery in the United States. J Hand Surg Am 2011;36(11):1835–40.
5. Matheron AS, Lequint T, Facca S, et al. Should we keep using the heating lamp in microsurgery? Chir Main 2011;30(5):323–6 [in French].
6. Barton B, Kleinert JM. The effect of caffeine on digital haemodynamics. J Hand Surg Br 1994;19(3):301–2.
7. Knight R, Pagkalos J, Timmons C, et al. Caffeine consumption does not have an effect on digital microvascular perfusion assessed by laser Doppler imaging on healthy volunteers: a pilot study. J Hand Surg Eur Vol 2015;40(4):412–5.
8. Zelken JA, Berli JU. Coffee, tea, and chocolate after microsurgery: why not? Ann Plast Surg 2015;74(2):139.
9. Brinkman JN, Derks LH, Klimek M, et al. Perioperative fluid management and use of vasoactive and antithrombotic agents in free flap surgery: a literature review and clinical recommendations. J Reconstr Microsurg 2013;29(6):357–66.
10. Ketchum LD. Pharmacological alterations in the clotting mechanism: use in microvascular surgery. J Hand Surg Am 1978;3(5):407–15.
11. Li X, Cooley BC. Effect of anticoagulation and inhibition of platelet aggregation on arterial versus venous microvascular thrombosis. Ann Plast Surg 1995;35(2):165–9 [discussion: 169–70].
12. Khouri RK, Cooley BC, Kenna DM, et al. Thrombosis of microvascular anastomoses in traumatized vessels: fibrin versus platelets. Plast Reconstr Surg 1990;86(1):110–7.
13. Buckley T, Hammert WC. Anticoagulation following digital replantation. J Hand Surg Am 2011;36(8):1374–6.
14. Morrison WA, McCombe D. Digital replantation. Hand Clin 2007;23(1):1–12.
15. Acland R. Thrombus formation in microvascular surgery: an experimental study of the effects of surgical trauma. Surgery 1973;73(5):766–71.
16. Khouri RK, Cooley BC, Kunselman AR, et al. A prospective study of microvascular free-flap surgery and outcome. Plast Reconstr Surg 1998;102(3):711–21.
17. Ashjian P, Chen CM, Pusic A, et al. The effect of postoperative anticoagulation on microvascular thrombosis. Ann Plast Surg 2007;59(1):36–9 [discussion: 39–40].
18. Nikolis A, Tahiri Y, St-Supery V, et al. Intravenous heparin use in digital replantation and revascularization: the Quebec provincial replantation program experience. Microsurgery 2011;31(6):421–7.
19. Conrad MH, Adams WP. Pharmacologic optimization of microsurgery in the new millennium. Plast Reconstr Surg 2001;108(7):2088–96 [quiz: 2097].
20. Ridha H, Jallali N, Butler PE. The use of dextran post free tissue transfer. J Plast Reconstr Aesthet Surg 2006;59(9):951–4.

21. Jallali N. Dextrans in microsurgery: a review. Microsurgery 2003;23(1):78–80.
22. Wechselberger G, Schoeller T, Ohler K, et al. Flap salvage in a "flow-through" flap by manual thrombectomy plus thrombolytic therapy. J Reconstr Microsurg 1998;14(2):127–9.
23. Lipton HA, Jupiter JB. Streptokinase salvage of a free-tissue transfer: case report and review of the literature. Plast Reconstr Surg 1987;79(6):977–81.
24. Tonks AM, Rees M. Streptokinase salvage of a rectus abdominis free flap. Plast Reconstr Surg 1995;95(5):933–4.
25. Fudem GM, Walton RL. Microvascular thrombolysis to salvage a free flap using human recombinant tissue plasminogen activator. J Reconstr Microsurg 1989;5(3):231–4.
26. Serletti JM, Moran SL, Orlando GS, et al. Urokinase protocol for free-flap salvage following prolonged venous thrombosis. Plast Reconstr Surg 1998; 102(6):1947–53.
27. Panchapakesan V, Addison P, Beausang E, et al. Role of thrombolysis in free-flap salvage. J Reconstr Microsurg 2003;19(8):523–30.
28. D'Arpa S, Cordova A, Moschella F. Pharmacological thrombolysis: one more weapon for free-flap salvage. Microsurgery 2005;25(6):477–80.
29. Buntic RF, Brooks D. Standardized protocol for artery-only fingertip replantation. J Hand Surg Am 2010;35(9):1491–6.
30. Furnas HJ, Lineaweaver W, Buncke HJ. Blood loss associated with anticoagulation in patients with replanted digits. J Hand Surg Am 1992;17(2):226–9.
31. Bauters TG, Buyle FM, Verschraegen G, et al. Infection risk related to the use of medicinal leeches. Pharm World Sci 2007;29(3):122–5.
32. van Alphen NA, Gonzalez A, McKenna MC, et al. Ciprofloxacin-resistant Aeromonas infection following leech therapy for digit replantation: report of 2 cases. J Hand Surg Am 2014;39(3):499–502.
33. Patel KM, Svestka M, Sinkin J, et al. Ciprofloxacin-resistant *Aeromonas hydrophila* infection following leech therapy: a case report and review of the literature. J Plast Reconstr Aesthet Surg 2013;66(1): e20–2.
34. Ridley TJ, Freking W, Erickson LO, et al. Incidence of treatment for infection of buried versus exposed Kirschner wires in phalangeal, metacarpal, and distal radial fractures. J Hand Surg Am 2017;42(7): 525–31.
35. van Leeuwen WF, van Hoorn BT, Chen N, et al. Kirschner wire pin site infection in hand and wrist fractures: incidence rate and risk factors. J Hand Surg Eur Vol 2016;41(9):990–4.
36. Lee SW, Lee DC, Kim JS, et al. Analysis of bone fixation methods in digital replantation. Arch Plast Surg 2017;44(1):53–8.
37. Hoffmann R, Buck-Gramcko D. Osteosynthesis in digital replantation surgery. Ann Chir Gynaecol 1982;71(1):14–8.
38. Tamai S. Twenty years' experience of limb replantation–review of 293 upper extremity replants. J Hand Surg Am 1982;7(6):549–56.
39. Nunley JA, Goldner RD, Urbaniak JR. Skeletal fixation in digital replantation. Use of the "H" plate. Clin Orthop Relat Res 1987;214:66–71.
40. Whitney TM, Lineaweaver WC, Buncke HJ, et al. Clinical results of bony fixation methods in digital replantation. J Hand Surg Am 1990;15(2):328–34.
41. Eggli S, Dietsche A, Vögelin E. Tenolysis after combined digital injuries in zone II. Ann Plast Surg 2005; 55(3):266–71.
42. Jupiter JB, Pess GM, Bour CJ. Results of flexor tendon tenolysis after replantation in the hand. J Hand Surg Am 1989;14(1):35–44.
43. Tamai S, Hori Y, Tatsumi Y, et al. Microvascular anastomosis and its application on the replantation of amputated digits and hands. Clin Orthop Relat Res 1978;(133):106–21.
44. Kleinert HE, Jablon M, Tsai TM. An overview of replantation and results of 347 replants in 245 patients. J Trauma 1980;20(5):390–8.
45. Silverman PM, Willette-Green V, Petrilli J. Early protective motion in digital revascularization and replantation. J Hand Ther 1989;2(2):84–101.
46. Silverman PM, Gordon L. Early motion after replantation. Hand Clin 1996;12(1):97–107.
47. Clarke H, Bonin RP, Orser BA, et al. The prevention of chronic postsurgical pain using gabapentin and pregabalin: a combined systematic review and meta-analysis. Anesth Analg 2012;115(2):428–42.
48. Lang RS, Gorantla VS, Esper S, et al. Anesthetic management in upper extremity transplantation: the Pittsburgh experience. Anesth Analg 2012; 115(3):678–88.

Secondary Surgery Following Replantation and Revascularization

Brent B. Pickrell, MD, Kyle R. Eberlin, MD*

KEYWORDS

- Secondary surgery • Revision surgery • Digital replantation • Digital revascularization
- Hand reconstruction

KEY POINTS

- Secondary surgery following digital replantation or revascularization is common and is often performed to improve range of motion, tendon gliding, sensibility, and/or contour.
- Patients offered revascularization or replantation should be informed about the likelihood of undergoing revision surgery after the index operation.
- Prevention of hand stiffness through aggressive edema control, proper hand positioning, and appropriate hand therapy may reduce the need for some secondary operations.
- Secondary surgery following replantation or revascularization requires patient compliance and well-defined operative goals.

INTRODUCTION

Through improved microsurgical techniques, successful digital replantation and revascularization has improved over time, with greater than 80% digital survival in many series.[1,2] Despite successful replantation and revascularization, however, most patients have impaired hand function and some may benefit from subsequent revision surgery. In some cases, primary repair of all injured structures may not be possible at the time of the index operation, making secondary surgery inevitable.[3] Mere survival of the replanted digit does not substantially benefit the patient without restoration of function.[4]

There are many reasons that patients undergo secondary procedures, including scar contracture, poor soft tissue coverage, tendon adhesions, joint stiffness, malunion or nonunion of fracture site or sites, and/or poor sensory recovery.[5] Current data suggest that the incidence of secondary procedures is around 50% after replantation but this varies widely from 2.9% up to 93.2%.[2,5–7] Rates of secondary surgery correlate to the level of amputation, with more proximal injuries having a higher incidence of secondary surgery.[8] Multiple digit amputations and avulsion injuries are also more likely to undergo secondary surgery, presumably from the wider zone of injury with more damaged structures.[5,6]

Although most hand surgeons report a decline in performing replantation over the past 10 years,[9] it is important for hand surgeons to be familiar with current techniques and trends to better counsel patients preoperatively when offering revascularization or replantation. Indeed, patients treated with an initial revascularization procedure can expect to undergo at least 1 secondary procedure.[6] Fufa and colleagues[10] reported an average of 1.7 procedures per replantation in their series of 121 successful replantations. Such information should be made known to the patient at

Disclosure statement: Dr B.B. Pickrell has no disclosures. Dr K.R. Eberlin is a consultant for AxoGen and Integra.
Division of Plastic and Reconstructive Surgery, Harvard Medical School, Massachusetts General Hospital, Wang Building, 55 Fruit Street, Boston, MA 02114, USA
* Corresponding author.
E-mail address: keberlin@mgh.harvard.edu

Hand Clin 35 (2019) 231–240
https://doi.org/10.1016/j.hcl.2019.01.004
0749-0712/19/

the time of the index procedure and should include a postoperative recovery and rehabilitation timeline.[11] In general, most secondary procedures are delayed until soft tissue equilibrium has been achieved, usually 3 to 6 months after the initial injury.

In this article, the authors present the most common secondary procedures performed after digital replantation or revascularization and discuss current techniques to improve outcomes.

TYPES OF SECONDARY SURGERY

Tendon Procedures

Secondary tendon procedures following replantation and revascularization include tenolysis, tendon reconstruction, tendon grafting, and tendon transfer, with tenolysis being most common.[4] In a review of the incidence of secondary surgery following digital replantation, Wang[4] noted that approximately half (47.2%) of postreplantation surgery involved tendon procedures.

Tenolysis

Tenolysis is indicated for the supple finger when passive range of motion (ROM) exceeds active ROM and progress with a well-supervised rehabilitation program has plateaued.[3] As with all types of tendon surgery, the soft tissues should be in good condition and scars should be pliable before proceeding.

Not all patients are candidates for tenolysis and, therefore, patient selection is a key component to optimize outcomes. Patients who are noncompliant with therapy after initial surgery are often poor candidates for tenolysis.[12] Because optimal results after tenolysis require immediate mobilization, any concomitant surgery that requires immobilization in the postoperative period should be done in a staged manner before tenolysis.[13] Therefore, soft tissue coverage and skeletal stability should be addressed before pursuing tenolysis and/or tendon reconstruction.

In the stiff finger following replantation, extensor tenolysis (with capsular release) is generally performed before flexor tenolysis and is often performed between 4 to 6 months postreplantation. A curvilinear or longitudinal incision is created over the dorsum of the finger centered at the site with maximal adhesions (usually at the site of prior tendon repair). Adhesions are first released between the tendon and overlying skin. Next, the deep aspect of the extensor mechanism is released, fully mobilizing the extensor tendon. This usually involves incising the transverse retinacular ligament at the level of the proximal interphalangeal (PIP) joint on both radial and ulnar aspects of the digit; the collateral ligaments are often elevated on their deep surface. This continues until the joint or joints have satisfactory passive motion and the tendons are sufficiently mobile.

For flexor tenolysis (performed 2–3 months or more after extensor tenolysis), a wide exposure is obtained either through a Bruner or midlateral incision but often follows the scar and surgical approach from the initial injury. The extent of adhesion and scarring is often more significant following replantation than following an isolated flexor tendon injury.[5] Release of all adhesions should be performed until healthy mobile tissue results.[14] A useful technique uses a small elevator that is passed through windows made in less critical parts of the sheath, deep to the pulley system.[12] Specialized tenolysis blades, if available, can help divide adhesions without compromising pulley integrity. Complete dissection of all adhesions between flexor digitorum profundus (FDP) and, if present, flexor digitorum superficialis tendons, and between the tendons and surrounding sheath, should ideally be completed until the tendons are freely mobile.[14] It is important to preserve the A2 and A4 pulleys and limit trauma to the flexor sheath because poor tissue handling may further contribute to adhesion formation. The surgeon should be prepared to perform a pulley reconstruction if the system is insufficient. If the flexor tendons appears unsalvageable secondary to poor healing, obliteration of a long segment of tendon sheath, or pulley insufficiency, consideration is made for staged tendon reconstruction. Longitudinal traction on the proximal end of the tendon to elicit finger flexion will help the surgeon identify any further adhesions. Alternatively, having the patient awake and involved during surgery, as popularized by Lalonde,[15] is particularly helpful to determine the extent of tenolysis required.

It is paramount that patients begin occupational therapy (ie, active ROM) immediately after tenolysis to maintain motion achieved intraoperatively, ideally within 24 hours. Reported outcomes following tenolysis after replantation are generally favorable. Jupiter and colleagues[16] supported flexor tenolysis after replantation of fingers, excluding replanted thumbs. The investigators performed tenolysis on average 10 months after replantation (range 5–19 months). Factors associated with poor results included crush or avulsion amputations, injuries to multiple digits, and fingers with significant PIP joint stiffness. Similarly, Yu and colleagues[5] demonstrated excellent or good functional recovery in 85% of subjects with total active motion increasing from 119° to 159° after tenolysis.

Secondary tendon reconstruction

Occasionally, secondary flexor tendon reconstruction following primary tendon repair will be required because some primary tendon repairs may gap, rupture, or develop extensive scarring within the fibroosseous tunnel such that effective tenolysis is not possible (**Fig. 1**). Both preoperative and intraoperative assessments are necessary to determine a patient's candidacy for single-stage versus 2-stage tendon reconstruction. However, given the frequent extensive soft tissue scarring accompanied by traumatic amputations, some patients may be better served through a 2-stage approach. This method was first described by Bassett and Carroll[17] in 1963 and later refined by Hunter in 1971.[18]

The first procedure of a staged reconstruction uses digital exploration, excision of scarred soft tissues and residual flexor tendon, reconstruction of the pulley system, and placement of a silicone implant (**Fig. 2**). This allows for concomitant correction of any joint contracture (ie, capsulotomy), reconstruction of critical pulleys, and formation of a mesothelial-lined pseudosheath around the silicone rod.[13] When encountered, any scarred tendons, sheath, or retinacula should be excised with care, leaving, if possible, a 1-cm distal stump of FDP tendon attached to the distal phalanx for later reattachment. Excised tendon material is used for pulley reconstruction, if required.

There are several techniques available for reconstruction of the pulley system but the simplest, preferred by the authors, is the use of remnant tendon that is generally available (see **Fig. 2**). If additional donor material is required, the palmaris longus can be used; however, one must consider the graft used during the second stage of surgery to avoid using critical autologous tendon that may be needed for the subsequent stage. Using the circumferential method first described by Bunnell,[19] the tendon graft encircles the middle and proximal phalanges beneath (deep to) the extensor tendon. This should be performed under direct visualization, with care taken to protect the adjacent neurovascular bundles. Other reconstructions involve weaving the graft into the pulley remnants. The repair is secured using nonabsorbable sutures. After the pulley system is reconstructed, the silicone tendon spacer is placed in the tendon sheath and affixed distally to the stump of the FDP tendon using a 3-0 polypropylene suture. The selection of the appropriately sized silicone implant is determined largely by the tightness of the pulleys. In the senior author's experience, a 3-mm or a 4-mm rod is satisfactory in most adult patients. It is important to ensure that the silicone rod glides smoothly and does not buckle with passive flexion before closure.[20]

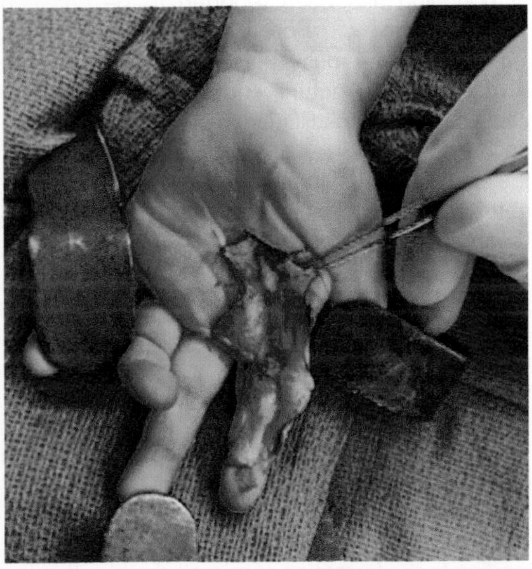

Fig. 1. Intraoperative view showing discontinuity of the index flexor tendon system following index finger revascularization and primary flexor tendon repair. Note the extensive scarring of the fibroosseous tunnel and significant peritendinous adhesions.

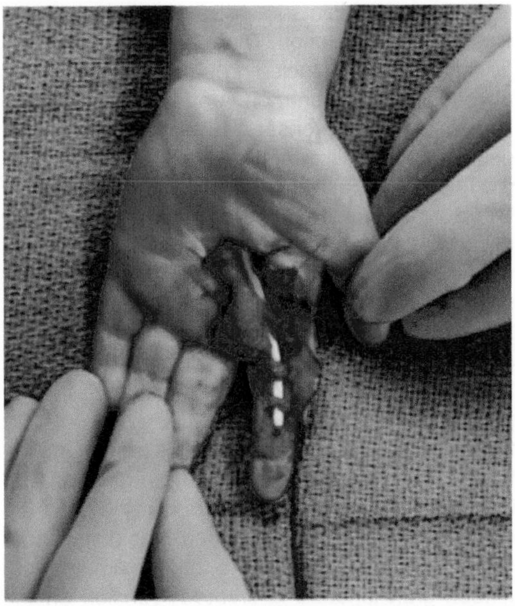

Fig. 2. Secondary flexor tendon reconstruction using a silicone rod secured deep to FDP insertion on distal phalanx. A2 and A4 pulley reconstruction using remnant FDP tendon.

The second stage involves replacement of the silicone implant with a tendon graft, which is commonly performed at least 3 months after the index operation. All wounds should be fully healed and supple and joints must be mobile before this stage of reconstruction. There are several options for suitable grafts, including palmaris longus and plantaris. Less common options include toe flexors or long extensors, extensor indicis proprius, and extensor digiti minimi.[20] Tendon allograft has also been described for this purpose.[21] When available, the authors prefer the ipsilateral palmaris longus tendon as a graft. However, when the proximal juncture of the graft-motor unit will be in the forearm, a longer graft is required and plantaris or a toe extensor is pursued. After graft harvest, the implant-FDP stump attachments are divided and the tendon graft is attached to the proximal end of the implant and is pulled distally through the newly created pseudosheath. Limiting trauma to the pseudosheath is advised. The implant is then removed and discarded, and the distal tendon juncture is secured. The distal finger wound is then closed, and the proximal motor tendon-graft juncture is created. Tension on the graft should be set so that the digit is flexed slightly more than its normal resting position with the wrist in a neutral position.

Bone Procedures

Successful functional results following replantation rely on adequate bone reduction, healing, and stability. Lower complication rates after revascularization have been associated with stable bony fixation,[22] whereas poor bony fixation can lead to stiffness, malunion, nonunion, or deformity.[23] Stable fracture fixation allows progressive tendon and joint motion commensurate with healing to prevent or minimize tendon adhesions and joint stiffness or contracture.[24] In this way, stable fracture fixation also helps to control pain, allow early active rehabilitation,[25] and protect vascular repairs.[24]

Bony problems following replantation can occur in as many of 30% to 50% of patients.[26,27] Secondary bone procedures following replantation are most commonly performed to address malunion; nonunion; or, less commonly, osteomyelitis.

Malunion

Malunion may occur secondary to primary bone misalignment, inadequate postsurgical immobilization, repeat trauma, and/or osseous resorption.[14] Whitney and colleagues[27] and Van Oosterom and colleagues[28] found that replantation was a risk factor for the development of malunion. Malunion can result in angulatory or rotatory deformities with concomitant stiffness, pain, and decreased grip strength.[29] Substantial digital overlap may also pose an aesthetic and/or functional problem.

Corrective osteotomies (closed or open) are the treatment of choice and are usually performed at the level of the malunion but may also be performed at the metacarpal level.[30] This allows multiplanar correction at the site of origin and permits additional soft tissue procedures (eg, capsulotomy), if desired.[13] Preoperatively, it is helpful to devise a template of the malunited phalanx to assess the dimensions of the wedge to be removed.[13] A closing wedge osteotomy is overall simpler and avoids the need for bone graft but shortens the digit.[29,31] In contrast, an opening wedge osteotomy secured with plate and screws is often accompanied by cancellous bone graft.[29,31]

Phalangeal osteotomy for malunions has produced acceptable results. Buchler and colleagues[29] achieved full correction in 76% and increased ROM in 89% of subjects. However, the investigators demonstrated that additional soft tissue injuries resulted in approximately one-half of the rate of excellent results (45% vs 83%) compared with those with isolated malunion.

Nonunion

Nonunion, observed less frequently than malunion,[13] usually occurs as a result of concomitant neurovascular injury during the initial trauma, bony deficiency, soft tissue injury, and/or infection,[13,28] and can be associated with tendon adhesions and joint contracture.[31] Radiographs alone may be unreliable in the diagnosis of nonunion; instability, deformity, and implant failure are more reliable clinical indicators.[31] A nonunion can be atrophic or hypertrophic, with most nonunion in the hand being atrophic (**Fig. 3**).[31] The incidence of nonunion has been reported to be between 10% and 31%[27,32,33] following digital replantation.

Fibrous tissue must be removed until there are acute, healthy fracture ends.[13] This is accomplished with an oscillating saw via a transverse cut through the irregular or atrophic aspects of the bone. If a resultant gap produces unacceptable shortening, intercalated corticocancellous bone grafting can be used.[13]

Osteomyelitis

Most cases of osteomyelitis following replantation are caused by direct inoculation of microorganisms that occurs after penetrating trauma or postoperative soft tissue infection.[34] Whereas intact bone cortex provides a mechanical barrier to pathogen penetration, traumatized bone is more easily infected. Local inflammation causes increased tissue pressure, lower pH, and lower oxygen tension, leading to the formation of microthrombi within the intraosseous vessels and bony necrosis.[34] A nidus of necrotic bone (ie, sequestrum) provides a harbor for pathogens because of its lack of vascularity and thus poor drug penetration.

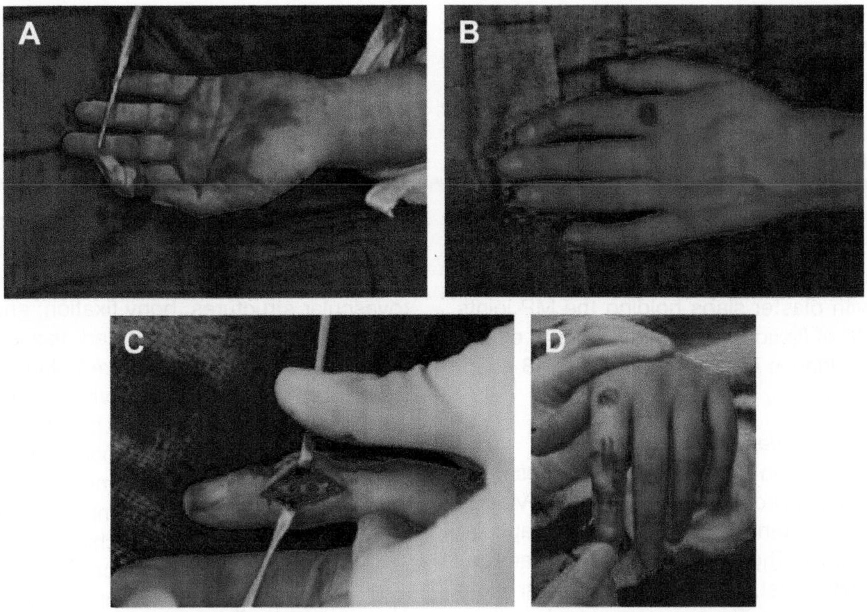

Fig. 3. (*A*) Initial injury. (*B*) Atrophic nonunion of middle phalanx with angulation of digit. (*C*) Intraoperative view of open reduction and internal fixation (ORIF). (*D*) Intraoperative view after ORIF and straightening of digit.

Aggressive bony debridement performed at the time of the index replantation or revascularization, particularly in the setting of comminuted fractures, and appropriate timing of soft tissue or bony reconstruction, are important factors for prevention of osteomyelitis.[35] When an infected sequestrum is present, operative intervention is required and all infected bone is debrided. The presence of implanted hardware affords additional protection to pathogens because many bacteria surround themselves with a protective barrier (biofilm) when localized to nonorganic surfaces. Management of osteomyelitis of the hand should consist of a combined surgical and medical approach to achieve the most favorable outcome.[34,36] Infected hardware should be removed, at least temporarily, if it is not well-fixed or if the screw holes are involved.

In patients with persistent or recurrent drainage after multiple debridements or in patients with failed reconstructions, amputation may be necessary.[37] In a study that included 46 subjects with osteomyelitis in the hand, the overall amputation rate was 39% (18 of 46 subjects), with 57% of subjects having a history of a traumatic or contaminated wound.[36] In subjects diagnosed or treated 6 months after the time of contamination or the onset of symptoms, there was an 86% amputation rate.

Joint Procedures

Joint stiffness secondary to joint contracture is very common following replantation and the etiologic factors are multifactorial.[38–41] Wang[4] noted that joint procedures were the second most common secondary procedures (18.9%) after digit replantation. The accumulation of inflammatory edema fluid or hematoma in the injured digit physically limits mobility and drives the hand to assume a characteristic posture, with the metacarpophalangeal (MP) joints in full extension and the PIP joints in 30° to 40° of flexion.[13] Although many MP and PIP joint contractures can be managed nonoperatively with edema control and hand therapy,[38] some joints will ultimately require surgical management.

The most common site of joint contracture after replantation or revascularization is the PIP joint. The operative intervention chosen is often capsulotomy or capsulectomy, particularly for PIP and MP joint contractures. In contrast, distal interphalangeal (DIP) joints contribute relatively little to overall finger ROM and joint stiffness is therefore better tolerated.[42] Similar to tenolysis, it is imperative that the patient be compliant and has a regimented hand therapy program scheduled postoperatively. Joints that are irrevocably injured and those with loss of articular cartilage may be better served with arthrodesis or arthroplasty (arthrodesis more common postreplantation).

Metacarpophalangeal joint

For MP joint contracture, we perform a dorsal curvilinear incision over the MP joint and incise a portion of the sagittal bands bilaterally to facilitate joint exposure. Thereafter, a transverse dorsal capsular incision is performed. Passive joint motion is then inspected for improvement and adequacy. If motion remains suboptimal after this maneuver (ie, <70°), limited division of dorsal collateral ligaments and/or release of volar plate adhesions can be performed. Repair of the dorsal extensor mechanism is then completed and the degree of flexion is rechecked before skin closure. Postoperatively, the patient is placed in a bulky dressing with plaster slabs holding the MP joints at 70° to 90° of flexion and the PIP joints in extension. Mobilization is initiated within 24 to 48 hours after the procedure.

Proximal interphalangeal joint

For PIP joint flexion contracture or stiffness, we prefer a dorsal approach similar to that previously described for extensor tenolysis (with capsular release) (**Fig. 4**). The transverse retinacular ligament is divided first, followed by the volar plate checkrein ligaments. The neurovascular bundle is visualized and protected. What proceeds next is usually dictated based on intraoperative assessment of the patient's on-table ROM. Using a sequential approach, the patient's ROM is assessed after each additional structure is divided to determine interval progress.[43] If motion is not improved after checkrein division, release of the accessory collateral ligament followed by the proper collateral ligament and the proximal portion of the volar plate can be performed.[43]

Soft Tissue Procedures and Scar Contractures

Secondary skin procedures after replantation or revascularization are often performed in a bimodal distribution and aim to address skin or soft tissue defects (early) or scar contractures (late).[4,5] Yu and colleagues[5] reported 92% of early secondary procedures in their series were performed for skin coverage. Similarly, Tark and colleagues[44] performed 79% of their secondary operations for soft tissue defects. Another series[42] consisting of 84% crush injuries reported that skin grafting was the most common secondary procedure performed during the first 2 months following replantation.

Many amputations that result from high-energy trauma can produce considerable soft tissue defects to the amputated part and nearby hand owing to an extensive zone of injury. Initially, focus is directed at identifying and repairing critical neurovascular structures, bony fixation, and debridement of all frankly devitalized tissue. Necrosis and resultant defects of injured skin may be the first problems noted after survival of the replanted part and warrant thoughtful planning[45] because function can be critically impaired when the soft tissue envelope is compromised.[46] Inadequate management can lead to amputation or permanent disability.[47] Although achieving early wound closure is desirable to reduce infection risk and optimize healing and motion, following severe crush or mangling injuries, and in the presence of significant contamination, it is often prudent to delay definitive soft tissue coverage until a stable wound has been achieved. This will sometimes require serial debridements separated by 24 to 48 hours[13] and intervening local wound care. We prefer early flap coverage to prevent desiccation and for the provision of healthy, well-vascularized soft tissues. Indeed, proper wound debridement remains fundamental before any definitive method of soft tissue coverage.[48]

Multiple techniques have been developed that serve as useful bridges until the wound and/or patient is ready for definitive soft tissue reconstruction. These include the use of negative-pressure therapy, allograft skin, or acellular dermal matrices (eg, Integra [Integra LifeSciences, Plainsboro, NJ]). When the wound is ready for definitive coverage, several options exist, including skin grafts, local advancement or rotational flaps, pedicled regional flaps, and free tissue transfer. Although skin grafts

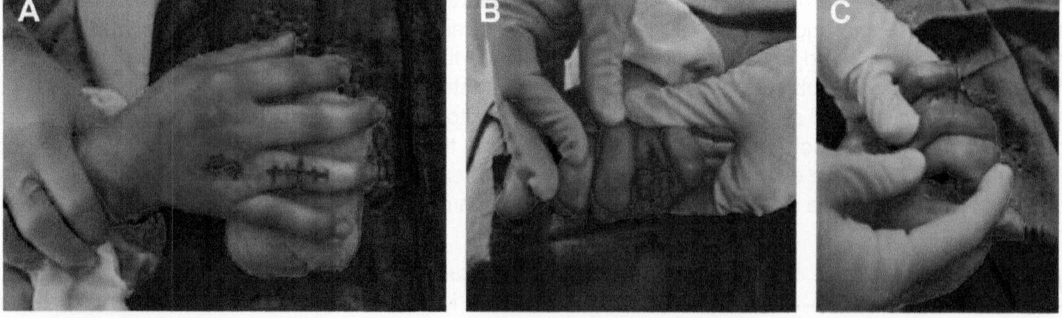

Fig. 4. (*A*) Dorsal approach to PIP joint. (*B, C*) On-table ROM assessment after division of transverse retinacular ligament.

will survive on a vascularized tissue bed, the exposure of nerve, tendon, or bone typically necessitates more robust vascularized soft tissue coverage. An optimal coverage should (1) be stable, durable, and able to withstand heavy demands of work; (2) allow free joint mobility; and (3) have an aesthetically acceptable appearance.[47] Additionally, coverage should be low-profile, supple over mobile areas (eg, joint and tendons), and have minimal shear characteristics on the volar aspect of the hand and fingers where friction is required for function.[13]

Skin grafts

Split-thickness skin grafts (STSGs) are often performed for defects involving the dorsum of the hand or digits. The authors preferentially harvest STSG from the lateral thigh, with thicknesses between 0.014 and 0.016 in. To guard against fluid collection and graft failure, so-called pie-crusting is used for wounds expected to bleed or produce exudate. Full-thickness skin grafts are preferred in areas prone to shear and load, such as the fingertips, palm, web spaces, and areas over joints, and are commonly harvested from the proximal ipsilateral extremity.[13] The increased thickness, compared with STSG, also affords improved cosmesis and less secondary contraction. For glabrous skin, the authors prefer the hypothenar area, which can be removed with a carefully planned ellipse to facilitate primary closure. Templating defects with an Esmarch bandage can be a helpful tool to ensure appropriate harvest dimensions.[49] Harvesting skin grafts from relatively inconspicuous areas is recommended.

After the graft is prepared, it is inset into the defect and sutured to the skin edges with absorbable 4-0 chromic sutures. Care is taken to ensure that maximal dermal contact with the underlying recipient bed is achieved. For concave defects on the hand (eg, first web space), we elect to secure our grafts with tie-over bolster dressings to prevent tenting of the graft. Mineral oil-soaked cotton wrapped in nonadherent petrolatum gauze can be easily molded into the concavity and then secured with nonabsorbable tied-over sutures placed in the surrounding skin. The bolster is left in place for 7 to 10 days.

Flaps

Flaps are traditionally indicated for coverage of wounds with exposed tendon (without peritenon), nerves, bone, blood vessels, joints, and hardware, often on the volar surface of the hand or digits. Many local, regional, and free flap options exist and for soft tissue coverage in the hand.[49,50]

Arterialized venous free flaps deserve special mention and have proven to be a reliable source of thin, pliable tissue for digital soft tissue coverage during replantation and revascularization. The primary advantages of venous flaps include ease of harvest, lack of donor site limitation, no sacrifice of a major periphery artery, and good postoperative contour.[48,51] This latter point may help to avoid secondary surgery for flap defatting or debulking.[52] Aside from use as pure skin flaps, these flaps can also be harvested as composite flaps with tendons and nerves or be used as flow-through bypass for digital revascularization.[52,53] One drawback to these flaps is the high incidence of postoperative congestion and edema. Epidermolysis may also occur. However, the flap congestion can be managed expectantly and usually begins to resolve after the first week postoperatively without further flap compromise.[52] A recent systematic review[54] of 756 flaps found a failure rate of 2.5% and early postoperative venous congestion in 60%. Similarly, Woo and colleagues[52] published a series of 154 venous flaps and achieved a 1.9% failure rate. When possible, we opt to harvest our venous flaps from the ipsilateral volar forearm.

Scar contracture

Scars that fail to soften with conservative measures and those with functional impairment should be evaluated for contracture release and resurfacing. For hypertrophic scars crossing digital creases, a simple Z-plasty may suffice if no skin deficit is present. Scar contracture may be particularly problematic in the web spaces, most notably the first web space. Adequate release of the web space depends on accurately identifying and treating the involved structures.[55] Skin deficiencies are treated with releasing incisions and can include a perpendicular linear incision or incisions incorporated into local flaps or Z-plasties. Release of the palmar fascia and adductor pollicis may be required. Contractures of the adductor pollicis, flexor pollicis brevis, or first dorsal interosseous muscles are treated with release of the origin or insertion and tendon-lengthening techniques. Restricted joint capsules or ligaments necessitate capsulotomies.[55]

Nerve Procedures

Secondary nerve reconstruction following replantation is most commonly performed for either an ongoing perceived sensory deficit or a symptomatic neuroma.

If there is a nerve gap at the time of the index replantation or revascularization that precludes a tension-free repair, options include immediate autograft or allograft nerve reconstruction, or, alternatively, secondary nerve reconstruction in a delayed fashion. In delayed cases, fibrosis and retraction of the nerve ends almost always prevents tension-free direct coaptation of the nerve ends, and interposition nerve grafting is most commonly required.[56]

It is our practice to perform autograft or allograft nerve reconstruction when the gap exceeds approximately 5 mm. Common autograft donor sources include anterior interosseous nerve, posterior interosseous nerve, medial and lateral antebrachial cutaneous (LABC) nerves, and sural nerve. Higgins and colleagues[57] investigated the different cross-sectional areas and fascicle number of donor nerves to provide guidelines for selection of nerve graft harvest based on the anatomic location of the nerve defect. The LABC nerve was noted to be the best match in caliber and fascicle number for digital nerve deficits between the MP joints and DIP joint, which are commonly encountered following replantation.

Processed nerve allografts have also shown promising results and have recently gained popularity in traumatic injuries. Means and colleagues[58] evaluated 20 digital nerve injuries randomized to either processed nerve allograft or hollow tube conduit and found subjects whose nerve reconstructions were performed with processed nerve allografts had significantly improved and more consistent functional sensory outcomes. Both options maintain benefits of no donor site morbidity and decreased operative time.

Neuromas may form following epineurial repair (neuroma-in-continuity) or following nerve transection without repair (terminal neuroma), and cause pain and tenderness that may limit activities of daily living.[59] Aside from functional impairment, patients suffering from painful neuromas may also be unable to maintain their job in the workforce.[60,61] Symptoms of a painful neuroma include sharp or burning pain, cold intolerance, or a shooting, electrical sensation elicited by direct pressure on the digit.[62–64] A recent review by Ives and colleagues[65] reported that as many as 26% of subjects who sustain amputations may form painful neuromas. Vlot and colleagues[64] noted that 6.6% of subjects who developed a painful neuroma after revision amputation underwent secondary surgery with a mean time to surgery of 11 months after their injury; in this way, replantation or revascularization may be superior to completion amputation.[64]

Surgical treatment of neuromas has been shown to significantly improve patient quality of life, self-reported pain, and depression.[63] With surgical intervention, the most common first step is neuroma resection. Thereafter, options include

1. Use of nerve allograft or autograft to reconnect severed proximal and distal stumps
2. Transposition into adjacent muscle or bone
3. Centro-central neurorrhaphy
4. Translocation of the nerve.[66]

Guse and Moran[67] reported that simple neuroma excision resulted in a high rate of reoperation (47%) and recommended against this technique. The investigators found that subjects who underwent neuroma excision with nerve repair had significantly improved postoperative Disability of the Arm, Shoulder, and Hand (DASH) scores compared with either muscle or bone transposition, and only required a single surgical procedure for neuroma management. Hazari and Elliot[68] reported 98% of nerve relocations achieved pain relief at the primary site and greater than 90% of nerves had no spontaneous pain, pain on movement, or hypersensitivity at the ultimate site of proximal relocation.

If the distal end of the transected nerve is available but primary tensionless repair is not possible, the authors recommend using allograft or autograft nerve for reconstruction. If there is no distal target, the damaged proximal stump should be moved to a less traumatized and less exposed environment.[14]

SUMMARY

Secondary surgery following replantation and revascularization is complex and aims to improve function, durability, sensibility, and contour of the reconstructed hand. Successful restoration of hand function relies on such procedures to improve long-term patient satisfaction. Hand surgeons who perform replantation must also be proficient in these techniques and understand their limitations, indications, and the importance of patient selection and postoperative compliance with ongoing hand therapy.

REFERENCES

1. Medling BD, Bueno RA Jr, Russell RC, et al. Replantation outcomes. Clin Plast Surg 2007;34:177–85.
2. Waikakul S, Sakkarnkosol S, Vanadurongwan V, et al. Results of 1018 digital replantations in 552 patients. Injury 2000;31:33–40.
3. Sabapathy SR, Bhardwaj P. Secondary procedures in replantation. Semin Plast Surg 2013;27:198–204.
4. Wang H. Secondary surgery after digit replantation: its incidence and sequence. Microsurgery 2002;22:57–61.

5. Yu JC, Shieh SJ, Lee JW, et al. Secondary procedures following digital replantation and revascularisation. Br J Plast Surg 2003;56:125–8.
6. Chinta M, Wilkens SC, Vlot MA, et al. Secondary surgery following initial replantation/revascularization or completion amputation in the hand or digits. Plast Reconstr Surg 2018;142(3):709–16.
7. Patradul A, Ngarmukos C, Parkpian V. Distal digital replantations and revascularizations: 237 digits in 192 patients. J Hand Surg Br 1998;23:578–82.
8. Pitzler D, Buck-Gramcko D. Secondary operations after replantation. Ann Chir Gynaecol 1982;71:19–27.
9. Payatakes AH, Zagoreos NP, Fedorcik GG, et al. Current practice of microsurgery by members of the American Society for Surgery of the hand. J Hand Surg 2007;32(4):541–7.
10. Fufa D, Calfee R, Wall L, et al. Digit replantation: experience of two U.S. academic level-I trauma centers. J Bone Joint Surg Am 2013;95(23):2127–34.
11. Yaffe B, Hutt D, Yaniv Y, et al. Major upper extremity replantations. J Hand Microsurg 2009;1(2):63–7.
12. Lilly SI, Messer TM. Complications after treatment of flexor tendon injuries. J Am Acad Orthop Surg 2006;14:387–96.
13. Green, David P, Wolfe SW. Green's operative hand surgery. Philadelphia: Elsevier/Churchill Livingstone; 2011.
14. Chiou GJ, Chang J. Refinements and secondary surgery after flap reconstruction of the traumatized hand. Hand Clin 2014;30:211–23.
15. Lalonde DH. Reconstruction of the hand with wide awake surgery. Clin Plast Surg 2011;38(4):761–9.
16. Jupiter JB, Pess GH, Bour CJ. Results of flexor tendon tenolysis after replantation in the hand. J Hand Surg 1989;14A:35–44.
17. Bassett AL, Carroll RF. Formation of tendon sheaths by silicone rod implants. Proceedings of the American Society for Surgery of the hand. J Bone Joint Surg 1963;45A:884–5.
18. Hunter JM, Salisbury RE. Flexor-tendon reconstruction in severely damaged hands. A two-staged procedure using a silicone-Dacron reinforced gliding prosthesis prior to tendon grafting. J Bone Joint Surg 1971;53A:829–58.
19. Bunnell S. Reconstructive surgery of the hand. Surg Gynecol Obstet 1924;34:259–74.
20. Freilich AM, Chhabra B. Secondary flexor tendon reconstruction, a review. J Hand Surg 2007;32A:1436–42.
21. Xie RG, Tang JB. Allograft tendon for second stage reconstruction. Hand Clin 2012;28(4):503–9.
22. Chen SH, Wei FC, Chen H, et al. Miniature plates and screws in acute complex hand injury. J Trauma 1994;37:237–42.
23. Gingrass RP, Fehring B, Matloub H. Intraosseous wiring of complex hand fractures. Plast Reconstr Surg 1980;66:383–94.
24. Sud V, Freeland AE. Skeletal fixation in digital replantation. Microsurgery 2002;22:165–71.
25. Jones JM, Schenk RR, Chesney RB. Digital replantation and amputation–comparison of function. J Hand Surg Am 1982;7:183–9.
26. Hoffman R, Buck-Gramcko D. Osteosynthesis in digital replantation surgery. Ann Chir Gynaecol 1982;71(1):14–8.
27. Whitney TM, Lineaweaver WC, Buncke HJ, et al. Clinical results of bony fixation methods in digital replantation. J Hand Surg Am 1990;15(2):328–34.
28. Van Oosterom FJT, Brete GJV, Ozdemir C, et al. Treatment of phalangeal fractures in severely injured hands. J Hand Surg Br 2001;26B(2):108–11.
29. Buchler U, Gupta A, Ruf S. Corrective osteotomy for post-traumatic malunion of the phalanges in the hand. J Hand Surg Br 1996;21:33–42.
30. Freeland AE, Lindley SG. Malunions of the finger metacarpals and phalanges. Hand Clin 2006;22(3):341–55.
31. Ring D. Malunion and nonunion of the metacarpals and phalanges. J Bone Joint Surg 2005;87:1380–8.
32. Pomerance J, Truppa K, Bilos ZJ, et al. Replantation and revascularization of the digits in a community microsurgical practice. J Reconstr Microsurg 1997;13(3):163–70.
33. Lee SW, Lee DC, Kim JS, et al. Analysis of bone fixation methods in digital replantation. Arch Plast Surg 2017;44:53–8.
34. Honda H, McDonald JR. Current recommendations in the management of osteomyelitis of the hand and wrist. J Hand Surg 2009;34A:1135–6.
35. McDonald LS, Bavaro MF, Hofmeister EP, et al. Hand infections. J Hand Surg Am 2011;36(8):1403–12.
36. Reilly KE, Linz JC, Stern PJ, et al. Osteomyelitis of the tubular bones of the hand. J Hand Surg 1997;22A:644–9.
37. Ferreira J, Fowler JR. Management of complications relating to complex traumatic hand injuries. Hand Clin 2015;31:311–7.
38. Weeks PM, Wray RC Jr, Kuxhaus M. The results of non-operative management of stiff joints in the hand. Plast Reconstr Surg 1978;61:58–63.
39. Curtis RM. Capsulectomy of the interphalangeal joints of the fingers. J Bone Joint Surg Am 1954;36(6):1219–32.
40. Curtis RM. Management of the stiff proximal interphalangeal joint. J Hand Surg Eur Vol 1969;1(1):32–7.
41. Kuczynski K. The proximal interphalangeal joint: anatomy and causes of stiffness in the fingers. J Bone Joint Surg Br 1968;50(3):656–63.

42. Yang G, McGlinn EP, Chung KC. Management of the stiff finger: evidence and outcomes. Clin Plast Surg 2014;41:501–12.
43. Hogan CJ, Nunley JA. Posttraumatic proximal interphalangeal joint flexion contractures. J Am Acad Orthop Surg 2006;14:524–33.
44. Tark KC, Kim YW, Lee YH, et al. Replantation and revascularization of hands: clinical analysis and functional results of 261 cases. J Hand Surg 1989; 14A:17–27.
45. Matsuzaki H, Kouda H. Secondary surgeries after digital replantations: a case series. Hand Surg 2012;17(3):351–7.
46. Friedrich JB, Katolik LI, Vedder NB. Soft tissue reconstruction of the hand. J Hand Surg 2009;34A: 1148–55.
47. Bashir MM, Sohail M, Shami HB. Traumatic wounds of the upper extremity: coverage strategies. Hand Clin 2018;34:61–74.
48. Cayci C, Carlsen BT, Saint-Cyr M. Optimizing functional and aesthetic outcomes of upper limb soft tissue reconstruction. Hand Clin 2014;30:225–38.
49. Miller EA, Friedrich J. Soft tissue coverage of the hand and upper extremity: the reconstructive elevator. J Hand Surg Am 2016;41(7):782–92.
50. Biswas D, Wysocki RW, Fernandez JJ, et al. Local and regional flaps for hand coverage. J Hand Surg Am 2014;39(5):992–1004.
51. De Lorenzi F, van der Hulst RR, den Dunnen WF, et al. Arterialized venous free flaps for soft-tissue reconstruction of digits: a 40-case series. J Reconstr Microsurg 2002;18(7):569–74.
52. Woo SH, Kim KC, Lee GJ, et al. A retrospective analysis of 154 arterialized venous flaps for hand reconstruction: an 11-year experience. Plast Reconstr Surg 2007;119(6):1823–38.
53. Yan H, Brooks D, Ladner R, et al. Arterialized venous flaps: a review of the literature. Microsurgery 2010; 30:472–8.
54. Wharton R, Creasy H, Bain C, et al. Venous flaps for coverage of traumatic soft tissue defects of the hand: a systematic review. J Hand Surg Eur Vol 2017;42(8):817–22.
55. Moody L, Galvez MG, Chang J. Reconstruction of first web space contractures. J Hand Surg Am 2015;40:1892–5.
56. Slutsky DJ. The management of digital nerve injuries. J Hand Surg Am 2014;39(6):1208–15.
57. Higgins JP, Fisher S, Serletti JM, et al. Assessment of nerve graft donor sites used for reconstruction of traumatic digital nerve defects. J Hand Surg 2002;27A:286–92.
58. Means KR, Rinker BD, Higgins JP, et al. A multicenter, prospective, randomized, pilot study of outcomes for digital nerve repair in the hand using hollow conduit compared with processed allograft nerve. Hand 2016;11(2):144–51.
59. Foo A, Sebastin SJ. Secondary interventions for mutilating hand injuries. Hand Clin 2016;32:555–67.
60. Goldstein S, Sturim H. Intraosseous nerve transposition for treatment of painful neuromas. J Hand Surg 1985;10:270–4.
61. Louis D, Hunter L, Keating T. Painful neuromas in long below-elbow amputees. Arch Surg 1980;115: 742–4.
62. Geraghty TJ, Jones LE. Painful neuromata following upper limb amputation. Prosthet Orthot Int 1996; 20(3):176–81.
63. Mackinnon SE. Evaluation and treatment of the painful neuroma. Tech Hand Up Extrem Surg 1997;1(3): 195–212.
64. Vlot MA, Wilkens SC, Chen NC, et al. Symptomatic neuroma following initial amputation for traumatic digital amputation. J Hand Surg Am 2018;43(1):86. e1-8.
65. Ives GC, Kung TA, Nghiem BT, et al. Current state of the surgical treatment of terminal neuromas. Neurosurgery 2018;83(3):354–64.
66. Brogan DM, Kakar S. Management of neuromas of the upper extremity. Hand Clin 2013;29(3):409–20.
67. Guse DM, Moran SL. Outcomes of the surgical treatment of peripheral neuromas of the hand and forearm. Ann Plast Surg 2013;71:654–8.
68. Hazari A, Elliot D. Treatment of end-neuromas, neuromas-in-continuity and scarred nerves of the digits by proximal relocation. J Hand Surg Br 2004;29B(4): 338–50.

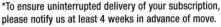

Printed and bound by CPI Group (UK) Ltd, Croydon, CR0 4YY

40318028

03040800C011

Printed and bound by CPI Group (UK) Ltd, Croydon, CR0 4YY
03/10/2024
01040306-0011